Foreword by Peter E. Lobie and Nam-Hyung Kim

# ORGANOIDS

## Advancements in Drug Discovery and Precision Medicine


Editors

**Boon-Cher Goh**
National University of Singapore, Singapore

**Chongyang Shen**
Chengdu University of Traditional Chinese Medicine, China

**Lingzhi Wang**
National University of Singapore, Singapore



World Scientific

NEW JERSEY • LONDON • SINGAPORE • BEIJING • SHANGHAI • HONG KONG • TAIPEI • CHENNAI • TOKYO

*Published by*

World Scientific Publishing Co. Pte. Ltd.
5 Toh Tuck Link, Singapore 596224
*USA office:* 27 Warren Street, Suite 401-402, Hackensack, NJ 07601
*UK office:* 57 Shelton Street, Covent Garden, London WC2H 9HE

Library of Congress Control Number: 2025030376

**British Library Cataloguing-in-Publication Data**
A catalogue record for this book is available from the British Library.

**ORGANOIDS**
**Advancements in Drug Discovery and Precision Medicine**



ISBN 978-981-98-1758-0 (hardcover)
ISBN 978-981-98-1759-7 (ebook for institutions)
ISBN 978-981-98-1760-3 (ebook for individuals)

For any available supplementary material, please visit
https://www.worldscientific.com/worldscibooks/10.1142/14430#t=suppl

Desk Editor: Shaun Tan Yi Jie

Typeset by Stallion Press
Email: enquiries@stallionpress.com

https://doi.org/10.1142/9789819817597_fmatter

# Foreword

The rapid evolution of organoid technology has revolutionized biomedical research, offering unprecedented opportunities in drug discovery and precision medicine. By bridging the gap between traditional cell cultures and complex *in vivo* models, organoids provide a physiologically relevant platform for studying disease mechanisms, testing therapeutic interventions, and personalizing treatment strategies.

This book, *Organoids: Advancements in Drug Discovery and Precision Medicine*, aims to serve as a comprehensive guide for researchers, clinicians, and industry professionals engaged in this transformative field.

Organoids have emerged as powerful tools, enabling scientists to recapitulate the structural and functional complexity of human organs *in vitro*. Their applications span high-throughput drug screening, toxicity testing, patient-specific disease modeling, and regenerative medicine. As the demand for predictive and personalized preclinical models continues to grow, organoid technology stands at the forefront of innovation — integrating advances in stem cell biology, tissue engineering, and computational science.

This book is structured to provide both foundational knowledge and cutting-edge insights into organoid research. The first section introduces the principles of organoid generation and advanced culture systems. Subsequent sections explore their applications in drug discovery, precision medicine, and emerging technologies such as single-cell omics, automation, and artificial intelligence. Each chapter — authored by leading experts in the field — offers methodological guidance, real-world case studies, and forward-looking perspectives to inspire further research and clinical translation.

This book will serve as a vital resource for students, scientists, and industry leaders alike — fostering collaboration and discovery in the quest to harness organoids for improved therapies and personalized healthcare. As the field continues to evolve, we eagerly anticipate the transformative impact of organoid technology on medicine and beyond.

Peter E. Lobie
Professor, Tsinghua Shenzhen International Graduate School,
Tsinghua University, China
Fellow, Royal Society of New Zealand

Nam-Hyung Kim
Professor, Chungbuk National University, Republic of Korea
Academician, Korean Academy of Science and Technology, Republic of Korea

https://doi.org/10.1142/9789819817597_fmatter

# About the Editors

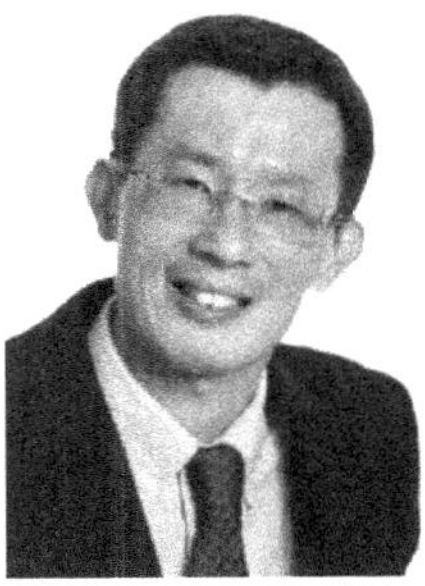

**Professor Boon-Cher Goh** is Chair Professor in the Department of Pharmacology at the Yong Loo Lin School of Medicine, National University of Singapore (NUS), where he is also Director of the NUS Centre for Cancer Research (N2CR); Senior Consultant in the Department of Hematology-Oncology at the National University Cancer Institute, Singapore (NCIS), where he is also Deputy Director of Research; Deputy Director of the Cancer Science Institute (CSI); and Group Chief (Physician Leadership and Organisation Development Office) of the National University Health System (NUHS). A pioneer of Singapore's clinical-trial ecosystem, he built the research infrastructure at NCIS into a leading clinical-research hub and, as Chair of the Cancer Therapeutics Research Group, strengthened Asia–Pacific research collaborations. His work spans pharmacogenetics, targeted therapies, and immuno-oncology, with an emphasis on precision medicine through pharmacogenetic biomarkers and patient-derived tumor organoids. His landmark studies — published in journals such as *Cell*, *Journal of Clinical Oncology*, and *The Lancet Oncology* — have reshaped therapeutic strategies worldwide. Recognized globally as a key opinion leader, he advises pharmaceutical companies on novel drug development and serves on the editorial boards of premier journals, including *Journal of Clinical Oncology* and *Annals of Oncology*. Through the seamless integration of scientific discovery and clinical practice, he continues to advance personalized cancer care around the world. He is a National Medical Research Council (NMRC)-accredited Distinguished Clinician Scientist.

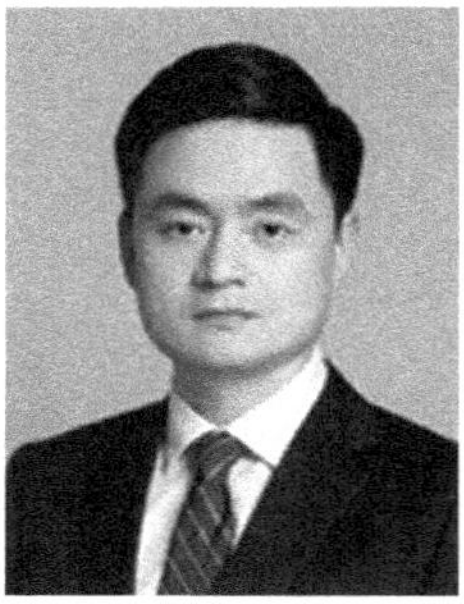

**Associate Professor Chongyang Shen** serves as a Principal Investigator at the Institute of Traditional Chinese Medicine and Stem Cell Research, Chengdu University of Traditional Chinese Medicine. With a Ph.D. from the West China School of Clinical Medicine, Sichuan University, he further honed his expertise as a Visiting Scholar (2018–2019) at the School of Medicine, Yale University, USA where he contributed to cutting-edge biomedical research. A recipient of competitive grants, he has successfully led two projects funded by the National Natural Science Foundation of China. His inventive contributions include 7 National Invention Patents, reflecting his commitment to translating research into practical solutions compliant with China's intellectual property regulations. His scholarly impact is underscored by over 30 peer-reviewed publications in high-impact journals such as *Advanced Functional Materials*, *ACS Materials Letters*, *Cancer Letters*, *Cell & Bioscience*, and *Stem Cell Research & Therapy*. His interdisciplinary work bridges traditional Chinese medicine with modern stem cell and materials science, positioning him at the forefront of biomedical innovation.

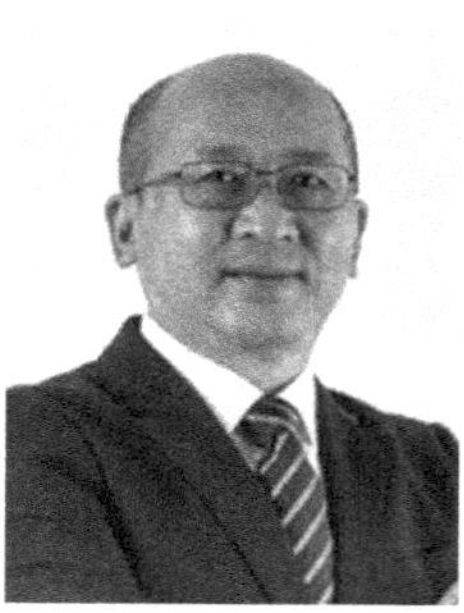

**Professor Lingzhi Wang** is the Principal Investigator of the Lung Cancer Therapy and Early Detection Laboratory at the National University of Singapore (NUS). He holds joint appointments at the NUS Centre for Cancer Research (N2CR) and the Department of Pharmacology at the Yong Loo Lin School of Medicine, NUS. With over 20 years of pioneering research experience, he is internationally recognized for his significant contributions to cancer pharmacology, biomarker discovery — including genetic biomarkers and patient-derived organoids — and the early diagnosis of lung cancer. His translational research effectively bridges basic science and clinical practice, advancing the frontiers of precision medicine and anticancer drug development. He has authored more than 170 peer-reviewed publications in high-impact journals such as *Annals of Oncology*, *Trends in Pharmacological Sciences*, and *Cell*. His work has garnered an h-index of 62 and over 10,000 citations. In recognition of his scientific excellence, he has received numerous prestigious awards, including the NMRC Excellent Scientist Award, the AAPS PhD Research Excellence Award, and a place on Stanford University's 2023 list of the World's Top 2% Scientists. Beyond his research, he serves on the editorial boards of several leading journals in pharmacology and oncology, contributing meaningfully to the global advancement of cancer research and improved treatment outcomes.

https://doi.org/10.1142/9789819817597_fmatter

# Contents

*Foreword* iii

*About the Editors* v

Chapter 1 Mastering Organoids: Fundamentals of Generation and Cultivation 1
*Huayang Xing, Suyao Xie, Yidan Chen, Jing Yue, Mohan Wu, Yang Wu*

Chapter 2 Advanced Organoid Culture Systems 26
*Yueyue Huangfu, Dengfeng Zhang, Jiaming Ye, Mingliang You, and Bingcheng Lin*

Chapter 3 Automation in Organoid-Based Precision Medicine 60
*Yanan Shi, Quanlin Xin, Wei Kang*

Chapter 4 Organoid Engineering Techniques for Drug Discovery and Development 78
*George Michael Nicolas, Ut Fai Chao, Shaohua Ma*

Chapter 5 Organoid-Driven Drug Discovery: Precision Screening and Target Validation 119
*Yunqi Man, Yanfei Liu, Qiwen Chen, Zhenbao Liu*

Chapter 6 Perspectives from a High-throughput Screening and Target Identification Laboratory 150
*Valentina Gonzalez-Pecchi, Elizabeth L. Zoeller, Matías I. Hepp, Sebastián Vera, Xiulei Mo, Kecheng Lei, Yuhong Du*

Chapter 7 Patient-Derived Organoids and Personalized Medicine 181
*Xiaoxiao Wang, Yufei Wang, Le Cheng, Zhaowu Ma, Xiaoguang Chen, Louis Zizhao Wang*

Chapter 8 Optimizing Organoid-Based Drug Sensitivity Testing: Essential Insights and Best Practices 220
*Yi Zhou, Ling Jiao, Wentao Yang, Xiaozhen Liu*

Chapter 9 Single-Cell Analysis and Omics Techniques 243
*Long Chen, Wei Jin, Xinrui Zhang, Jun Zhang, Liming Chen*

Chapter 10 Artificial Intelligence and Machine Learning in Organoid Technology 281
*Hong Kai Lee, Min Qiu, Yijun Chen*

Chapter 11 Ethical and Regulatory Considerations 311
*Khatri Simran, Win Lwin Thuya, Cao Yang, Yifeng Ren, Malia Alexandra Foo, Fengming You*

*Index* 337

https://doi.org/10.1142/9789819817597_0001

Chapter 1

# Mastering Organoids: Fundamentals of Generation and Cultivation

Huayang Xing[1,2,3,*], Suyao Xie[3], Yidan Chen[2], Jing Yue[2], Mohan Wu[4], Yang Wu[4]

[1]*Innovative Institute of Chinese Medicine and Pharmacy, Chengdu University of Traditional Chinese Medicine, Chengdu 61000, China*

[2]*Hangzhou Cancer Institute, Hangzhou Cancer Hospital, Hangzhou 310002, China*

[3]*Department of R&D, Hangzhou AimingMed Medical Technology Co., Ltd., Hangzhou 310000, China*

[4]*School of Biomedical Engineering, Harbin Institute of Technology (Shenzhen), Shenzhen 518055, China*

**Abstract:** This chapter offers a foundational overview of organoid biology, beginning with the classification and derivation of organoids from gastrointestinal, neural, pulmonary, hepatic, and tumor tissues. By examining the biological underpinnings and methodological approaches to organoid culture, readers will gain a comprehensive understanding of the versatility and scientific value of these models. Special emphasis is placed on tumor organoids, which have become indispensable in cancer research. Their ability to mirror patient-specific tumor heterogeneity positions them as valuable assets in precision medicine, drug screening, and treatment response prediction. The chapter also includes a detailed, step-by-step protocol for establishing tumor organoids — from tissue isolation to cryopreservation — accompanied by illustrative guidance to support reproducibility and implementation in research laboratories. In addition, cartilage organoids are introduced as a promising frontier in tissue engineering, with potential applications in regenerative medicine and the study of cartilage-related diseases. By integrating cutting-edge techniques and emerging applications, this chapter serves as a practical and insightful guide for researchers, clinicians, and students looking to harness the full potential of organoid technology in both basic and translational science.

**Keywords:** organoids, culture protocol, tumor, tissue engineering

*Corresponding author. Email: arielreally@gmail.com

## Key Points

1. Introduction to organoids: The definition and types of organoids are presented to provide a foundational understanding of this innovative technique.
2. Comprehensive overview: A detailed summary of organoid biology and their various sources is provided, offering insights into the versatility and potential of organoid models.
3. Tumor organoids: The applications of tumor organoids in cancer research, personalized medicine, and drug testing are discussed.
4. Protocol: A step-by-step protocol for establishing tumor organoids is outlined, with key illustrations to guide readers through the process.
5. Organoids in tissue engineering: Cartilage organoids are introduced as a cutting-edge approach in tissue engineering, highlighting their potential for regenerative medicine.

## 1.1 Introduction

Organoids represent a groundbreaking advancement in biomedical research, providing 3D, physiologically relevant models that closely resemble human tissues in both structure and function. As an innovative *in vitro* system, organoids are derived from various stem cell sources — including adult stem cells, embryonic stem cells, and human pluripotent stem cells — and can recapitulate the complexity of organ-specific architecture and cellular diversity [1]. These models have rapidly gained traction as powerful tools for investigating tissue development, disease mechanisms, and individualized therapeutic responses [2].

## 1.2 Organoid Definition and Types

### 1.2.1 *Organoid Definition*

An organoid is a 3D, self-organized cell-based *in vitro* model, derived from stem cells or progenitor cells. It can reconstitute the architecture, cellular composition, and functionality of the original organ to a significant extent [6].

Key features of organoids include:

(1) Self-organization: Organoids can self-organize into structures that mimic specific tissues or organs with the specific growth factors added in the culture medium.
(2) Multicellular composition: They include multiple cell types like those found in the original organ, enabling more accurate modeling of organ function.
(3) Physiological relevance: Organoids often exhibit functionalities, such as secretion, absorption, or response to stimuli, similar to their *in vivo* counterparts.

Organoids have applications in disease modeling, drug discovery, precision medicine, developmental biology, and regenerative medicine, making them indispensable tools in translational research [7–9].

### 1.2.2 *Types and Sources of Organoids*

Organoids can generally be classified into three categories based on their source of origin:

(1) Organoids derived from human pluripotent stem cells (hPSCs)
   - These include organoids of the brain, kidney, liver, intestine, heart, skin, and ear.
   - hPSCs can be directed to differentiate into organ-specific structures using established protocols [2, 6, 10].

(2) Organoids derived from adult stem cells (ASCs)
   - ASCs are utilized to generate organoids from tissues that contain resident progenitor cells.
   - Examples include organoids of the intestine, colon, lung, pancreas, stomach, and esophagus [6, 10].

(3) Tumor organoids
   - These organoids are established from cancer patient-derived samples, including surgical tissues, biopsies, endoscopic specimens, and malignant effusions.
   - A detailed protocol for generating tumor organoids from tissue samples is provided in Section 1.4.

A comprehensive summary of the types of organoids and their sources is provided in Table 1.1, which focuses exclusively on organoids derived from human or mouse tissues/cells, excluding those from other species such as pigs or snakes.

**Table 1.1** Published organoid models from various organs and hPSCs.

| Substructures/ Organs | Source | Cell/Tissue Types | Disease Model |
|---|---|---|---|
| Appendix [11, 12] | ASCs | Epithelial cell, enterocyte, mucosal-associated invariant T cell | Tumor, acute appendicitis |
| Brain [13–16] | hPSCs | Forebrain, midbrain, whole brain, cortex, hippocampus and choroid plexus | Autism, microcephaly, Alzheimer's disease, glioblastoma (from tumor tissue) |
| Bladder [17, 18] | ASCs | Urothelial stem/basal cell, luminal cell | Tumor |
| Colon [19, 20] | hPSCs/ASCs | Lgr5+ stem cell, villus cell, goblet cell, enteroendocrine cell | Tumor, inflammatory bowel disease |
| Ear [21] | hPSCs | Outer epithelium, functional hair cell, mesenchymal, neuronal cell | NA |
| Esophagus [22, 23] | ASCs | Fibroblast, immune cell, basaloid cell, epithelial cell | Tumor, esophagitis |
| Heart [24] | hPSCs | Cardiomyocytes (cTnT), stromal cells (CD90), endothelial cells (CD31), pericytes (NG2), and epicardial cells (WT1) | NA |
| Intestine [25–27] | hPSCs/ASCs | Lgr5+ stem cell, Paneth cell, villus cell, goblet cell, enteroendocrine cell | Cystic fibrosis, inflammatory bowel disease, infectious diseases and host-microbe interactions |
| Kidney [28–30] | hPSCs | Stromal, endothelial, nephron cell, ureteric epithelium, renal vesicle, distal tubule, loop of Henle, proximal tubule and podocyte | Tumor (from tumor tissue), nephrotoxicity, kidney injury |
| Liver [31, 32] | hPSCs/ASCs | Lgr5+ stem cell, bile dutal cell, hepatocyte, cholangiocyte | Tumor, cystic fibrosis, Alagille syndrome |
| Lung [33–35] | hPSCs/ASCs | basal, ciliated, club cell small/large airway, alveolar organoid | Tumor, cystic fibrosis, viral infection |
| Mammary [36] | ASCs | Mature luminal, luminal progenitor, basal/stem cell | Tumor |
| Ocular [37] | hPSCs | Retinal cell, corneal, limbal, conjunctival epithelial cell | NA |

Table 1.1 (*Continued*)

| Substructures/ Organs | Source | Cell/Tissue Types | Disease Model |
|---|---|---|---|
| Pancreas [38–41] | hPSCs/ASCs | Lgr5+ stem cell, acinar cell, ductal cells, endocrine cell | Tumor |
| Reproductive (Female) [42–44] | ASCs | Endometrial, cervical, ovarian cancer organoids | Tumor |
| Reproductive (Male) [45] | ASCs | Epididymal, prostate, testicular organoids | Tumor, fertility, infection |
| Salivary gland [46] | ASCs | C-kit+ progenitor cell | Radiation-induced hyposalivation |
| Skin [47] | hPSCs/ASCs | Epidermal keratinocyte, dermal fibroblast, hair-bearing skin organoid (in a co-culture model with epidermis and dermis) | Tumor, skin plasticity and regeneration |
| Stomach [48, 49] | hPSCs/ASCs | LGR5+ stem cell, surface/antral mucous cell, endocrine cell | Tumor, *Helicobacter pylori* infection |
| Tongue [50] | ASCs | Squamous epithelial cell, stratum corneum | Tumor, lingual regeneration |

## 1.3 Applications of Tumor Organoids

Tumor organoids, also known as patient-derived organoids, can be generated from primary patient tumor samples under specific *in vitro* conditions. These organoids preserve the histological structure and functional characteristics of the original tumors while exhibiting stable proliferation in a 3D culture system [51]. As illustrated in Figure 1.1, tumor organoids have been widely adopted to personalized medicine, new drug discovery, tumor modeling, tumorgenesis mechanisms exploration, immunotherapy evaluation and translational research.

### 1.3.1 *Personalized Strategies for Enhancing Treatment Outcomes*

Tumor organoids serve as a vital platform for advancing personalized medicine. By enabling the *in vitro* testing of various drug combinations and the simulation of radiation therapy protocols, tumor organoids facilitate the identification of the most

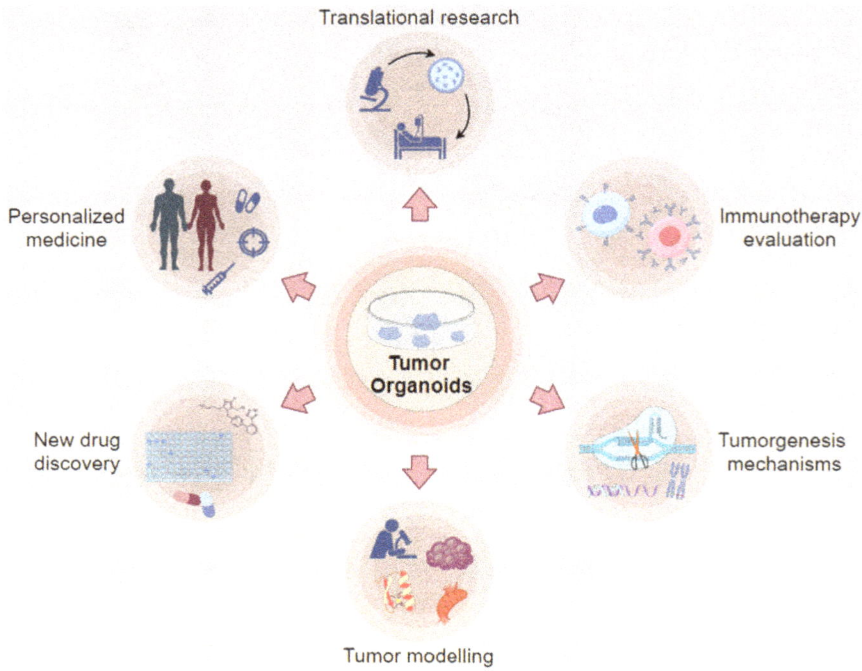


**Figure 1.1** Applications of tumor organoids. Owing to tumor organoids' excellent performance in simulating the *in vivo* tumor microenvironment and heterogeneity, tumor organoids are widely used in fundamental research, drug development, and personalized medicine, as elaborated in Section 1.3.

effective treatment regimen for individual patients [52, 53]. This approach not only significantly enhances the treatment precision and improves outcome but also minimizes unnecessary side effects that patients might experience during therapy [54].

### 1.3.2 *Drug Screening and Validation in Drug Development*

In the early stages of new drug development, tumor organoids offer a powerful model for simulating drug responses across various tumor subtypes and genetic backgrounds. These 3D cultures closely replicate the complexity of human tumors, allowing researchers to assess the efficacy and toxicity of candidate compounds in a physiologically relevant context. By leveraging organoid models, researchers can rapidly identify and prioritize promising therapeutic candidates, thereby streamlining the drug development pipeline, enhancing translational relevance, and reducing both time and cost associated with preclinical testing [55].

### 1.3.3 *Basic Science Research and Tumor Heterogeneity Reproduction*

Tumor organoids retain the genetic characteristics and heterogeneity of their original tumors, effectively bridging the gap between patient-derived cells and patient-derived xenografts. This fidelity enables researchers to reconstruct key aspects of tumor initiation, progression, and interactions with the tumor microenvironment in a controlled *in vitro* setting [56, 57]. By studying organoids derived from patients, scientists can gain valuable insights into the dynamic behavior of tumor cells, including their evolutionary adaptations and resistance mechanisms in response to environmental pressures. As such, tumor organoids represent an indispensable tool for advancing our understanding of tumor biology and heterogeneity in basic science research.

### 1.3.4 Tumor Molecular Mechanism Investigation

Tumor organoids offer a robust and physiologically relevant platform for investigating the molecular mechanisms underlying tumor initiation, progression, and treatment resistance. By integrating gene editing techniques, tumor organoids can provide direct insights into the impact of genetic variations on cell behavior. This strategy not only reveals the molecular mechanisms driving tumor onset and progression but also provides a scientific basis for the development of new targeted therapy drugs. Tumor organoids can also develop drug-resistant subpopulations over long-term cultures. By studying these resistant cells in organoids, researchers can uncover the adaptation mechanisms of tumors under drug pressure, such as gene mutations, drug efflux, and DNA repair mechanisms, thereby offering new strategies to overcome drug resistance [56].

### 1.3.5 Immunotherapy Effectiveness Evaluation

The use of tumor organoids in immunotherapy research is increasingly prevalent. By co-culturing organoids with immune cells, the interaction between immune cells and tumor cells in the tumor microenvironment can be simulated, helping researchers better understand immune escape mechanisms and the impact of the tumor microenvironment on immune responses [58, 59]. Additionally, organoid models show great potential in evaluating the effectiveness and safety of innovative therapies, such as CAR-T cell treatment, providing substantial support for developing more effective immunotherapy strategies.

### 1.3.6 Accelerating Translational Research

Tumor organoids play a pivotal role in accelerating translational research by bridging the gap between basic science discoveries and clinical application. Their ability to closely mimic the genetic, architectural, and functional characteristics of human tumors allows for more accurate predictions of treatment responses and disease progression in patients. This makes organoid models invaluable for testing novel therapeutic strategies, refining drug formulations, and identifying biomarkers for patient stratification. By enabling faster, more reliable preclinical testing, tumor organoids expedite the transition from experimental research to clinical trials, ultimately shortening the timeline for bringing new, effective therapies to patients [60–63].

As a cutting-edge technology and valuable *in vitro* model, tumor organoids provide essential support for studying tumor biology while playing a pivotal role in advancing personalized medicine, accelerating drug development, and optimizing treatment strategies. With ongoing advancements in cultivation techniques and gene editing technologies, the potential applications of tumor organoids are expected to expand significantly, offering new avenues of hope for cancer patients.

## 1.4 Protocol of Tumor Organoid Establishment

### 1.4.1 *Materials and Reagents*

MasterAim® Tumor Organoid Culture Medium (AimingMed, Hangzhou, China), MasterAim® Primary Enhancer (AimingMed, Hangzhou, China), MasterAim® Tissue Preservation Medium (AimingMed, Hangzhou, China), MasterAim® Anti-Adherence Solution (AimingMed, Hangzhou, China), MasterAim® Tissue Dissociation Medium (AimingMed, Hangzhou, China), MasterAim® Organoid Cryopreservation Medium (AimingMed, Hangzhou, China), Penicillin–Streptomycin (Gibco, USA), D-PBS (Dulbecco's Phosphate-Buffered Saline) (Gibco, USA), Red Blood Cell Lysis Buffer

(Sangon, China), Myco-Lumi™ Luminescence Mycoplasma Detection Kit (Beyotime, China), Matrigel (Low Growth Factor, Phenol Red-Free, Corning, USA), TrypLE Express Enzyme (1X, Phenol Red, Gibco, USA); 3.5 cm and 10 cm culture dishes, 24-well plates (Tissue culture-treated for dome embedding; recommended in order: Corning #3524, Greiner Bio-one #662160, Thermo Scientific #142475), cut 1 mL pipette tips, Pasteur pipettes, 15 mL and 50 mL centrifuge tubes, pipette tips (1 mL, 200 μL, 10 μL), pipettes (10 mL, 25 mL, 50 mL).

## 1.4.2 *Experimental Procedures*

**Tips:**

- All pipettes, pipette tips, and other plastic consumables that are in contact with tissues or organoids must be pre-rinsed with MasterAim® Anti-Adherence Solution.
- Pre-cool the washing solutions used during sample processing.
- Perform operations on ice whenever possible to maintain the activity of the samples.

### 1.4.2.1 *Reagent Preparation*

- Washing Solution: DPBS + 1% Penicillin–Streptomycin, pre-cooled for use.
- Tumor Organoid Culture Medium Preparation: Take the MasterAim® Tumor Organoid Basal Medium and MasterAim® Tumor Organoid Medium Supplement out of −20°C and thaw at 4°C. Transfer all medium supplements into the basal medium and mix thoroughly to prepare the complete organoid culture medium.
- It is recommended to aliquot the complete medium and store at −20°C. After opening, keep it at 4°C and use within two weeks to avoid repeated freeze-thaw cycles.
- For primary organoid construction, add 1X MasterAim® Primary Enhancer to the culture medium. For passaged organoids, use the complete tumor organoid medium directly.
- The complete organoid medium does not contain antibiotics. Add antibiotics as needed based on experimental requirements.

#### 1.4.2.2 *Sample Collection*

- Informed consent from the patient must be obtained before collecting clinical samples.
- Patient samples should be preserved in MasterAim® Tissue Preservation Medium at 4°C and shipped to the lab within 48 hours.

#### 1.4.2.3 *Tissue Preparation before Digestion*

i. Upon arrival, based on the tissue size, transfer the tissue to a 3.5 cm or 10 cm culture dish placed on an ice plate, containing 2–8°C cold washing solution (approximately 1–2 mL).
ii. Measure the length and width of the tissue sample using a ruler and take photos to document the tissue quality.
iii. Tissue preparation: Remove fat and necrotic tissue as much as possible, retaining only the lesion. If uncertain, leave it intact. When processing both normal and tumor organoids, prioritize normal tissue processing.
iv. Tissue cleansing: Place the tissue into a 50 mL Falcon tube and wash it with 10–15 mL of washing solution, repeating 5–10 times until the solution becomes clear.

**Tips:**

- For digestive tract tissues (e.g., nasopharynx, oral cavity, stomach, or intestinal samples), increase washing frequency to 20 times.
- Collect the washing and transport solutions if needed, centrifuge and check for cell presence. If significant cell pellet is observed, wash the tissue at least 5 more times and collect the cell pellet.
- The washing step helps remove microorganisms that could cause contamination, as well as unwanted cells (e.g., blood cells, dead cells, cell debris). To avoid contamination later, increase the washing frequency to 10 or more times if needed.
- Sample cryopreservation: If the tissue is larger than 0.5 cm in diameter or requires freezing, divide it into portions. Use one portion for organoid culture and store the other in a labeled cryovial. Store the tissue in a −80°C freezer or liquid nitrogen (approximately the size of a mung bean).

### 1.4.2.4 *Tissue Dissociation*

i. Sample cutting: Remove most of the washing solution and transfer the sample to an Eppendorf tube or culture dish. Add 200 μL of washing or dissociation solution and mince the sample with scissors.
ii. Cut the tissue into 0.5–1 $mm^3$ pieces and ensure the fragments are evenly sized. The mincing step is crucial for subsequent digestion, so the tissue should be minced as uniformly as possible.
iii. Observe a small amount of the solution with the tissue under a microscope to check for cell leakage and photograph the sample for records.
iv. **Step I Dissociation:** Use a pre-rinsed Pasteur pipette to transfer the minced tissue from the Eppendorf tube to a 15 mL centrifuge tube. Add 4–8 mL of MasterAim® Tissue Dissociation Medium I (depend on the tissue volume) and digest the tissue in a water bath with shaking at 37°C for 30–60 mins, checking every 20 minutes for large cell releases. The digestion time may be adjusted based on the tissue's condition (Figure 1.2A1, no cells were observed in the residual tissue).
   - During microscopic observation after mincing, if large numbers of cells are seen to release, this indicates that the sample is relatively easy to digest, and digestion time may need to be shortened. For samples with high fibrosis levels, yield may be lower, and digestion time can be extended as needed.
v. **Step II Dissociation:**
   a) After digestion with Tissue Dissociation Medium I, add 8–16 mL of washing solution (twice the volume of the digestion solution) to terminate the digestion.
   b) Centrifuge at 300 g for 5 minutes, discard the supernatant, and add 2 mL of MasterAim® Tissue Dissociation Medium II and digest the tissue in a water bath with shaking at 37°C for 10–15 mins.
   c) Under the microscope, check whether the cell clusters have been further digested into smaller clusters. Generally, when most clusters in the field of view consist of 5–20 cells, stop the digestion (Figure 1.2A2, most cell clumps have been digested into small cell clusters). For esophageal cancer, digest to a single cell suspension instead of cell clusters.
vi. After completing digestion, add 4 mL of washing solution (twice the volume of the digestion solution) to stop the digestion. Centrifuge at 300 g for 5 minutes and collect the cells.

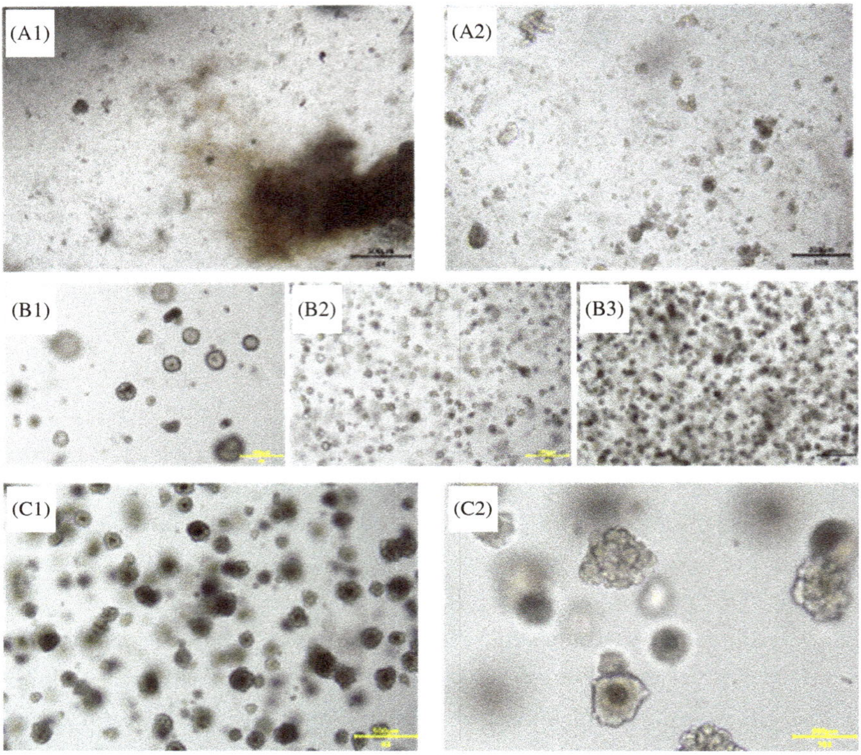


**Figure 1.2** Representative images during the process in establishing tumor organoids. Illustration of tissue condition after Tissue Dissociation Medium I (A1) and II (A2); Examples of organoid seeding density (B1: low density, B2: recommended density, B3: high density); C1/2: Examples of tumor organoids' morphology pre-passaging. Scale bar = 500 μm in A1/2, B1/2/3 and C1, scale bar = 200 μm in C2.

vii. Discard the supernatant, add 2 mL of washing solution to resuspend the cells.

viii. (Optional) Skip this step for small samples, i.e., biopsy or endoscopic samples. Pre-rinse a 100 μm cell strainer with 2 mL of Anti-Adherence Solution, then filter the cell suspension through it, collecting the filtrate in a pre-moistened 50 mL Falcon tube (including tube walls). Rinse the cell suspension tube multiple times with washing solution, filtering each time. Centrifuge the filtrate at 300 g for 5 minutes.

ix. Carefully discard the supernatant without disturbing the cell pellet. Use a pipette tip to aspirate the very bottom layer of liquid to avoid contact with the pellet.

x. (Optional) If the pellet contains a significant amount of red blood cells (reddish color), add 1–2 mL of red blood cell lysis buffer. Adjust the volume based on pellet size and pipette up and down several times with a 1 mL pipette tip. Incubate at room temperature for 6 minutes, then add 4–6 mL of washing solution to resuspend the cells and centrifuge at 300 g for 5 minutes.

#### 1.4.2.5 *Establishment of Tumor Organoids*

i. Cell counting: Resuspend the cell pellet obtained in the previous step in 1 mL of washing solution and count the cell clusters using an automatic or manual cell counter. Each 50 μL gel droplet requires approximately 400–1,000 cell clusters (around 200,000–300,000 cells).
ii. Resuspend the cell pellet obtained in the previous step in Matrigel according to the cell count. Use a mixture of 1 part culture medium to 1.5–2 parts Matrigel. Pay attention to the temperature at this step; if the temperature is too high, the gel may solidify or generate bubbles, leading to loss of organoids.
iii. Take 50 μL of the organoid-Matrigel suspension and add it to the center of a 24-well plate (pre-warmed at 37°C for 30 minutes). To prevent bubbles during seeding, press the pipette to the first stop only (do not press to the bottom). The seeded droplet should form a solid dome at the center of each well.
iv. Allow dome to solidify at 37°C for 5 minutes, then invert it and let it sit for 25 minutes to allow the dome to solidify in the inverted position.
v. Using a pipette, gently add 600 μL of 37°C pre-warmed MasterAim® Tumor Organoid Culture Medium to each well along the sidewall (for P0, add 1X MasterAim® Primary Enhancer). Avoid adding the medium directly onto the dome.
vi. Add D-PBS to any wells without domes to maintain humidity during incubation.
vii. Cover the plate and incubate at 37°C with 5% $CO_2$.
viii. Change the medium every 2–4 days and monitor the growth, documenting with photos until ready for passaging. Generally, the organoids need to be passaged after 7–21 days post-seeding.
ix. The recommended organoid seeding density is shown in Figure 1.2B2, and morphology of tumor organoids before passaging in Figure 1.2C1/C2.

**Tips:**

- Use chilled pipette tips and cold culture medium for dome seeding. The matrix gel should be thawed on ice in advance.
- Do not seed organoids in the outermost wells of the plate.
- When changing or adding medium, avoid touching the dome. To prevent cross-contamination, use a different pipette tip for each well when removing liquid.

### 1.4.2.6 *Passaging of Tumor Organoids*

i. Remove the culture medium and add 0.5 mL of TrypLE per well (using a 24-well plate as an example). Use a 1 mL pipette tip to pipette up and down 6–10 times to break up the dome. To minimize organoid loss, it is recommended to collect all organoids together for digestion. (Increase the volume of TrypLE as needed based on the quantity of organoids.)
ii. Incubate at room temperature for 5–10 minutes (or in a 37°C incubator for 5 minutes).
iii. Observe the organoids under a microscope. If the organoid fragments are still too large or the structure remains intact, increase the incubation time.

**Tips:**

- In the initial organoid culture, fibroblast growth may appear on the bottom of the culture plate. During passaging, avoid scraping the plate bottom to help remove these cells in the next generation culture.
- During organoid cluster passaging, each cell cluster typically contains about 5–20 cells, with a size of 20–50 μm. For esophageal cancer, passaging requires digestion into single cells.
- Transfer the cells into a centrifuge tube containing 6 mL of pre-cooled DPBS-PS (pre-rinsed). Centrifuge at 300 g for 5 minutes and collect the organoids.
- Repeat steps i–viii in Section 1.4.2.5.

### 1.4.2.7 *Cryopreservation of Tumor Organoids*

i. Check organoid growth status and determine if the sample meets the cryopreservation standards and the number of cryopreservation tubes needed. Photograph the organoids and print labels.

ii. Place the cryobox in a 4°C refrigerator for later use.
iii. Collect 1 mL of culture supernatant from the organoid culture before freezing and use a Myco-Lumi™ Luminescence Mycoplasma Detection Kit or Mycoplasma PCR Detection Kit for mycoplasma testing. Refer to the product manual for specific procedures.
iv. Carefully remove the culture medium from the wells, then gently rinse the domes twice with cold DPBS. After rinsing, remove the DPBS.
v. Add 0.5 mL of TrypLE Express Enzyme (1X) per well (24-well plate) and gently pipette to disperse the domes. Under a microscope, observe the digestion process, and when organoids reach a size of 40–60 μm, add DPBS in a volume at least twice that of the digestion solution to stop digestion.
vi. Transfer the cell suspension to a 15 mL centrifuge tube (pre-rinsed), gently pipette to mix without creating bubbles, and centrifuge at 300 g for 5 minutes. Discard the supernatant.
vii. Add 1 mL of DPBS to resuspend the cells, then mix gently. Take 10 μL of the suspension and mix with 10 μL of AO/PI staining solution in a 1:1 ratio and count viable cells.
viii. After counting, centrifuge at 300 g for 5 minutes and discard the supernatant.
ix. Resuspend the pellet in organoid cryopreservation solution, mix gently without creating bubbles, and aliquot 1 mL into each labeled cryovial.
x. Place the cryovials in a controlled-rate freezing container at -80°C overnight, and transfer to liquid nitrogen storage for long-term storage.

#### 1.4.2.8 *Thawing of Tumor Organoids*

i. Label a 15 mL centrifuge tube and add 9 mL of pre-warmed DMEM/F12 medium to the tube.
ii. Thaw the cryovial: Take out the cryovial and immediately place it in a 37°C water bath for rapid thawing. Gently shake the cryovial to dissolve it within 1–2 minutes (stop thawing when only small ice particles remain inside).
iii. Open the cryovial and use a 1 mL pipette tip to transfer the thawed cell suspension to the previously prepared 15 mL centrifuge tube. Centrifuge at 1200 rpm for 5 minutes. Use a 1 mL pipette tip to carefully remove the supernatant, and switch to a smaller pipette tip if needed to remove any remaining supernatant without disturbing the cell pellet.

iv. Resuspend the cell pellet in 1 mL of pre-warmed DMEM/F12 medium (perform resuspension gently, as freshly thawed cells are fragile) and proceed with cell counting.
v. During thawing, recount the number of viable cells. Adjust the working volume as needed to maintain a 1:2 ratio of medium to Matrigel. It is recommended to seed at least 20,000 viable cells per 50 μL dome.
vi. Repeat steps iii–vii in Section 1.4.2.5.
vii. Observe organoid growth the next day without changing the medium. After three days, perform a half or full medium change depending on the organoid growth status.

## 1.5 Cartilage Organoids in Tissue Engineering

Cartilage is an embryonic skeleton unique to vertebrates, playing a crucial role in support and protection within the body. Damage to cartilage can result from trauma, cancer resection, aging, or congenital diseases. Unlike most tissues, cartilage is avascular, aneural, and alymphatic, which limits its ability to regenerate after injury [64]. Severe cartilage injury may lead to joint diseases like osteoarthritis, significantly impacting a patient's quality of life [5]. Therefore, developing effective treatments for cartilage defects and promoting cartilage regeneration is an urgent need in bone tissue engineering, with substantial clinical relevance.

Organoid technology has seen rapid development in recent years, due to its ability to precisely simulate the structural and functional intricacies of human organs at a small scale [65]. Cartilage organoids refer to 3D cell clusters formed by the differentiation of stem cells (e.g., embryonic stem cells, induced pluripotent stem cells (iPSC), ASCs, and mesenchymal stem cell) through *in vitro* cultivation [5], aiming to mimic the histological characteristics and physiological function of cartilage tissue [66] (Figure 1.3A). Based on the recapitulation of developmental events during embryogenesis and articular cartilage regeneration [67], cartilage organoids can serve as disease models to understand the pathogenesis of cartilage-related diseases and provide an advanced platform for drug development and toxicity testing. For example, Sun *et al.* [68] generated 3D-cultured synovial mesenchymal stromal cell (SMSC) organoids and showed that SMSC organoids led to decreased miR-138 expression and higher expression of its target gene FOXC1, leading to better chondrogenic and anti-arthritic properties of the SMSC organoids compared to 2D cultured SMSCs, which indicated

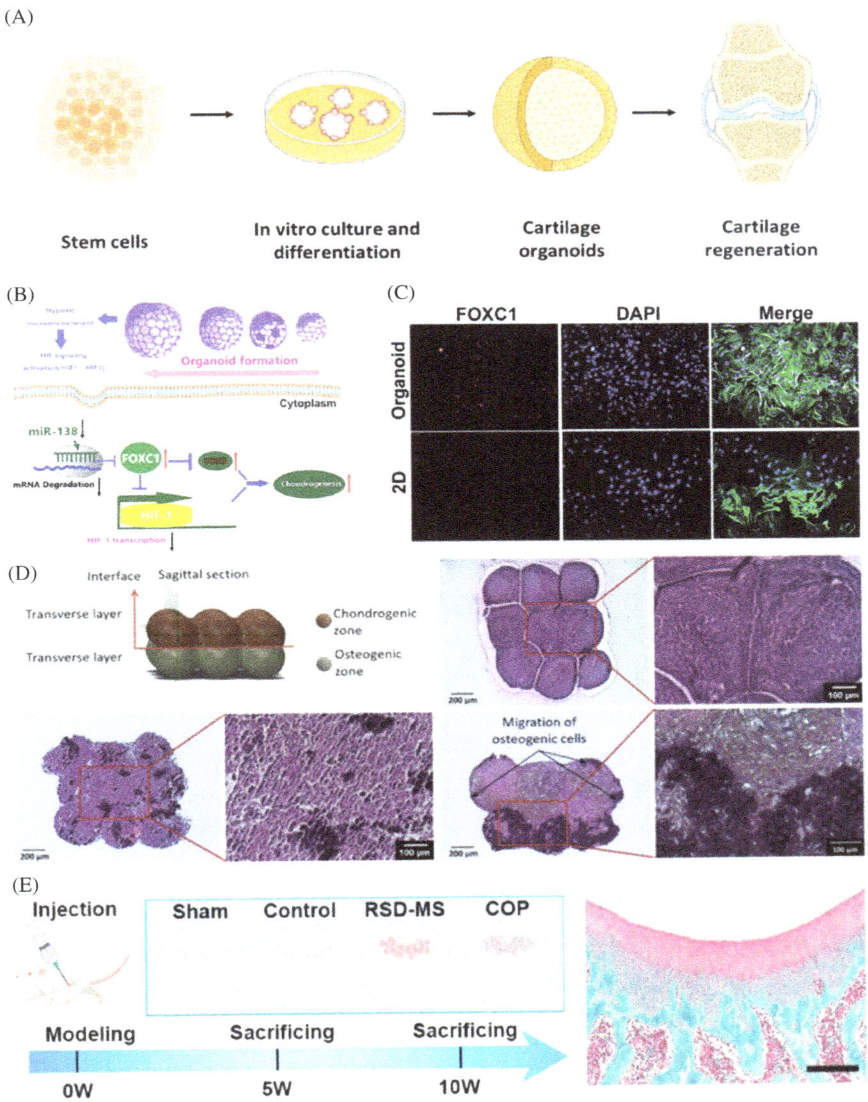


**Figure 1.3** Preparation and application of cartilage organoids. (A) The formation process of cartilage organoids. (B) Schematic representation of how miR-138/FOXC1/HIF signaling pathway might mediate chondrogenesis and the therapeutic effects of SMSC organoids in osteoarthritis. Adapted with permission from [68]. (C) FOXC1 expression (red) with immunostaining in cultured SMSC organoids (green for cytoskeleton). Adapted with permission from [68]. (D) The construction of the osteochondral interface based on organoid microspheres. Adapted with permission from [72]. (E) Scheme of cartilage defect modeling and treatment protocol and representative Safranin O/Fast Green staining of femur cartilage at 10 weeks after treatment based on cartilage organoid precursors. Adapted with permission from [74].

its potential in cartilage regeneration and osteoarthritis therapy (Figure 1.3B–C). Thorup *et al.* [69] developed an ectopic cartilage formation assay, which enabled the efficient screening of molecules with cartilage regeneration potential by evaluating cartilage organoids derived from nude mice. Therefore, the application of cartilage organoids reduces the need for animal experiments, shortens the time required to explore disease mechanisms and drug screening, and allows for the evaluation of the differentiation potential of cartilage cells from different donors, facilitating personalized medicine.

In addition to serving as disease models and being used for drug screening tools, cartilage organoids have the potential to integrate into host tissue, aiding in the repair and regeneration of damaged cartilage [70]. Thus, constructing cartilage organoids as transplant material for cartilage regeneration offers a novel approach to tissue engineering. Wu *et al.* [71] developed a hybrid approach integrating extrusion-based and aspiration-assisted bioprinting techniques to generate zonally stratified cartilage, achieving the construction of bioprinted cartilage that harmonizes anatomical similarity with biological functions. Furthermore, aspiration-assisted bioprinting technology was used for positioning of chondrogenic and osteogenic organoids to build the osteochondral interface, where two types of spheroids tightly fused with their respective morphology maintained [72], which has made a significant contribution to the *in vitro* construction of transplantable cartilage tissue (Figure 1.3D). Abe *et al.* [73] created cartilage organoids derived from cynomolgus monkey iPSC, showing that allogeneic iPSC-derived cartilage organoids survived and integrated, which further remodeled the articular cartilage in a primate model of chondral defects in the knee joints. Shen *et al.* [74] utilized microfluidic technology, combining silk methacrylate, supramolecular DNA hydrogel techniques, and photopolymerization technology, to fabricate RGD-SF-DNA hydrogel microspheres (RSD-MSs). Bone mesenchymal stem cells were seeded onto RSD-MSs for *in vitro* chondrogenic induction, leading to the creation of cartilage organoid precursors. In *in vivo* experiments, the repair ability of cartilage organoid precursors was validated, providing an innovative strategy and material choice for cartilage tissue engineering (Figure 1.3E).

Consequently, the integration of cartilage organoids with tissue engineering techniques offers a novel solution for regenerative medicine of cartilage. Additionally, customizing scaffolds and loading patients' cells eliminates immune rejection and better meets the specific needs of individual patients, advancing the development of personalized medicine.

In summary, this chapter offers a concise overview of organoid technology, emphasizing its applications in tumor modeling. It highlights key advancements such as organoid biobank development for high-throughput drug screening and the use of patient-derived organoids as predictive tools in precision medicine. Organoids enable detailed modeling of tumor heterogeneity and cancer progression, while integration with gene editing and tissue engineering expands their potential in regenerative and personalized therapies.

Despite significant progress, challenges remain, including the lack of standardized protocols, limited reproducibility, and difficulty replicating the tumor microenvironment at scale. Continued efforts to standardize methods and integrate organoids into clinical workflows are critical to realizing their full impact in cancer research and precision oncology.

## Key Opinion Points

1. The term "organoids" is often misused in this field, and scientists should use it more cautiously to ensure clarity and consistency. Clear definitions and standardized criteria are essential for maintaining scientific rigor and fostering effective communication within the research community.
2. The establishment of various types of organoids has been widely documented; however, the process remains labor-intensive and time-consuming. Automation presents a promising opportunity to streamline and optimize this process, enhancing consistency and standardization.
3. Integrating organoids with tissue engineering provides a novel approach for tissue regeneration.

## References

1. Fatehullah A, Tan SH, Barker N. Organoids as an in vitro model of human development and disease. Nature Cell Biol. 2016;18(3):246–254.
2. Clevers H. Modeling development and disease with organoids. Cell. 2016;165(7): 1586–1597.

3. Tuveson D, Clevers H. Cancer modeling meets human organoid technology. Science. 2019;364(6444):952–955.
4. Bleijs M, van de Wetering M, Clevers H, Drost J. Xenograft and organoid model systems in cancer research. EMBO J. 2019;38(15):e101654.
5. Yu Y, Wang J, Li Y, Chen Y, Cui W. Cartilaginous organoids: advances, applications, and perspectives. Adv NanoBiomed Res. 2023;3(1):2200114.
6. Zhao Z, Chen X, Dowbaj AM, Sljukic A, Bratlie K, Lin L, *et al.* Organoids. Nat Rev Methods Primers. 2022;2(1):94.
7. Lancaster MA, Huch M. Disease modelling in human organoids. Dis Model Mech. 2019;12(7):dmm039347.
8. Wensink GE, Elias SG, Mullenders J, Koopman M, Boj SF, Kranenburg OW, *et al.* Patient-derived organoids as a predictive biomarker for treatment response in cancer patients. NPJ Precis Oncol. 2021;5(1):30.
9. Kim J, Koo BK, Knoblich JA. Human organoids: model systems for human biology and medicine. Nat Rev Mol Cell Biol. 2020;21(10):571–584.
10. Ahammed B, Kalangi SK. A decade of organoid research: progress and challenges in the field of organoid technology. ACS Omega. 2024;9(28):30087–30096.
11. Drost J, Clevers H. Organoids in cancer research. Nat Rev Cancer. 2018;18(7):407–418.
12. Fujii M, Sato T. Somatic cell-derived organoids as prototypes of human epithelial tissues and diseases. Nat Mater. 2021;20(2):156–169.
13. Takahashi T. Organoids for drug discovery and personalized medicine. Annu Rev Pharmacol Toxicol. 2024;64:453–472.
14. Xia Y, Kong HJ. Tissue and organoids: from homeostasis to disease development. Annu Rev Biomed Eng. 2023;25:47–69.
15. Gunti S, Hoke ATK, Vu KP, London D, Karpiouk A, Ogden SC, *et al.* 3D brain organoids: a new frontier in disease modeling and drug screening. Cells. 2021;10(10):2601.
16. Wang Y, Hu J, Chen X, Li J, Wang Z, Yang P, *et al.* Organoids and organs-on-chips: insights into predicting drug toxicity. Acta Pharm Sin B. 2021;11(7):1789–1807.
17. Wiedenmann S, Breunig M, Merkle J, von Toerne C, Georgiev T, Moussus M, *et al.* Single-cell-resolved differentiation of human induced pluripotent stem cells into pancreatic duct-like organoids on a microwell chip. Nat Biomed Eng. 2021;5(8):897–913.
18. Dekkers JF, Berkers G, Kruisselbrink E, Vonk AM, de Jonge HR, Janssens HM, *et al.* Characterizing responses to CFTR-modulating drugs using rectal organoids derived from patients with cystic fibrosis. Nat Med. 2016;22(8):940–946.
19. Zhang Z, Xu M, Zhang B, Zhang X, Zhang Y, Xu Y, *et al.* Tumor-repopulating cells induce PD-1 expression in CD8+ T cells by transferring kynurenine and AhR activation. Cancer Cell. 2018;33(3):480–494.e7.

20. Vlachogiannis G, Hedayat S, Vatsiou A, Jamin Y, Fernández-Mateos J, Khan K, *et al.* Patient-derived organoids model treatment response of metastatic gastrointestinal cancers. Science. 2018;359(6378):920–926.
21. Sachs N, Papaspyropoulos A, Zomer-van Ommen DD, Heo I, Böttinger L, Klay D, *et al.* Long-term expanding human airway organoids for disease modeling. EMBO J. 2019;38(4):e100300.
22. Han Y, Yang L, Cao H, Liang Y, Jiang Y, Zhang J, *et al.* The generation of lung organoids from human pluripotent stem cells. Am J Physiol Lung Cell Mol Physiol. 2021;320(5):L887–L905.
23. Seino T, Kawasaki S, Shimokawa M, Tamagawa H, Toshimitsu K, Fujii M, *et al.* Human pancreatic tumor organoids reveal loss of stem cell niche factor dependence during disease progression. Cell Stem Cell. 2018;22(3):454–467.e6.
24. Gao D, Vela I, Sboner A, Iaquinta PJ, Karthaus WR, Gopalan A, *et al.* Organoid cultures derived from patients with advanced prostate cancer. Cell. 2014;159(1):176–187.
25. Fendler A, Bauer D, Busch J, Jung K, Wulf-Goldenberg A, Kunz S, *et al.* Toward precision medicine in prostate cancer: single-cell analysis of patient-derived organoids to predict drug response. J Exp Clin Cancer Res. 2020;39(1):64.
26. Karthaus WR, Hofree M, Choi D, Linton EL, Turkekul M, Bejnood A, *et al.* Regenerative potential of prostate luminal cells revealed by single-cell analysis. Science. 2020;368(6490):497–505.
27. Wang S, Gao D, Chen Y, Liu G. The potential of organoids in urological cancer research. Nat Rev Urol. 2017;14(7):401–414.
28. Artegiani B, Hendriks D, Beumer J, Kok R, Zheng X, Joore I, *et al.* Fast and efficient generation of knock-in human organoids using homology-independent CRISPR-Cas9 precision genome editing. Nat Cell Biol. 2020;22(3):321–331.
29. Marsee A, Roos FJ, Verstegen MMA, Gehart H, Hu H, Oosterhoff LA, *et al.* Building consensus on definition and nomenclature of hepatic, biliary, and pancreatic organoids. Cell Stem Cell. 2021;28(5):816–832.
30. Takahashi Y, Sekine K. Organoids for modeling development and disease: moving from Petri dishes to bioreactors. Curr Opin Biotechnol. 2021;70:72–78.
31. Sato T, Vries RG, Snippert HJ, van de Wetering M, Barker N, Stange DE, *et al.* Single Lgr5 stem cells build crypt–villus structures in vitro without a mesenchymal niche. Nature. 2009;459(7244):262–265.
32. Chua CW, Shibata M, Lei M, Toivanen R, Barlow L, Bergren SK, *et al.* Single luminal epithelial progenitors can generate prostate organoids in culture. Nat Cell Biol. 2014;16(10):951–961.
33. Clevers H. What is an adult stem cell? Science. 2015;350(6266):1319–1320.

34. Sachs N, de Ligt J, Kopper O, Gogola E, Bounova G, Weeber F, *et al.* A living biobank of breast cancer organoids captures disease heterogeneity. Cell. 2018;172(1–2): 373–386.e10.
35. Boj SF, Hwang CI, Baker LA, Chio II, Engle DD, Corbo V, *et al.* Organoid models of human and mouse ductal pancreatic cancer. Cell. 2015;160(1–2):324–338.
36. Dutta D, Heo I, Clevers H. Disease modeling in stem cell-derived 3D organoid systems. Trends Mol Med. 2017;23(5):393–410.
37. van de Wetering M, Francies HE, Francis JM, Bounova G, Iorio F, Pronk A, *et al.* Prospective derivation of a living organoid biobank of colorectal cancer patients. Cell. 2015;161(4):933–945.
38. Skardal A, Shupe T, Atala A. Organoid-on-a-chip and body-on-a-chip systems for drug screening and disease modeling. Drug Discov Today. 2016;21(9):1399–1411.
39. Dutta D, Clevers H. Organoid culture systems to study host–pathogen interactions. Curr Opin Immunol. 2017;48:15–22.
40. Dedhia PH, Bertaux-Skeirik N, Zavros Y, Spence JR. Organoid models of human gastrointestinal development and disease. Gastroenterology. 2016;150(5):1098–1112.
41. Spence JR, Mayhew CN, Rankin SA, Kuhar MF, Vallance JE, Tolle K, *et al.* Directed differentiation of human pluripotent stem cells into intestinal tissue in vitro. Nature. 2011;470(7332):105–109.
42. Forbester JL, Goulding D, Vallier L, Hannan N, Hale C, Pickard D, *et al.* Interaction of Salmonella enterica serovar Typhimurium with intestinal organoids derived from human induced pluripotent stem cells. Infect Immun. 2015;83(7):2926–2934.
43. In J, Foulke-Abel J, Estes MK, Zachos NC, Kovbasnjuk O, Donowitz M. Human mini-guts: new insights into intestinal physiology and host–pathogen interactions. Nat Rev Gastroenterol Hepatol. 2016;13(11):633–642.
44. Leslie JL, Huang S, Opp JS, Nagy MS, Kobayashi M, Young VB, *et al.* Persistence and toxin production by Clostridium difficile within human intestinal organoids result in disruption of epithelial paracellular barrier function. Infect Immun. 2015;83(1):138–145.
45. Ettayebi K, Crawford SE, Murakami K, Broughman JR, Karandikar U, Tenge VR, *et al.* Replication of human noroviruses in stem cell–derived human enteroids. Science. 2016;353(6306):1387–1393.
46. Hill DR, Huang S, Nagy MS, Yadagiri VK, Fields C, Mukherjee D, *et al.* Bacterial colonization stimulates a complex physiological response in the immature human intestinal epithelium. eLife. 2017;6:e29132.
47. Bartfeld S, Bayram T, van de Wetering M, Huch M, Begthel H, Kujala P, *et al.* In vitro expansion of human gastric epithelial stem cells and their responses to bacterial infection. Gastroenterology. 2015;148(1):126–136.e6.

48. Williamson IA, Arnold JW, Samsa LA, Gaynor L, DiSalvo M, Cocchiaro JL, *et al.* A high-throughput organoid microinjection platform to study gastrointestinal microbiota and luminal physiology. Cell Mol Gastroenterol Hepatol. 2018;6(3):301–319.
49. Sato T, Stange DE, Ferrante M, Vries RG, Van Es JH, Van den Brink S, *et al.* Long-term expansion of epithelial organoids from human colon, adenoma, adenocarcinoma, and Barrett's epithelium. Gastroenterology. 2011;141(5):1762–1772.
50. Yui S, Nakamura T, Sato T, Nemoto Y, Mizutani T, Zheng X, *et al.* Functional engraftment of colon epithelium expanded in vitro from a single adult Lgr5+ stem cell. Nat Med. 2012;18(4):618–623.
51. Nadkarni RR, Abed S, Cox BJ, Yeung RS. Organoids as a model system for studying human polycystic kidney disease. Kidney Int. 2019;95(6):1299–1304.
52. Cruz NM, Song X, Czerniecki SM, Gulieva RE, Churchill AJ, Kim YK, *et al.* Organoid cystogenesis reveals a critical role of microenvironment in human polycystic kidney disease. Nat Mater. 2017;16(11):1112–1119.
53. Takasato M, Er PX, Becroft M, Vanslambrouck JM, Stanley EG, Elefanty AG, *et al.* Directing human embryonic stem cell differentiation towards a renal lineage generates a self-organizing kidney. Nat Cell Biol. 2014;16(1):118–126.
54. Kim YK, Refaeli I, Brooks CR, Jing P, Gulieva RE, Hughes MR, *et al.* Gene-edited human kidney organoids reveal mechanisms of disease in podocyte development. Stem Cells. 2017;35(12):2366–2378.
55. Freedman BS, Brooks CR, Lam AQ, Fu H, Morizane R, Agrawal V, *et al.* Modelling kidney disease with CRISPR-mutant kidney organoids derived from human pluripotent epiblast spheroids. Nat Commun. 2015;6:8715.
56. Czerniecki SM, Cruz NM, Harder JL, Menon R, Annis J, Otto EA, *et al.* High-throughput screening enhances kidney organoid differentiation from human pluripotent stem cells and enables automated multidimensional phenotyping. Cell Stem Cell. 2018;22(6):929–940.e4.
57. van den Berg CW, Ritsma L, Avramut MC, Wiersma LE, van den Berg BM, Leuning DG, *et al.* Renal subcapsular transplantation of PSC-derived kidney organoids induces neo-vasculogenesis and significant glomerular and tubular maturation in vivo. Stem Cell Reports. 2018;10(3):751–765.
58. Garreta E, Prado P, Tarantino C, Oria R, Fanlo L, Martí E, *et al.* Fine tuning the extracellular environment accelerates the derivation of kidney organoids from human pluripotent stem cells. Nat Mater. 2019;18(4):397–405.
59. Takasato M, Er PX, Chiu HS, Maier B, Baillie GJ, Ferguson C, *et al.* Kidney organoids from human iPS cells contain multiple lineages and model human nephrogenesis. Nature. 2015;526(7574):564–568.

60. Czerniecki SM, Annis J, Otto EA, Lu L, Sussman CR, Williams C, *et al.* High-throughput screening of kidney organoids for drug nephrotoxicity. bioRxiv. 2017:190173.
61. Tumurbaatar B, Ahn SM, Song Y, Kim YK, Kwon SH. Human kidney organoids generated from urine-derived cells reveal avascular and immature phenotypes that can be modulated by engineering approaches. Biomaterials. 2022;280:121273.
62. Kumar SV, Er PX, Lawlor KT, Motazedian A, Scurr M, Ghobrial I, *et al.* Kidney micro-organoids in suspension culture promote maturation of nephron progenitors, lifting the curse of planar cell polarity in organoid development. bioRxiv. 2019:564252.
63. Schutgens F, Rookmaaker MB, Margaritis T, Rios A, Ammerlaan CM, Jansen J, *et al.* Tubuloids derived from human adult kidney and urine for personalized disease modeling. Nat Biotechnol. 2019;37(3):303–313.
64. Dekkers JF, Wiegerinck CL, de Jonge HR, Bronsveld I, Janssens HM, de Winter-de Groot KM, *et al.* A functional CFTR assay using primary cystic fibrosis intestinal organoids. Nat Med. 2013;19(7):939–945.
65. Firth AL, Dargitz CT, Qualls SJ, Menon T, Wright R, Singer O, *et al.* Generation of multiciliated cells in functional airway epithelia from human induced pluripotent stem cells. Proc Natl Acad Sci USA. 2014;111(17):E1723–E1730.
66. Dye BR, Hill DR, Ferguson MA, Tsai YH, Nagy MS, Dyal R, *et al.* In vitro generation of human pluripotent stem cell derived lung organoids. eLife. 2015;4:e05098.
67. Chen YW, Huang SX, de Carvalho AL, Ho SH, Islam MN, Volpi S, *et al.* A three-dimensional model of human lung development and disease from pluripotent stem cells. Nat Cell Biol. 2017;19(5):542–549.
68. Nikolić MZ, Sun D, Rawlins EL. Human lung development: recent progress and new challenges. Development. 2018;145(16):dev163485.
69. Nikolić MZ, Caritg O, Jeng Q, Johnson JA, Sun D, Howell KJ, *et al.* Human embryonic lung epithelial tips are multipotent progenitors that can be expanded in vitro as long-term self-renewing organoids. eLife. 2017;6:e26575.
70. McCauley KB, Hawkins F, Serra M, Thomas DC, Jacob A, Kotton DN. Efficient derivation of functional human airway epithelium from pluripotent stem cells via temporal regulation of Wnt signaling. Cell Stem Cell. 2017;20(6):844–857.e6.
71. Dye BR, Dedhia PH, Miller AJ, Nagy MS, White ES, Shea LD, *et al.* A bioengineered niche promotes in vivo engraftment and maturation of pluripotent stem cell-derived human lung organoids. eLife. 2016;5:e19732.
72. Sachs N, Papaspyropoulos A, Zomer-van Ommen DD, Heo I, Bottinger L, Klay D, *et al.* Long-term expanding human airway organoids for disease modeling. EMBO J. 2019;38(4):e100300.

73. Jacob A, Morley M, Hawkins F, McCauley KB, Jean JC, Heins H, *et al.* Differentiation of human pluripotent stem cells into functional lung alveolar epithelial cells. Cell Stem Cell. 2017;21(4):472–488.e10.
74. Leibel SL, McVicar RN, Winquist AM, Niles WD, Snyder EY, Wang Y, *et al.* Reversal of β-cell-like features in lung-derived induced pluripotent stem cells by Pdx1 silencing. Diabetes. 2011;60(5):1383–1394.

https://doi.org/10.1142/9789819817597_0002

Chapter 2

# Advanced Organoid Culture Systems

**Yueyue Huangfu[1], Dengfeng Zhang[1], Jiaming Ye[1,*], Mingliang You[2], and Bingcheng Lin[1]**

[1]*Hangzhou Organ-on-Chip Technology Co., Ltd., 310000, Hangzhou, Zhejiang Province, China*

[2]*Hangzhou AimingMed Technologies Co., Ltd., 310000, Hangzhou, Zhejiang Province, China*

**Abstract:** Organoid technology has emerged as a transformative platform for simulating hard-to-access organs and investigating the physiological development and pathogenesis of diseases. It offers new insights into personalized medicine, drug screening and disease mechanisms. Traditional methods rely on matrix gels and bioactive media to guide stem cells to self-organize into 3D structures. However, challenges such as insufficient standardization, limited reproducibility and the absence of vascular, immune and neural components limit their ability to accurately recapitulate the dynamic organ microenvironment. These limitations prevent the faithful reproduction of organ-specific morphology and function, making it difficult to study developmental processes and signaling pathways. In recent years, interdisciplinary approaches integrating organ-on-chip and 3D printing technologies have significantly advanced organoid culture systems, improving reproducibility, maturation and biomimicry. This chapter systematically reviews and summarizes the rapid advances in organoid construction based on advanced culture systems in recent years. By exploring future development directions, it is expected that these cutting-edge organoid culture systems and construction technologies will be rapidly and widely applied in clinical practice and drug development, contributing to the improvement of human health and the diagnosis and treatment of diseases.

**Keywords:** microfluidic chip, organ-on-chip, 3D bioprinting, organoid-on-chip

---

[*]Corresponding author. Email: yejiaming723@126.com

## Key Points

1. The latest advances in combining organoid technology with organ-on-chip and 3D printing technologies are summarized, as well as their potential applications in biomedicine.
2. A description of the development process of organoid-on-chip technology and the construction process has been presented.
3. The advantages and disadvantages of organoids, organ-on-chip and organoid-on-chip technologies are compared and analyzed.
4. The technical limitations and future directions of combining organoids with organ-on-chip and 3D printing technologies are also discussed.

## 2.1 Introduction

Organoids represent a highly promising platform for modeling organs that are challenging to access for tissue sampling and for unraveling the developmental processes of organogenesis. Remarkable progress has been made in constructing physiopathological models for various human organs (Figure 2.1A), including the kidney, heart, and brain, thereby providing innovative and more realistic frameworks for personalized medicine, drug screening, and the investigation of pathophysiological mechanisms [1–6].

Traditional organoid construction employs matrix gels and specialized media enriched with stimulatory factors to provide biochemical and biophysical cues that closely mimic the human body, thereby facilitating the self-assembly of stem cells into 3D structures characterized by remarkable architectural complexity [7]. This widely employed method is relatively straightforward to implement; however, the variability of additives in the culture medium leads to low standardization and poor reproducibility, as shown in Figure 2.1B. Furthermore, the absence of appropriate vascular, immune, and neural components hinders accurate replication of the complex and dynamic microenvironment present during organ development, thereby limiting the reproduction of organ-specific morphological features and functions. These limitations hinder the reproduction of organ-specific morphology and functions, complicating research into organ morphogenesis, differentiation, and signaling [8].

To address these challenges, researchers in stem cell and developmental biology are collaborating with engineers and physicists to develop advanced culture systems aimed

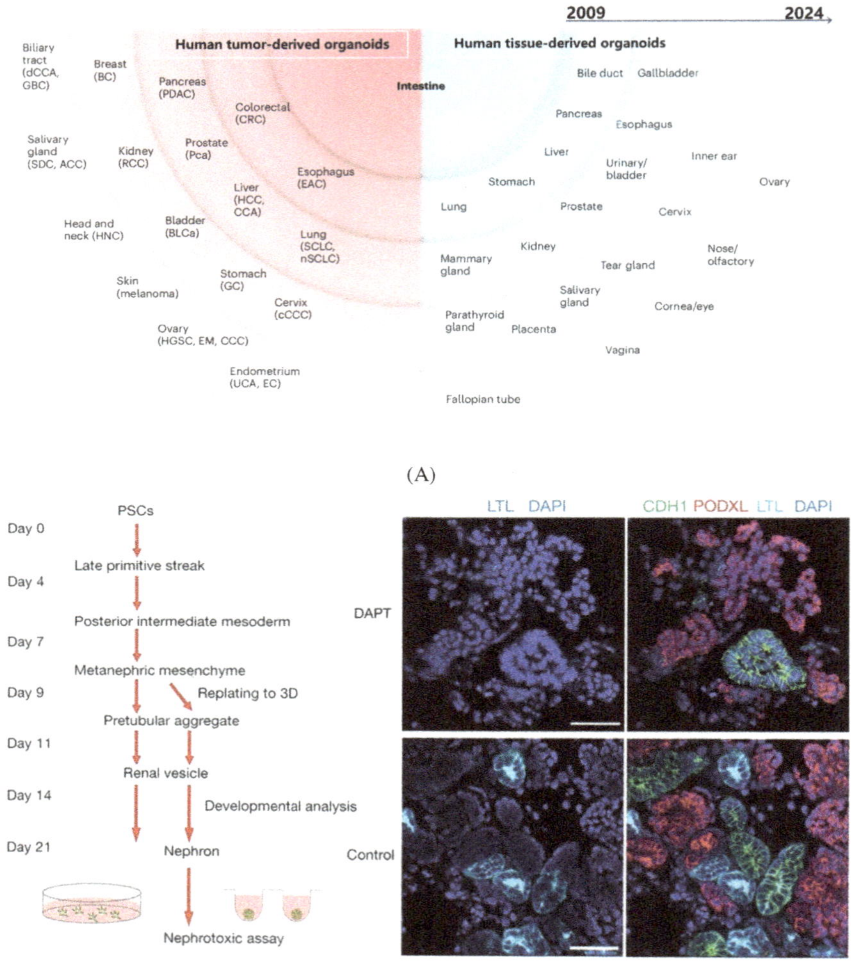


**Figure 2.1** Organoids and conventional construction. (A) Discovery of different types of epithelial organoids. Reproduced with permission from [1]. (B) Recapitulating kidney development and injury through kidney organoids. Reproduced with permission from [2].

at improving the reproducibility, maturation, and biomimetic properties of organoids. In particular, organoid culture systems developed in recent years through the integration of organ-on-chip and 3D printing [9–12] technologies have enabled researchers to achieve several significant breakthroughs [13]. Notably, in 2022, the U.S. Food and

Drug Administration (FDA) approved an investigational therapy for clinical trials for the first time based entirely on preclinical efficacy data derived from organoid-on-chip modeling of autoimmune demyelinating neuropathies, in conjunction with existing safety data [14]. This milestone highlights the pivotal role of organoid-on-chip platforms in rare disease modeling and drug development, underscoring their potential to transform biomedical research and therapeutic innovation.

## 2.2 Microfluidic and Organ on Chips

### 2.2.1 *Microfluidic Chip*

Microfluidics is a rapidly evolving interdisciplinary technology combining chemistry, fluid physics, microelectromechanical systems, materials science, and biological engineering. This cutting-edge field employs microchannels with dimensions ranging from a few to hundreds of microns to process or manipulate extremely small fluid volumes of fluids ($10^{-9}$ to $10^{-18}$ liters), combining the processes of separation, reaction, and detection within a small-scale microdevice occupying only a few square centimeters. This technology is commonly referred to as "microfluidic-on-chips", "microfluidic chips", or "lab-on-a-chip" [15, 16], as shown in Figure 2.2A. Its applications span various fields, including engineering, physics, chemistry, and biology (Figure 2.2B), with its scope continually expanding and yielding far-reaching implications [17, 18].

Microfluidics is distinguished by its ability to conserve samples and reagents, deliver high-resolution and sensitive separation and detection, reduce costs, and provide rapid analysis. Initially applied in analytical methods such as capillary electrophoresis, this technology leverages the unique physical behaviors of fluids at the microscale. Unlike their macroscale counterparts, microscale fluids demonstrate distinct inertial effects, convective and diffusive transport, and interfacial tension properties. For example, when water flows from two converging microchannels, it moves in parallel in a laminar state, with mixing occurring exclusively through molecular diffusion at the fluid interfaces. This phenomenon has facilitated the development of interfacial synthesis techniques. Additionally, a variety of strategies have been devised to manipulate microscale fluids using boundary effects, such as electrophoretic phenomena and fluid-structure interactions [19].

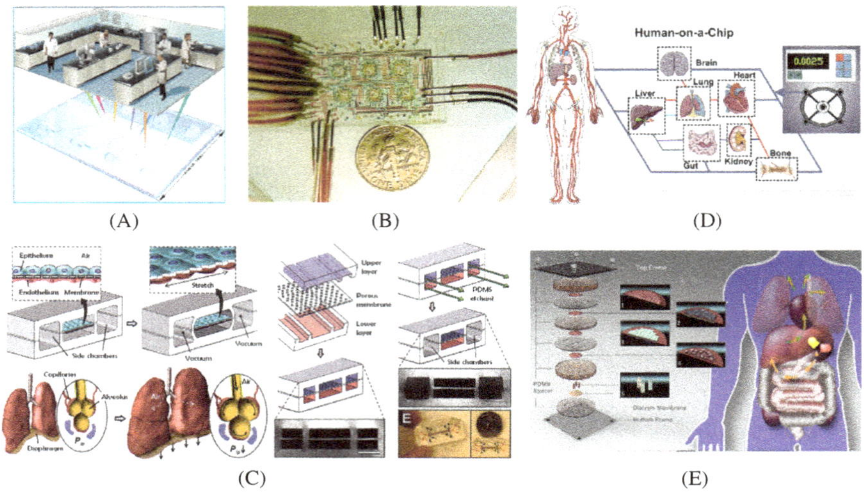


**Figure 2.2** Microfluidic and organ on chips. (A) Conceptual diagram of a "lab-on-a-chip" system. Reproduced with permission from [16]. (B) A microfluidic device facilitating long-term culture and monitoring ultra-low-density bacterial consortia at single-cell resolution. Reproduced with permission from [18]. (C) A biomimetic microsystem that reconstitutes the critical functional alveolar-capillary interface of the human lung, initially referred to as an "organ-on-chip". Reproduced with permission from [31]. (D) "Human-on-a-chip" system facilitates tissue-tissue and organ-organ interactions. Reproduced with permission from [50]. (E) A laminated microfluidic device to mimic the drug ADME response test *in vivo*. Reproduced with permission from [51].

The foundational concepts of microfluidics can be traced back to the 1970s, when photolithography was employed to fabricate gas chromatographs on silicon wafers, which subsequently evolved into various applications such as microfluidic capillary electrophoresis and microreactors [20]. It was not until the 1990s that microfluidics experienced a resurgence, driven by the advancement of open-tubular and miniaturized liquid chromatographs constructed on silicon wafers [21]. Simultaneously, Manz *et al.* [22] first introduced the concept of a miniature total analysis system in 1990, highlighting the "micro" and "total" aspects of this analytical framework. The following year, they developed a chemical analysis system on a glass chip that employed electroosmotic pumping and electrophoretic separation to differentiate sample components [23]. In 2001, the journal *Lab on a Chip* was established and quickly garnered numerous high-quality research submissions, solidifying its position as the leading publication in the field of microfluidics. In 2003, *Forbes* magazine recognized microfluidics as one of the 15 most significant inventions poised to influence the future of humanity. The following year, *Business 2.0* magazine identified microfluidics as one of seven technologies anticipated to transform the future landscape. Today, microfluidics has transitioned from an analytical tool into a burgeoning multidisciplinary field with rapidly expanding applications across biology, chemistry, medicine, and various other domains.

The primary materials employed in the fabrication of microfluidic chips include silicon wafers, glass, polydimethylsiloxane (PDMS), polymethylmethacrylate (PMMA), polytetrafluoroethylene, and paper substrates. Notably, PDMS has emerged as a pivotal material for cellular research owing to its exceptional biocompatibility, suitable stiffness, and favorable light and gas permeability. Microfluidic chip processing methods primarily encompass the following techniques:

1) Photolithography, which represents the foundational technology in microfluidic chip fabrication, utilizing photoresist, masks, and ultraviolet light for microfabrication. This mature process has been extensively employed to create microstructures on silicon, glass, and quartz substrates;
2) Molding, suitable for polymer-based microfluidic chips such as PDMS, fabricates microstructures using photolithography to create molds into which polymer materials are poured for curing;
3) Thermocompression, applicable to thermoplastic polymers like PMMA and polycarbonate, replicates microchannels through a four-step process involving heating, heat retention, cooling, and demolding;
4) LIGA (Lithographite, Galano formung and Abformung) technology combines photolithography with electroforming and plastoforming techniques for the fabrication of microdevices from various polymers, metals, metal alloys, and ceramics;
5) Laser etching technology employs precise laser control to fabricate microchannels and microholes in materials including plastics, metals, and ceramics;
6) Finally, 3D printing constructs 3D objects from computer-aided design models by adding raw materials layer by layer — this method simplifies the manufacturing process of microfluidic chips while offering a diverse range of material options [16].

A comprehensive microfluidic system generally comprises the following essential components: 1) an area for the introduction of reagents and samples (which may include liquids, gases, powders, or biological materials); 2) a liquid movement and reaction zone (encompassing mixing, separation, droplet formation [24], etc.); 3) pumping and valve mechanisms (such as Quake [25, 26] and Tesla valves [27, 28]); and 4) additional devices (including integrated detectors and microelectrodes [29, 30]). Given their characteristics of miniaturization, ease of manipulation, and diverse processing methodologies, microfluidic chips have increasingly garnered the attention of biologists. Consequently, alongside advancements in developmental biology, the evolution and application of organ-on-chips technology have been significantly accelerated.

### 2.2.2 *Organ-on-Chip*

Organ-on-chips (OoCs) are microfluidic chip-based models meticulously designed to replicate the smallest functional units of human tissues or organs *in vitro*. Therefore, prior to the development of an OoC system, it is essential to achieve a thorough understanding of the critical physiological microenvironment, which includes various cell types as well as extracellular biochemical and physical stimuli. Subsequently, microfluidic technology can be utilized to recreate this microenvironment *in vitro* with high fidelity, thereby enabling the creation of biomimetic microsystems capable of accurately predicting organ responses. Notably, Ingber *et al.* [31] pioneered the lung chip (Figure 2.2C) — initially referred to as "organ-on-chip" — which employs upper and lower chambers separated by a PDMS porous membrane to simulate the air-liquid interface of alveolar epithelial cells while replicating mechanical stimuli during respiration through membrane stretching. This innovative approach effectively mimics a complex integrated organ-level response when exposed to bacterial agents and inflammatory cytokines within the alveolar space.

In classical organ-on-chip systems featuring adjacent microchannels separated by porous membranes or microgroove structures, the inoculation of various cell types facilitates independent cellular growth while permitting the free diffusion of secretions, thereby enabling interactions among different cells. Furthermore, the utilization of pumps or alternative methods to drive fluid flow within microchannels provides cells with real-time access to fresh nutrients and facilitates the timely removal of accumulated metabolic waste products. The shear forces generated by fluid flow can influence cytoskeletal rearrangement through mechanotransduction, thereby affecting cellular morphology and structure under physiological conditions. In epithelial cells, functional proteins exhibit a regionalized distribution in response to fluid shear stress, leading to the establishment of a polarized cell structure aligned from the apical surface towards the basement membrane, while concurrently contributing to the formation of a denser epithelial barrier [32–36]. Shear forces induced by fluid flow in intestine-on-a-chip systems can enhance microvilli formation, thereby increasing the surface area. Additionally, these systems incorporate intestinal commensal bacteria, regulate oxygen gradients, and apply periodic mechanical forces to simulate conditions analogous to intestinal peristalsis [37–39]. Numerous challenges in drug development within the field of neurology have arisen due to the limited predictive accuracy of animal models and 2D culture systems. OoC technology presents a promising alternative to address these limitations. By integrating various brain-relevant cell types, such as endothelial cells, neurons, and glial cells into these chips, OoC technology can effectively replicate the human blood-brain barrier — a selective permeability barrier essential for maintaining homeostasis within the central nervous system — thereby enabling researchers to create more accurate models that reflect both structural and functional characteristics of brain tissue [40–43]. In oncology research, OoCs facilitate the assessment of drug efficacy, simulate tumor metastasis, and enable the development of personalized tumor models. These advanced systems provide a more physiologically relevant environment compared to traditional *in vitro* methods, allowing for better prediction of how tumors will respond to various therapeutic agents. By incorporating multiple cell types that mimic the tumor microenvironment, OoC platforms can replicate complex interactions between cancer cells and surrounding stromal cells, immune cells, and extracellular matrix components [44–48].

The origins of organ-on-chip technology can be traced back to 2003, when researchers first endeavored to integrate cell culture with microfluidics to create a prototype of organ-on-chip. In 2010, the National Center for Advancing Translational Sciences (NCATS) launched the OoC Drug Screening Initiative, a collaborative effort involving the FDA, the National Institutes of Health, and the Defense Advanced Research Projects Agency aimed at developing a series of organ chips that accurately replicate human organs. By 2016, NCATS had established a partnership with the Center for the Advancement of Science in Space to explore new funding opportunities for advancing organ-on-chip technology. In 2023, the FDA announced that animal models would no longer be required for new drug development [49]. OoC technology is also experiencing significant growth in other regions; for instance, the European Medicines Agency and Center for Drug Evaluation (China) are actively developing appropriate policies and standards to facilitate the healthy advancement of this technology while ensuring its efficacy and safety in clinical trials and medical practice.

The emergence of various regulatory guidelines has highlighted the extensive application potential of OoC technology, encompassing drug screening, mechanism of efficacy and toxicity studies, disease modeling, precision medicine, as well as the identification and discovery of biomarkers. However, the human body constitutes a highly intricate biological system in which interactions and feedback mechanisms among multiple organs are of paramount importance. For instance, upon administration, oral medications undergo the ADMET (absorption, distribution, metabolism, excretion, toxicity) process; furthermore, the stability of the internal environment and the progression of various diseases involve multiple organ systems. From this perspective, the organ-on-a-chip model may be perceived as an oversimplification, thereby necessitating the development of multiorgan-on-a-chip (Figure 2.2D) or human-on-a-chip systems [50].

In 2016, Bingcheng Lin's group developed a laminated microfluidic device capable of mimicking the ADME response of drugs (Figure 2.2E). This device serves as a reliable tool for simultaneously evaluating anti-tumor activity, hepatotoxicity, and pharmacokinetics, accurately reflecting hepatic drug metabolism, drug distribution in target tissues, and the employed administration methods [51]. In the same year, the research team developed a multi-organ bionic microfluidic model to investigate cancer metastasis [52]. Primary cells isolated from various organs were utilized to replicate each organ and the flow of breast and salivary gland cancer cells through the chambers, thereby simulating the dynamic adhesion of circulating tumor cells (CTCs) to the endothelium *in vivo*. It was observed that engineered CTCs exhibited varying lung metastatic potential within the microfluidic model, consistent with findings obtained from nude mouse models. Subsequently, the researchers simulated liver and bone metastasis of CTCs using this microfluidic model, thereby confirming its applicability in studying multi-organ cancer metastasis.

To date, OoC technology has achieved significant advancements in academia. However, its full implementation in industrial settings remains hindered by several technological barriers. One potential breakthrough resides within the pharmaceutical industry, where OoC technology can alleviate the high failure rate of drug development, optimize the selection of drug candidates, and consequently expedite the preclinical testing process for new therapeutics. Looking forward, it is anticipated that OoCs — when integrated with artificial intelligence and designed to be plug-and-play, highly versatile, fully automated, and compatible with standard laboratory practices — will transform biological and medical research by providing comprehensive and personalized models.

### 2.2.3 *Organoid-on-Chip*

OoC technology has developed biomimetic *in vitro* models by providing monolayers of cells with an extracellular microenvironment that simulates physiological conditions. In biology, organoids, which exploit the self-organizing properties of pluripotent or adult stem cells to create multicellular constructs that mimic the structures and functions of native organs, are emerging as a promising approach to *in vitro* modelling of human organs [53–56]. The organoid-on-a-chip (Figure 2.3A) represents an advanced *in vitro* model that integrates the advantages of these two technologies, featuring more biomimetic tissue or organ structures and more precise extracellular microenvironments [56–60].

Deguchi *et al.* [61] employed OoC technology to reproduce interstitial flow (Figure 2.3B), facilitating the differentiation of human pluripotent stem cells into intestinal epithelial and non-epithelial cells for constructing an *in vivo*-like multilayered small intestine tissue comprising mucus, intestinal epithelial, mesenchymal cell, and extracellular matrix layers. This system can be utilized for drug metabolism and infectious disease studies. The authors discovered that slow interstitial flow (with a bottom passage medium flow rate of 30 μL/h from day 5 to 24) can promote the structural and functional maturation of intestine epithelium, inducing alignment of the basement membrane and mesenchymal cell layers, supporting structural integrity of the intestinal epithelium, facilitating establishment of cellular polarity, increasing mucin accumulation, and enhancing expression of intestinal markers. Homan *et al.* [13] reported a microfluidic perfusion platform (Figure 2.3C) capable of applying physiological shear

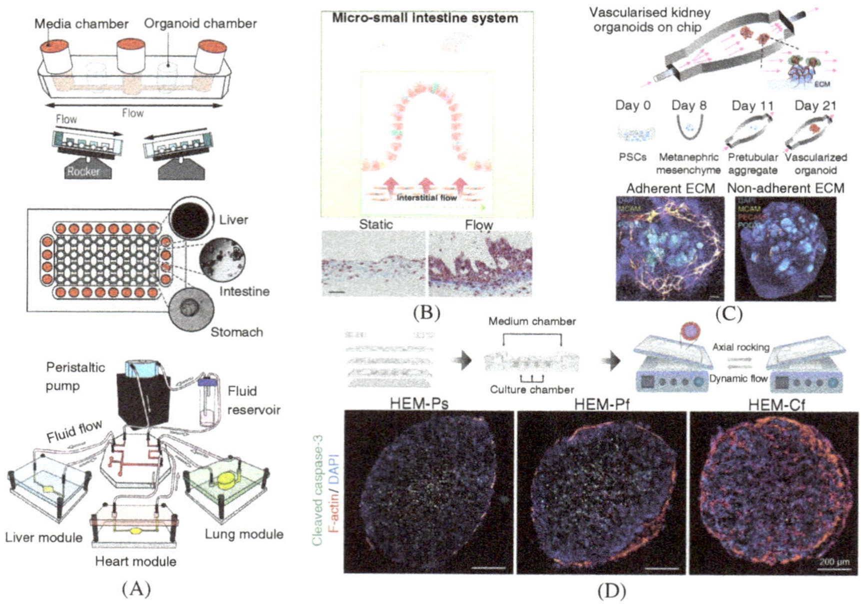


**Figure 2.3** Modeling organoid-on-chips. (A) Modeling organoid-on-chips facilitates tissue-tissue and organ-organ interactions. Reproduced with permission from [60]. (B) Schematic representation of the micro-small intestine system. Reproduced with permission from [61]. (C) Enhanced vascularization observed in engineered renal organoids through dynamic extracellular matrix coupling and microfluidic perfusion. Reproduced with permission from [13]. (D) A perfusable culture system based on *in vivo*-like heart micro-environments. Reproduced with permission from [62].

stress during kidney organoid culture. Their experimental results demonstrated that vascularized kidney organoids cultured under dynamic flow conditions displayed enhanced maturation of podocyte and tubular compartments, along with improved cellular polarity and adult-specific gene expression profiles, relative to static controls.

Min *et al.* [62] developed a perfusion culture system by integrating native heart-like cellular and extracellular components with dynamic flow that mimics the *in vivo* cardiac microenvironment, thereby enhancing the efficiency of human myocardial tissue preparation. The structure of the culture chip is illustrated in Figure 2.3D, featuring three adjacent organoid culture chambers at the center and two medium chambers positioned at either end, each linked to a microchannel that facilitates continuous medium flow from the end chambers through the central organoid culture chambers via ongoing oscillation of rocking perfusion, thereby enabling a dynamic perfusion culture for the cells. Dynamic culture within microfluidic chips significantly improved the viability and contractility, and enhanced synchronized contractions of cardiac tissues, potentially leading to a higher level of myocardium regeneration, facilitating the maturation of the cells comprising the cardiac tissues, promoting cell-cell interactions for electrical synchronization by preventing apoptosis, and encouraging the formation of gap junctions. The researchers subsequently employed the system for drug evaluation, modeling cardiac fibrosis, and facilitating cardiac tissue transplantation in rats, demonstrating considerable potential as a viable alternative to existing human *in vitro* cardiac models and future therapeutic strategies for cardiac regeneration.

Hiratsuka *et al.* [63] cultured kidney organoids derived from autosomal recessive polycystic kidney disease (ARPKD) on gelatin-fibrin substrates and employed flow perfusion using OoC technology to replicate physiological functions and pathological changes, providing a more realistic experimental platform for studying ARPKD. The authors concluded that flow-induced mechanosensory signaling is a critical factor in the pathogenesis of ARPKD. Utilizing this model, they identified 229 signaling pathways not detected by static models and pinpointed potential therapeutic targets validated in patient kidney samples. Furthermore, the authors tested two FDA-approved drugs along with one investigational drug currently undergoing clinical trials that could target and inhibit cyst formation. This study underscores the significant potential of organoid microarray models in elucidating complex disease mechanisms for therapeutic testing and discovery. The construction of organoid-on-chip systems significantly differs from the cultivation of organoids in traditional culture plates, primarily encompassing the steps of microarray design and fabrication, collagen modification, cell inoculation, fluid perfusion, cell differentiation, marker detection, and drug testing; the specific sequence may vary depending on the experimental objectives. Using this work as a case study, the detailed process for constructing organoid microarrays is outlined as follows:

1. *Engineered extracellular matrix preparation*: Type A gelatin (300 bloom) and fibrinogen were enzymatically cross-linked using transglutaminase and thrombin, respectively. Cross-linking was achieved by dissolving 2% (wt%) gelatin, fibrinogen (10 mg/mL), 2.5 mM calcium chloride, and transglutaminase (2 mg/mL) in phosphate-buffered saline, followed by incubation at 37°C for 15 minutes. Subsequently, 1 mL of this solution was rapidly mixed with thrombin to

achieve a final concentration of 2 U/mL. The resulting mixture was then quickly poured onto the microfluidic chip and allowed to gel for approximately 5 minutes at room temperature before undergoing further solidification in an incubator at 37°C for an additional 3 hours. Finally, the microfluidic chip was further solidified at room temperature for another 3 hours.

2. *Chip modification and organoid seeding*: Medium covering three-quarters of the extracellular matrix was passed through the chips, followed by inoculation of 14-day differentiated organoids in designated areas for attachment to the extracellular matrix. The lid of the chip was placed on the seal and secured with screws; subsequently, the chambers were filled with medium consisting of ARMPI supplemented with GlutaMAX, 1% double antibody (Gibco), and 1.5% heat-inactivated fetal bovine serum (Gibco). The system was then cultured dynamically until day 35. All media were pre-equilibrated in a cell culture incubator for at least 2 hours prior to chip assembly and organoid inoculation. The kidney organoid chips were subsequently positioned in the incubator for a resting period of 30 minutes. The inlet perfusion line was connected to a peristaltic pump and perfused at a rate of 42.7 μL/min overnight within the incubator. On day 2 (day 15 of organoid differentiation), the perfusion rate was increased to 4.27 mL/min, and the culture medium in the reservoir was changed every two to three days.
3. *Drug testing*: The dosing concentration of each drug was initially determined through continuous drug concentration gradient testing conducted on days 16 to 35 of organoid differentiation. Once the concentrations were established, the drugs were added to the external medium reservoir during medium renewal on days 2 and 3, followed by continuous drug testing from days 16 to 35 of organoid differentiation.
4. *Detection and Analysis*: A comprehensive assessment of organoid maturity, model construction simulation, and the effects of drug stimulation was conducted using techniques such as immunofluorescence labeling, next-generation sequencing, single-cell RNA sequencing, quantitative reverse transcription PCR, and immunohistochemistry, tailored to meet specific research needs.

As illustrated in Figure 2.4 [64], the integration of organoids with OoC systems to develop organoid-on-chip platforms offers substantial potential, while presenting significant technical challenges. This interdisciplinary approach requires concerted

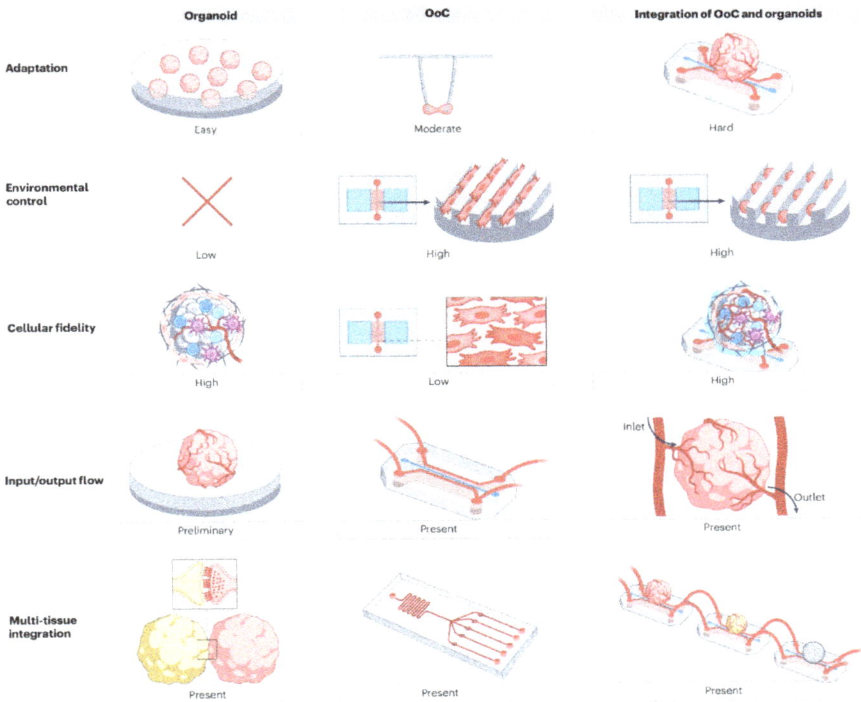


**Figure 2.4** Advances and challenges of organoids and OoC integration systems. Reproduced with permission from [64].

efforts across multidisciplinary scientific and engineering domains to advance this emerging field. To effectively underscore the technological advantages of organoid-on-chip systems, it is imperative to develop integrated and automated platforms for their construction. Such advancements are crucial as they not only streamline workflows but also enhance the reproducibility and reliability of experimental outcomes. Furthermore, there is an increasing demand for high-throughput drug screening in pharmaceutical research. The integration of automation can facilitate high-throughput methodologies, enabling more extensive data collection and analysis. Vascularized organoid chips are particularly noteworthy because they accurately replicate the complex architecture and functionality of human tissues compared to traditional models. Multi-organoid-on-chip systems represent a significant innovation by allowing interactions among various organ types on a single platform, thereby providing insights into systemic responses to pharmacological agents or disease states. Investigating highly biocompatible and low-adsorption materials for chip fabrication is essential to minimize interference during experiments while ensuring that biological samples remain viable over extended periods. Additionally, enhancements in standardization practices for organoid chips will improve comparability across diverse studies and laboratories, fostering collaboration within the scientific community.

## 2.3 Integration of 3D Bioprinting and Organoids for Disease Modeling

3D printing has found applications across diverse fields, including food production, biomedicine, dentistry, healthcare, architecture, and aerospace [65–67]. The technology of 3D bioprinting facilitates the biofabrication of complex intrinsic spatial structures through precise layer-by-layer positioning and deposition of biomaterials, biochemical reagents, and living cells. As a leading technology for simulating human physiology at present, organoids represent a significant advancement in modern biomedical research [68]. However, their applicability is constrained by insufficient precision in tissue composition and high structural variability. Computer-assisted 3D bioprinting allows for precise control over the fabrication process to generate organoids with uniform dimensions and reduced batch-to-batch variability while enabling automated mass production that provides high-throughput *in vitro* models for drug screening and therapeutic development. Furthermore, 3D bioprinting can enhance organoid development and maturation by modulating the biochemical microenvironment; it holds promise for addressing the limitation that artificially assembled organoids often lack vascularization. The synergistic integration of 3D bioprinting technology with organoid systems represents a promising strategy poised to significantly impact drug discovery and personalized medicine.

### 2.3.1 *3D Bioprinting Technology*

The emergence of biocompatible functional materials has enabled the transition of 3D printing from cell-free processes to cell-laden printing that accurately mimics natural tissues. This progress has markedly accelerated the application of 3D printing in the biomedical domain, particularly in fundamental research and specific clinical applications such as tissue engineering, disease model development, and drug screening.

3D bioprinting is an advanced biomanufacturing technology that innovatively integrates 3D printing with biomaterials. The process of 3D bioprinting can be broadly outlined as follows: with the assistance of a computer, cells, growth factors, and "bioink" consisting of a mixture of various biomaterials are deposited or cured in layers according to a specific spatial arrangement to form a tissue or organ substitute with a 3D structure. Essentially, 3D bioprinting represents an extension of additive manufacturing technology. By incorporating individual characteristics, it enables the layer-by-layer deposition of cells and non-cellular components onto a substrate while precisely positioning and distributing biological materials and cells. This technology effectively replicates the complex interactions between cells and their surrounding microenvironment while mimicking the physical, chemical, and mechanical properties of natural tissues to achieve a high degree of fidelity in reproducing target tissues or organs [69].

As shown in Figure 2.5, inkjet printing, extrusion printing, laser-assisted printing, and stereolithography (SLA) represent the four predominant bioprinting technologies currently in widespread use [70]. Inkjet bioprinting is a technique that physically manipulates an aqueous solution of bioink to generate droplets and employs a nozzle to eject these droplets onto a receiving substrate [71]. The technology is an improvement

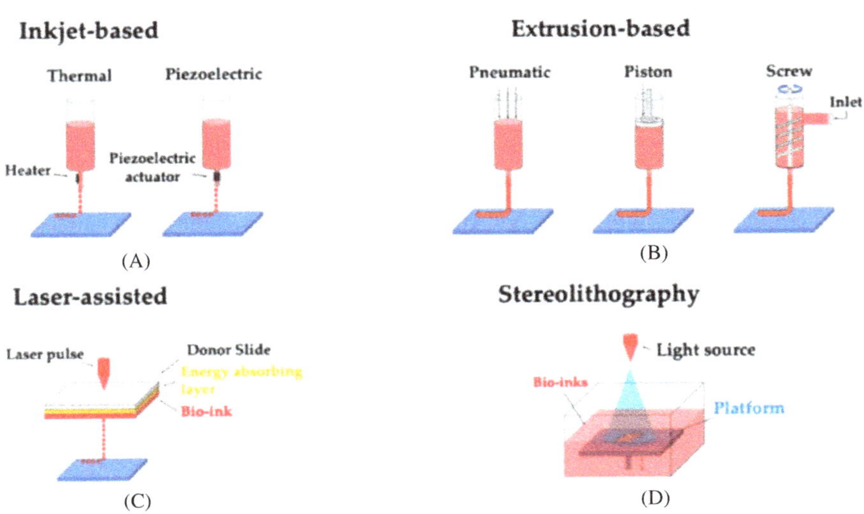


**Figure 2.5** Four main bioprinting methods. Reproduced with permission from [70]. (A) Inkjet bioprinting. (B) Extrusion bioprinting. (C) Laser-assisted bioprinting. (D) Stereolithography bioprinting.

based on traditional 2D inkjet printing. It replaces the ink in the 2D printer cartridges with bioink, substitutes the paper with an electronically controlled lift platform, and adds a *z*-axis to the original 2D *x*-*y* axes [72]. Specifically, bioink is extruded through pneumatic pressure pulses generated either by heating a thermal actuator or via piezoelectric pressure produced by a piezoelectric actuator, resulting in droplets of controllable size that are deposited onto the substrate through a nozzle. These droplets subsequently form continuous patterns and solidify [73, 74]. Bioinkjet printing has the advantages of fast printing speed, low cost, simple operation and wide availability. However, due to its low droplet directionality, uneven droplet sizes, and frequent nozzle clogging, it is only suitable for printing materials with low cell density ($<1 \times 10^6$ cells/mL) and low viscosity (<15 mPa/s). Inkjet printing with low viscosity and low cell concentration may result in poor structural integrity and low cell encapsulation efficiency, making it unsuitable for large-scale 3D structure fabrication.

Extrusion bioprinting is a pressure-driven technology that currently represents the most widely utilized form of bioprinting. Unlike the liquid droplets employed in inkjet printing, extrusion printing uses an air pump or mechanical screw plunger to extrude bioink into a continuous filament, which is then deposited onto a substrate through a nozzle or needle. The extruded bioink cures and serves as the foundational layer for subsequent material deposition. Under precise computer control, a micro-extrusion head traverses along the *z*-axis to construct specific 3D structural models by sequentially layering materials atop one another [75]. Extrusion printers are equipped with multiple print heads capable of simultaneously or alternately delivering various bioinks, including formulations that encapsulate different cell types. This is particularly useful for creating complex multi-layered and multi-regional structures [76]. The technique can be adapted for bioprinting at high cell densities and accommodates virtually any viscosity while providing excellent control over both cell distribution and structural morphology. However, in this type of contact-based printing where external forces are applied, shear stresses generated during the process may adversely affect cellular morphology and viability [77].

Laser-assisted bioprinting comprises three components: the donor slide, the laser pulse, and the receiver slide. This technique relies on a laser pulse traversing a transparent donor slide that is coated with a laser-absorbing material and cell suspension to eject droplets of cell suspension onto a receiving substrate [78]. Unlike inkjet and extrusion printing methods, this approach eliminates direct contact between the dispensing nozzle and the bioink, thereby preserving cell viability. The technology enables precise localization of multiple cell types with high accuracy and resolution; however, its printing speed is moderate. Laser-assisted printing technology faces limitations due to the high cost of equipment, complexities associated with controlling the laser printing system, as well as issues related to low stability and scalability. Additionally, the side effects of laser irradiation on cells remain incompletely understood.

SLA is a technology that uses liquid photosensitive resin as the raw material and employs visible or ultraviolet light to precisely scan layer by layer according to a preset pattern to construct 3D objects. The principle is that the photosensitive resin in the scanned area undergoes a photopolymerization reaction, transforming from a fluid to a solid [79]. At the conclusion of the printing process, any unreacted resin on the surface is washed away and subsequently placed in a UV curing oven to enhance the mechanical properties of the structure. SLA technology operates as a non-contact printing method, avoiding issues related to cell or material clogging that affect other bioprinting technologies while eliminating negative shear forces encountered in nozzle-based printing. As one of the more established and widely adopted 3D printing technologies, SLA offers significant advantages regarding print efficiency, accuracy, and surface quality. It provides high resolution along with rapid and precise manufacturing capabilities across a broad range of ink viscosities (1–300 mPa/s) [80]. However, concerns regarding UV irradiation effects on cellular DNA, limited availability of photosensitive biomaterials, and increased cytotoxicity associated with SLA must be addressed.

Cell-loaded bioinks serve as the fundamental raw material for 3D bioprinting, designed to replicate the extracellular matrix found in tissues and provide structural support for cell growth and development. Typically, these bioinks are flowable liquids that can be easily extruded and rapidly solidified to maintain their shape through physical or chemical stimuli. When the liquid bioink undergoes gelation, the ink can undergo cross-linking reactions and encapsulate the cells. The physical properties of bioinks significantly influence printability, manufacturing fidelity, and mechanical stress on cellular components [81]. An effective bioink must exhibit appropriate rheological characteristics (including shear thinning behavior, storage modulus, and viscosity), along with desirable mechanical properties, biodegradability, biocompatibility, permeability to oxygen and nutrients, rapid gelation post-printing, and shape integrity [82].

Among the various types of bioinks, hydrogels are the most widely utilized. A hydrogel is a polymeric material characterized by a 3D network structure formed through the gelation of hydrophilic polymers with high water absorption capacity in aqueous environments [83]. Gelation occurs via physical or chemical cross-linking mechanisms. Physical cross-linking primarily involves hydrogen bonding, electrostatic interactions, crystallization, and hydrophobic interactions, whereas chemical cross-linking is typically achieved through the formation of covalent bonds (Figure 2.6) [84, 85].

Hydrogels exhibit robust mechanical properties and are capable of retaining or adsorbing substantial amounts of water without disintegrating or dissolving. They demonstrate

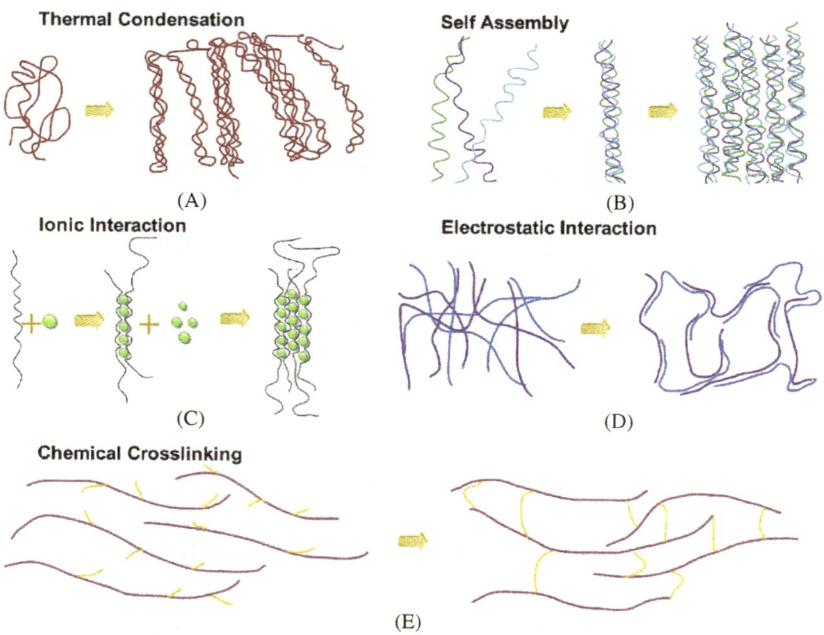


**Figure 2.6** Cross-linking of hydrogels. Reproduced with permission from [85]. (A)–(D) Physical cross-linking: (A) Thermal condensation. (B) Molecular self-assembly. (C) Ionic gelation. (D) Electrostatic interaction. (E) Chemical cross-linking.

excellent water absorption, biodegradability, biocompatibility, and high plasticity, positioning them as prime candidates for 3D bioprinting materials. On the one hand, hydrogels are considered an excellent carrier for encapsulating and delivering cells, providing an ideal chamber for the uniform distribution of cells, which is beneficial for their proliferation, migration, and metabolic activities. On the other hand, the porous structure of hydrogels has excellent oxygen permeability and high porosity, allowing them to serve as carriers and delivery systems for hydrophilic therapeutics in drug therapy research.

Hydrogels can be derived from a diverse array of natural or synthetic hydrophilic polymers. Natural hydrophilic polymers refer to biopolymers that are sourced and extracted from nature, including polysaccharides, peptides, proteins, etc. Among these, agarose, collagen, alginate, and gelatin are the most commonly utilized natural materials [86]. Natural biopolymers exhibit high water content, exceptional biocompatibility, and favorable biodegradability while facilitating the transport of metabolic wastes and nutrients, providing a critical microenvironment for sustaining the physiological activities of diverse cell types. Furthermore, natural biopolymers can be easily loaded with bioactive molecules and cells to promote cell adhesion, proliferation, and differentiation [87]. These characteristics are crucial for determining whether 3D bioprinted objects can be applied within a biological organism, and they are not easily replicated in synthetic materials.

Natural biopolymers have many advantages, but they also have shortcomings such as insufficient physicochemical properties and weak immunogenicity, which limit their further application. Solely utilizing natural polymeric materials may lead to relatively weak mechanical properties that are insufficient to support multilayer scaffold structures. In contrast, synthetic polymer materials offer enhanced mechanical strength and printability, effectively compensating for these deficiencies. Polyethylene glycol, polyacrylamide, polyacrylic acid, and polyvinyl alcohol are some of the most common synthetic hydrophilic polymer materials. Synthetic biomaterials demonstrate superior mechanical properties and long-term structural stability while typically exhibiting lower hydrophilicity and cellular compatibility. Based on the fact that both natural bioinks and synthetic bioinks are not perfect, most bioinks used for 3D bioprinting are currently formed by mixing natural polymers with synthetic hydrophilic polymers. For instance, a composite hydrogel bioink formed by mixing methacrylated gelatin (GelMA), oxidative hyaluronic acid, and dopamine-conjugated hyaluronic acid (HA-DA) can provide adequate mechanical scaffold support after cross-linking, rendering the printing process highly controllable and stable while significantly enhancing the practicality of constructing multilayer scaffolds [88].

### 2.3.2 *Organoids and 3D Bioprinting*

Based on the different subjects utilized for 3D bioprinting, organoid bioprinting can be categorized into two distinct groups. The first group involves the bioprinting of undifferentiated stem cells, and the second group the bioprinting of already differentiated stem cells or organoids themselves. Tebon *et al.* [89] precisely controlled the deposition of tumor cells in a well plate using an extrusion-based printing method to construct tumor organoids. The general process is briefly outlined as follows: on ice, the medium and matrix gel were mixed in a 3:4 ratio for gel dilution, and then human mammary stem cells were added to create a single-cell suspension. After vortex mixing, the syringe was transferred and the bubbles removed. Then, the mixture was transferred to a bioprinter cartridge and placed in a rotary incubator at 17°C for 30 min. During this incubation period, the printer was sterilized using UV irradiation and the print head preheated. Following incubation, calibration of the printer commenced by extruding a small volume of material at pressures between 10–15 kPa. A subsequent extrusion at 40 kPa removed any gelatinized material pins and ensured smooth material flow during extrusion. The bioink was then extruded into each well of the 96-well plate at pressures ranging from 7–15 kPa, taking approximately four minutes to produce prints (<200 μm) on the bottom surface of one well (Figure 2.7). Upon completion of printing, the plates were incubated at 37°C for no less than 30 minutes to allow solidification of the matrix. Finally, 100 μL of human mammary stem cell culture medium was added to each well for cell proliferation and differentiation. The bioprinted tumor organoids maintained consistency with manually seeded 3D cultures in terms of cell viability, histological characteristics, and transcriptome levels, while also improving organoid throughput and structural consistency.

Research showed that digital light processing printing technology could effectively aggregate GelMA hydrogel microspheres containing bone marrow-derived stem cells into bone repair organoids. The 3D bioprinting bone repair organoid was more effective for rapid bone regeneration in rabbit bone defect sites compared to traditional

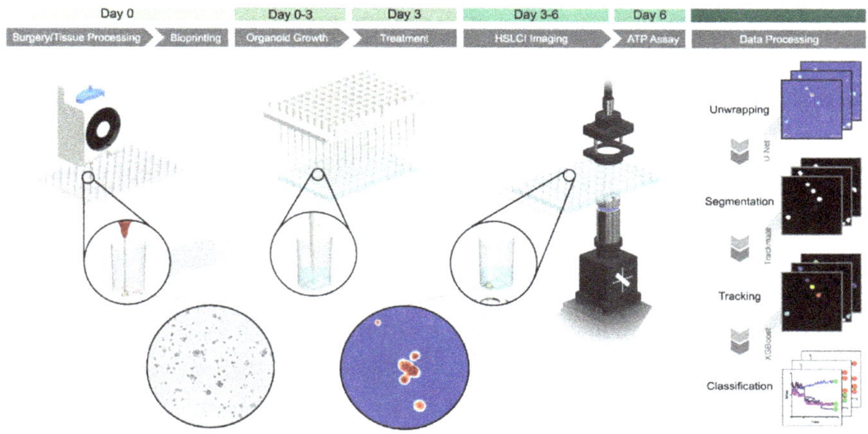


**Figure 2.7** Extrusion-based bioprinting is employed to deposit single-layer Matrigel constructs into a 96-well plate, allowing for the monitoring of organoid model establishment and growth through imaging. Reproduced with permission from [89].

treatment strategies using mesenchymal stem cell aggregates [90]. Reid *et al.* [91] found that 3D printing could precisely control the 3D assembly of human mammary epithelial cells, resulting in human mammary organoids with high fidelity and controllable spatial structures. These constructed mammary organoids outperformed randomly self-assembled 3D organoids regarding assembly efficiency, reproducibility, and scalability.

Despite the presence of various cell types, organoids remain incomplete. Current organoid culture systems are unable to fully replicate the specific physiological microenvironments present in natural tissue organs, including tissue-tissue interfaces, vascular networks, resident immune cells, and signals that promote organogenesis [92]. The developmental conditions for organoids are relatively complex, and artificially cultured organoids often lack precise control over their microenvironment, leading to poor reproducibility and high variability between batches. Furthermore, deficiencies such as the absence of organ-specific morphological features and uncontrolled size limit the physiological relevance and reliability of organoids in therapeutic applications [93]. In contrast, 3D bioprinting can produce organoids with good morphological uniformity by precisely controlling the 3D spatial arrangement of bioink and cells. Additionally, 3D bioprinting can offer biochemical and biophysical cues to support organoid development and maturation. Non-invasive techniques such as high-resolution fluorescence confocal or multiphoton microscopy can be employed for post-printing imaging observation and data analysis to characterize the morphology and function of printed tissues. The application of 3D printing technology to automate the production of organoids has significant potential to address many challenges associated with traditional organoid culture.

Bioprinting technology offers the potential to construct vascularized tissues and holds promise for addressing the current challenge of non-vascularized constructs. Lee *et al.* [94] generated a multiscale vascular system model from images of human coronary arteries and their branches scanned by magnetic resonance imaging, and created a thermoreversible support channel composed of gelatin microparticle slurry according to the model. Then, they used the reversible embedding of suspended hydrogels bioprinting technology to extrude collagen bioink containing fibronectin and pro-angiogenic factors into the mold according to the model. The thermoreversible support bath can dissolve at 37°C, resulting in a vascular structure with good mechanical properties and high fidelity. The development of these porous microstructures facilitates infiltration and microvascularization of endothelial and perivascular cells, resulting in multi-scale vascular structures characterized by favorable mechanical properties and high fidelity. Furthermore, it has been reported that vascularized tissues containing cells can also be fabricated using multi-material 3D bioprinting techniques. The efficacy of this method in generating vascular structures is attributed to the use of sacrificial inks composed of triblock copolymers that are printed via an extrusion process; they are then liquefied to leave hollow channels suitable for seeding with endothelial cells, thereby enabling integration of a vascular network within the tissue that supplies nutrients while facilitating oxygen transport and waste removal essential for tissue growth and development [95].

The integration of stem cell biology with microengineering technology to develop organoid-on-chip systems represents a valuable approach for drug screening and disease modeling. Chip systems are beneficial for the formation of organoids and the expansion of 3D cultures, enabling real-time imaging and *in situ* tracking. Wang *et al.* [96] successfully constructed liver organoids using human induced pluripotent stem cells in perfusable microcolumn chips, which exhibited good morphological and functional properties and can be effectively used for drug hepatotoxicity testing. The application of 3D bioprinting technology in microfluidic chips or well-plate organoid construction enables the automated production of highly consistent organoids, enhancing reproducibility essential for basic research and preclinical drug safety evaluation [97]. Lawlor *et al.* [98] rapidly generated kidney organoids in 96-well plates (one organoid per well) through cell extrusion bioprinting, resulting in kidney organoids characterized by high reproducibility, fine resolution, high throughput, and good consistency. This demonstrates that 3D bioprinting holds significant promise for developing high-throughput tissue culture platforms and improving the accuracy of drug screening.

Despite the considerable potential demonstrated by 3D bioprinting across various applications, the technology continues to face several limitations, including a narrow range of printable materials, insufficient resolution, slow printing speed, and unsuitability for large-scale production. Over the years, researchers have been dedicated to finding materials for 3D bioprinting to meet the demand for constructing various types of biological tissues, but the types of bioinks available remain limited. Conventional 3D printing materials must possess appropriate resolution, printability, processability, structural stability, and a certain degree of shape fidelity. In contrast, bioinks must also exhibit characteristics such as cross-linkability, the ability to support cell growth and differentiation, desirable mechanical properties compatible with various native tissues, and biocompatibility [99].

To address this limitation, scientists have researched and developed various new types of bioinks to fulfill the requirements of 3D bioprinting across various application scenarios. Hossein *et al.* [100] introduced a novel composite plant-based ink primarily composed of papaya seed mucilage and infused with an appropriate proportion of cellulose nanofibrils, which offers advantages such as renewability, sustainability, environmental friendliness, and cost-effectiveness. This ink is suitable for supporting cell attachment, survival, and proliferation while enabling high-fidelity 3D printing of multilayer lattice structures, meeting the criteria for soft tissue engineering scaffold materials. Cheng and Hsu [101] innovatively proposed a dual cross-linking system comprising gelatin methacryloyl and dialdehyde-functionalized polyurethane, which can form self-healing hydrogels and injectable cryogels at two different temperature states. The self-healing hydrogel formed at room temperature demonstrated good stackability, high resolution, wet adhesion, and transparency. The frozen cryogel produced at low temperatures exhibited high compressibility, injectability, and excellent biocompatibility. Xia *et al.* [102] developed a GelMA-HA-Arg-Gly-Asp functional hydrogel with adjustable mechanical properties, specifically designed for cochlear organoid culture. The composite hydrogel could promote the proliferation and differentiation of cochlear progenitor cells, which was beneficial for the formation of inner ear sensory epithelium. The study indicated that functional bioink can provide signaling stimuli for organoid growth and development, promoting organogenesis. Graham *et al.* [103] designed a freeform bioprinting material that supports freeform 3D bioprinting (Figure 2.8). It was a MAGIC matrix comprised of an inert alginate microgel granular support and a viscous basement membrane interstitium. The MAGIC matrix was used for 3D bioprinting to achieve high-throughput generation of complex organoids such as the intestine, mammary gland, blood vessels, salivary glands, and brain. Compared to conventional pure Matrigel, the organoids generated from MAGIC demonstrate significant improvements in size, shape, maturation time, and efficiency during morphogenesis. This innovative composite matrix enabled diverse types of 3D bioprinting while holding potential for fabricating complete 3D microphysiological systems.

The resolution of 3D printing is intricately linked to the printability of bioinks, which is influenced by the rheological properties of the bioinks [104]. The rheological properties of bioinks are affected by the physical characteristics of each component, including cell volume fraction, intercellular interactions, spatial arrangement of cells, and the rate of ink gelation [105]. Bioinks with a high cell volume fraction exhibit increased cross-linking and stiffness, but they may interfere with cell proliferation,

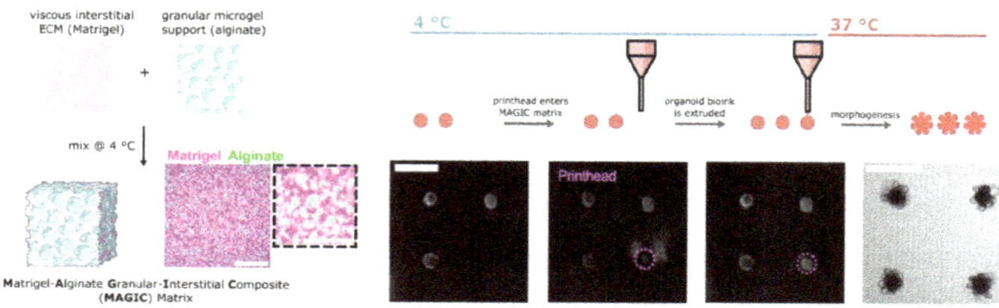


**Figure 2.8** MAGIC extracellular matrix is used for extrusion bioprinting and construct uniform and complex organoid architectures. Reproduced with permission from [103].

migration, and matrix deposition. In contrast, bioinks with lower cell volume fractions compromise shape fidelity and lack sufficient printability. Hydrogels typically exhibit shear-thinning or stimuli-responsive properties. Shear-thinning hydrogels can be printed under shear stress and regain their mechanical properties after extrusion. Stimuli-responsive hydrogels undergo gelation upon exposure to physical or chemical stimuli after printing. Nevertheless, shear-thinning hydrogels face challenges related to extended recovery time, which may result in reduced print fidelity. Stimuli-responsive hydrogels are limited by gelation kinetics. Slow gelation may lead to improper dispersion following printing while rapid gelation could cause nozzle clogging during fabrication [106]. It has been demonstrated that varying physicochemical factors such as pH, temperature, and collagen concentration within the gel constitutes an effective strategy for controlling gelation rates and enhancing print fidelity. Wang *et al.* [107] showed that the gelation process of hydrogels formed from a composite of pea protein and hydroxypropyl starch was significantly influenced by pH levels. The structure, strength, and printability of these hydrogels could be modulated by altering pH values. At pH 3, the hydrogel formed a layered structure; at pH 5, they form granuled aggregation networks; at pH 7 and 9, porous structures were observed; and at pH 11, a honeycomb structure emerged. Rapid adjustment of pH could control the gelation rate of collagen, thereby developing a suspended hydrogel that prints collagen fibers with a resolution of 20 micrometers. This method effectively improved the defect of the hydrogel being too soft and prone to sagging, and enhanced the fidelity and resolution of the printing [94].

In traditional manufacturing processes, production costs typically decrease as output volume increases. Generally, mass production and processing become straightforward and efficient following the completion of initial mold fabrication [108]. For 3D printing technology, it is not suitable for mass production and can only manufacture a few small parts or a small number of slightly larger parts. It shows the disadvantages of being slow and requiring long working hours when it comes to large-scale production [109]. The production of large objects through 3D bioprinting presents specific difficulties and challenges primarily due to constraints imposed by the size of printer and the capacity of the ink reservoir [110].

Overall, the design and development of novel bioprinting materials still have significant challenges ahead. Future bioprinting materials should exhibit a diverse array of desirable properties, including physical characteristics (such as expansion ratio, porosity, and degradability), chemical attributes (including chemical composition and resistance to various chemicals), mechanical properties (such as tensile/compressive strength, elongation, toughness), rheological behaviors (including shear modulus and viscosity), cellular functions (such as attachment, migration, growth, and differentiation), and biocompatibility. Furthermore, the extended operational hours required for mass production and the current limitations in producing large components must be addressed through the advancement of 3D printing technologies.

## 2.4 Future Directions and Emerging Trends

Organoid technology, as a cutting-edge domain in biomedical research, is at the forefront of advancing personalized medicine and drug development. This technology enables the cultivation of miniature organ models with 3D structures *in vitro*, effectively simulating the functions and pathological states of actual organs, thereby providing novel insights for disease research and treatment.

Looking forward, organoid technology is anticipated to integrate profoundly with advanced technologies such as artificial intelligence, gene sequencing and gene editing, and single-cell RNA sequencing to propel personalized medicine and facilitate precise therapeutic responses to drugs; establish multi-organ co-culture systems while incorporating pharmacokinetic simulation techniques to replicate the concentration distribution of compounds across various human organs for evaluating drug toxicity and efficacy; further enhance vascularization in organoid construction to improve model accuracy and longevity while more accurately mimicking the complexity of human organs and tumor microenvironments — applying these advancements within regenerative medicine and oncology fields such as tissue and organ repair; and develop integrated devices aimed at optimizing and standardizing organoid culture systems to bolster their stability, fidelity, reproducibility, and scalability.

Nevertheless, the advancement of organoid technology encounters several challenges including technological standardization, ethical considerations, as well as improving simulations of complex human environments. As these issues are progressively addressed, it is expected that organoid technology will assume an increasingly significant role in regenerative medicine, disease modeling, and drug development — ultimately yielding revolutionary impacts on human health.

## Key Opinion Points

1. Organoid + Organ-on-Chip = Game Changer
   Combines biomimicry, reproducibility, and dynamic microenvironments for better drug/disease modeling.
2. 3D Bioprinting Fixes Organoid Flaws
   Enables precision, scalability, and vascularization; reduces batch variability.
3. Vascularization is Critical
   Needed for nutrient/waste exchange; solved via perfusion chips or sacrificial bioprinting.
4. Industry Adoption Lags Behind Research
   Standardization, scalability, and regulatory hurdles slow clinical/pharma translation.
5. Future: Multi-Organ Systems + Artificial Intelligence
   Multi-organ chips for systemic studies; artificial intelligence for data-driven drug discovery and personalized medicine.

## References

1. Verstegen MMA, *et al.* Clinical applications of human organoids. Nat Med. 2025;31:409–421.
2. Morizane R, *et al.* Nephron organoids derived from human pluripotent stem cells model kidney development and injury. Nat Biotechnol. 2015;33:1193–1200.
3. Richards DJ, *et al.* Human cardiac organoids for the modelling of myocardial infarction and drug cardiotoxicity. Nat Biomed Eng. 2020;4:446–462.
4. Tan H-Y, Cho H, Lee LP. Human mini-brain models. Nat Biomed Eng. 2020;5:11–25.
5. Lancaster MA, Knoblich JA. Generation of cerebral organoids from human pluripotent stem cells. Nat Protoc. 2014;9:2329–2340.
6. Wimmer RA, *et al.* Human blood vessel organoids as a model of diabetic vasculopathy. Nature. 2019;565:505–510.
7. Fatehullah A, Tan SH, Barker N. Organoids as an in vitro model of human development and disease. Nat Cell Biol. 2016;18:246–254.
8. Hofer M, Lutolf MP. Engineering organoids. Nat Rev Mater. 2021;6:402–420.
9. Ayan B, *et al.* Aspiration-assisted bioprinting for precise positioning of biologics. Sci Adv. 2020;6:eaaw5111.
10. Reid JA, Mollica PA, Bruno RD, Sachs PC. Consistent and reproducible cultures of large-scale 3D mammary epithelial structures using an accessible bioprinting platform. Breast Cancer Res. 2018;20:122.

11. Brassard JA, Nikolaev M, Hubscher T, Hofer M, Lutolf MP. Recapitulating macro-scale tissue self-organization through organoid bioprinting. Nat Mater. 2021;20:22–29.
12. Bernal PN, *et al.* Volumetric bioprinting of organoids and optically tuned hydrogels to build liver-like metabolic biofactories. Adv Mater. 2022;34:e2110054.
13. Homan KA, *et al.* Flow-enhanced vascularization and maturation of kidney organoids in vitro. Nat Methods. 2019;16:255–262.
14. Rumsey JW, *et al.* Classical complement pathway inhibition in a "human-on-chip" model of autoimmune demyelinating neuropathies. Adv Ther. 2022;5:2200030.
15. Nunes JK, Stone HA. Introduction: Microfluidics. Chem Rev. 2022;122:6919–6920.
16. Lin B, Qin J. Schematic Illustration of Microfluidic Lab-on-a-Chip (图解微流控芯片实验室). Beijing: Science Press; 2008.
17. Whitesides GM. The origins and the future of microfluidics. Nature. 2006;442:368–373.
18. Balagaddé FK, *et al.* Long-term monitoring of bacteria undergoing programmed population control in a microchemostat. Science. 2005;309:137–140.
19. Squires TM, Quake SR. Microfluidics: Fluid physics at the nanoliter scale. Rev Mod Phys. 2005;77:977–1026.
20. Reyes DR, Iossifidis D, Auroux PA, Manz A. Micro total analysis systems. 1. Introduction, theory, and technology. Anal Chem. 2002;74:2623–2636.
21. Manz A, *et al.* Design of an open-tubular column liquid chromatograph using silicon chip technology. Sens Actuators B Chem. 1990;1:249–255.
22. Manz A, Graber N, Widmer HM. Miniaturized total chemical analysis systems: A novel concept for chemical sensing. Sens Actuators B Chem. 1990;1:244–248.
23. Harrison DJ, *et al.* Micromachining a miniaturized capillary electrophoresis-based chemical analysis system on a chip. Science. 1993;261:895–897.
24. Ghosh A, Ganguly R, Schutzius TM, Megaridis CM. Wettability patterning for high-rate, pumpless fluid transport on open, non-planar microfluidic platforms. Lab Chip. 2014;14:1538–1550.
25. Hansen CL, Skordalakes E, Berger JM, Quake SR. A robust and scalable microfluidic metering method that allows protein crystal growth by free interface diffusion. Proc Natl Acad Sci U S A. 2002;99:16531–16536.
26. Thorsen T, Maerkl SJ, Quake SR. Microfluidic large-scale integration. Science. 2002;298:580–584.
27. Han Q, *et al.* The role of Tesla valves in microchannel flow boiling. Int J Heat Mass Transf. 2024;234:126148.
28. Hong CC, Choi JW, Ahn CH. A novel in-plane passive microfluidic mixer with modified Tesla structures. Lab Chip. 2004;4:109–113.

29. Dungchai W, Chailapakul O, Henry CS. Electrochemical detection for paper-based microfluidics. Anal Chem. 2009;81:5821–5826.
30. Xu S, *et al.* Soft microfluidic assemblies of sensors, circuits, and radios for the skin. Science. 2014;344:70–74.
31. Huh D, *et al.* Reconstituting organ-level lung functions on a chip. Science. 2010; 328:1662–1668.
32. Wilmer MJ, *et al.* Kidney-on-a-chip technology for drug-induced nephrotoxicity screening. Trends Biotechnol. 2016;34:156–170.
33. Qu Y, *et al.* A nephron model for study of drug-induced acute kidney injury and assessment of drug-induced nephrotoxicity. Biomaterials. 2018;155:41–53.
34. Benam KH, *et al.* Small airway-on-a-chip enables analysis of human lung inflammation and drug responses in vitro. Nat Methods. 2016;13:151–157.
35. Buckley CE, St Johnston D. Apical-basal polarity and the control of epithelial form and function. Nat Rev Mol Cell Biol. 2022;23:559–577.
36. Lee J, Kim K, Kim S. Kidney on chips. Methods Cell Biol. 2018;146:85–104.
37. Wu J, *et al.* An intelligent intestine-on-a-chip for rapid screening of probiotics with relief-enteritis function. Adv Mater. 2024;36:e2408485.
38. Grant J, *et al.* Establishment of physiologically relevant oxygen gradients in microfluidic organ chips. Lab Chip. 2022;22:1584–1593.
39. Bein A, *et al.* Microfluidic organ-on-a-chip models of human intestine. Cell Mol Gastroenterol Hepatol. 2018;5:659–668.
40. Pediaditakis I, *et al.* Modeling alpha-synuclein pathology in a human brain-chip to assess blood-brain barrier disruption. Nat Commun. 2021;12:5907.
41. Palma-Florez S, *et al.* BBB-on-a-chip with integrated micro-TEER for permeability evaluation of multi-functionalized gold nanorods against Alzheimer's disease. J Nanobiotechnol. 2023;21:115.
42. Chin E, Goh E. Blood-brain barrier on a chip. Methods Cell Biol. 2018;23:159–182.
43. Zakharova M, *et al.* Multiplexed blood-brain barrier organ-on-chip. Lab Chip. 2020; 20:3132–3143.
44. Liu Z, *et al.* A pathomimetic colorectal tumor-on-a-chip for in vitro reconstitution of the primary colorectal cancer. Adv Mater Technol. 2023;8:2200758.
45. Mathur L, Ballinger M, Utharala R, Merten CA. Microfluidics as an enabling technology for personalized cancer therapy. Small. 2020;16:e1904321.
46. Hachey SJ, *et al.* An in vitro vascularized micro-tumor model of human colorectal cancer recapitulates in vivo responses to standard-of-care therapy. Lab Chip. 2021;21:1333–1351.
47. Horejs C. A tumour chip for drug screening. Nat Rev Mater. 2020;5:786.

48. Del Piccolo N, *et al.* Tumor-on-chip modeling of organ-specific cancer and metastasis. Adv Drug Deliv Rev. 2021;175:113798.
49. Wadman M. FDA no longer has to require animal testing for new drugs. Science. 2023;379:127–128.
50. Picollet-D'hahan N, Zuchowska A, Lemeunier I, Le Gac S. Multiorgan-on-a-Chip: A systemic approach to model and decipher inter-organ communication. Trends Biotechnol. 2021;39:788–810.
51. An F, *et al.* A laminated microfluidic device for comprehensive preclinical testing in the drug ADME process. Sci Rep. 2016;6:25022.
52. Kong J, *et al.* A novel microfluidic model can mimic organ-specific metastasis of circulating tumor cells. Oncotarget. 2016;7:78421–78432.
53. Zhao Z, *et al.* Organoids. Nat Rev Methods Primers. 2022;2:94.
54. Clevers H. Modeling development and disease with organoids. Cell. 2016;165: 1586–1597.
55. Lancaster MA, *et al.* Cerebral organoids model human brain development and microcephaly. Nature. 2013;501:373–379.
56. Lancaster MA, Knoblich JA. Organogenesis in a dish: modeling development and disease using organoid technologies. Science. 2014;345:1247125.
57. Fang G, Chen YC, Lu H, Jin D. Advances in spheroids and organoids on a chip. Adv Funct Mater. 2023;33:2215043.
58. Nikolaev M, *et al.* Homeostatic mini-intestines through scaffold-guided organoid morphogenesis. Nature. 2020;585:574–578.
59. Wang Y, Wang L, Zhu Y, Qin J. Human brain organoid-on-a-chip to model prenatal nicotine exposure. Lab Chip. 2018;18:851–860.
60. Park SE, Georgescu A, Huh D. Organoids-on-a-chip. Science. 2019;364:960–965.
61. Deguchi S, *et al.* Construction of multilayered small intestine-like tissue by reproducing interstitial flow. Cell Stem Cell. 2024;31:1315–1326.e1318.
62. Min S, *et al.* Versatile human cardiac tissues engineered with perfusable heart extracellular microenvironment for biomedical applications. Nat Commun. 2024;15:2564.
63. Hiratsuka K, *et al.* Organoid-on-a-chip model of human ARPKD reveals mechanosensing pathomechanisms for drug discovery. Sci Adv. 2022;8:eabq0866.
64. Zhao Y, *et al.* Integrating organoids and organ-on-a-chip devices. Nat Rev Bioeng. 2024;2:588–608.
65. Jiang H, *et al.* 3D food printing: main components selection by considering rheological properties. Crit Rev Food Sci Nutr. 2018;59:2335–2347.
66. Rajabi M, McConnell M, Cabral J, Ali MA. Chitosan hydrogels in 3D printing for biomedical applications. Carbohydr Polym. 2021;260:117768.

67. Khorsandi D, *et al.* 3D and 4D printing in dentistry and maxillofacial surgery: Printing techniques, materials, and applications. Acta Biomater. 2021;122:26–49.
68. Corrò C, Novellasdemunt L, Li VSW. A brief history of organoids. Am J Physiol Cell Physiol. 2020;319:C151–C165.
69. Handral KH, Tay SH, Chan WW, Choudhury D. 3D Printing of cultured meat products. Crit Rev Food Sci Nutr. 2020;62:272–281.
70. Lam EHY, Yu F, Zhu S, Wang Z. 3D bioprinting for next-generation personalized medicine. Int J Mol Sci. 2023;24:6357.
71. Gudapati H, Dey M, Ozbolat I. A comprehensive review on droplet-based bioprinting: Past, present and future. Biomaterials. 2016;102:20–42.
72. Murphy SV, Atala A. 3D bioprinting of tissues and organs. Nat Biotechnol. 2014; 32:773–785.
73. Saunders RE, Gough JE, Derby B. Delivery of human fibroblast cells by piezoelectric drop-on-demand inkjet printing. Biomaterials. 2008;29:193–203.
74. Xu T, Jin J, Gregory C, Hickman JJ, Boland T. Inkjet printing of viable mammalian cells. Biomaterials. 2005;26:93–99.
75. Placone JK, Engler AJ. Recent advances in extrusion-based 3D printing for biomedical applications. Adv Healthc Mater. 2017;7:1701161.
76. Valot L, Martinez J, Mehdi A, Subra G. Chemical insights into bioinks for 3D printing. Chem Soc Rev. 2019;48:4049–4086.
77. Kačarević ŽP, *et al.* An introduction to 3D bioprinting: Possibilities, challenges and future aspects. Materials (Basel). 2018;11:2199.
78. Ovsianikov A, *et al.* Laser printing of cells into 3D scaffolds. Biofabrication. 2010;2: 014104.
79. Melchels FP, Feijen J, Grijpma DW. A review on stereolithography and its applications in biomedical engineering. Biomaterials. 2010;31:6121–6130.
80. Raman R, *et al.* High-resolution projection microstereolithography for patterning of neovasculature. Adv Healthc Mater. 2015;5:610–619.
81. Schwab A, *et al.* Printability and shape fidelity of bioinks in 3D bioprinting. Chem Rev. 2020;120:11028–11055.
82. Agostinacchio F, Mu X, Dirè S, Motta A, Kaplan DL. In situ 3D printing: opportunities with silk inks. Trends Biotechnol. 2021;39:719–730.
83. Abdollahiyan P, Oroojalian F, Mokhtarzadeh A, de la Guardia M. Hydrogel-based 3D bioprinting for bone and cartilage tissue engineering. Biotechnol J. 2020;15:2000095.
84. He X, Lu Q. Design and fabrication strategies of cellulose nanocrystal-based hydrogel and its highlighted application using 3D printing: A review. Carbohydr Polym. 2023; 301:120351.

85. Unagolla JM, Jayasuriya AC. Hydrogel-based 3D bioprinting: A comprehensive review on cell-laden hydrogels, bioink formulations, and future perspectives. Appl Mater Today. 2020;18:100479.
86. Leberfinger AN, Ravnic DJ, Dhawan A, Ozbolat IT. Concise review: Bioprinting of stem cells for transplantable tissue fabrication. Stem Cells Transl Med. 2017;6:1940–1948.
87. Xu J, *et al.* 3D printing for bone-cartilage interface regeneration. Front Bioeng Biotechnol. 2022;10:828921.
88. Li Q, *et al.* 3D printing of microenvironment-specific bioinspired and exosome-reinforced hydrogel scaffolds for efficient cartilage and subchondral bone regeneration. Adv Sci (Weinh). 2023;10:2303650.
89. Tebon PJ, *et al.* Drug screening at single-organoid resolution via bioprinting and interferometry. Nat Commun. 2023;14:5160.
90. Tasoglu S, Demirci U. Bioprinting for stem cell research. Trends Biotechnol. 2013;31: 10–19.
91. Mertz L. Bioprinting for precision medicine. IEEE Pulse. 2019;10:16–21.
92. Gungor-Ozkerim PS, *et al.* Bioinks for 3D bioprinting: an overview. Biomater Sci. 2018;6:915–946.
93. Ji S, Guvendiren M. Recent advances in bioink design for 3D bioprinting of tissues and organs. Front Bioeng Biotechnol. 2017;5:23.
94. Chimene D, *et al.* Advanced bioinks for 3D printing: A materials science perspective. Ann Biomed Eng. 2016;44:2090–2102.
95. Mandrycky C, Wang Z, Kim K, Kim DH. 3D bioprinting for engineering complex tissues. Biotechnol Adv. 2016;34:422–434.
96. Ma X, *et al.* 3D bioprinting of functional tissue models for personalized drug screening and in vitro disease modeling. Adv Drug Deliv Rev. 2018;132:235–251.
97. Ramesh S, *et al.* Three-dimensional bioprinting of a cell-laden bone matrix for personalized bone regeneration. ACS Appl Mater Interfaces. 2021;13:5732–5744.
98. Bhise NS, *et al.* A liver-on-a-chip platform with bioprinted hepatic spheroids. Biofabrication. 2016;8:014101.
99. Lee A, Hudson AR, Shiwarski DJ, *et al.* 3D bioprinting of collagen to rebuild components of the human heart. Science. 2019;365:482–487.
100. Ong CS, *et al.* Bioprinting of endothelial cells with decellularized extracellular matrix in hydrogels for vasculature development. Biofabrication. 2017;9:045009.
101. Zhang YS, *et al.* 3D bioprinting for tissue and organ fabrication. Ann Biomed Eng. 2017;45:148–163.

102. Li J, *et al.* 3D bioprinting of hydrogels for tissue engineering: Rational design and emerging applications. Mater Sci Eng R Rep. 2020;140:100543.
103. Daly AC, Davidson MD, Burdick JA. 3D bioprinting of high cell-density heterogeneous tissue models through spheroid fusion within self-healing hydrogels. Nat Commun. 2021;12:753.
104. Jodat YA, *et al.* Human-derived organ-on-a-chip for personalized drug development. Curr Pharm Des. 2018;24:5471–5486.
105. Shin Y, Han S, Jeon JS, Yamamoto K, Zervantonakis IK, *et al.* Microfluidic assay for simultaneous culture of multiple cell types on surfaces or within hydrogels. Nat Protoc. 2012;7:1247–1259.
106. Yazdi AA, *et al.* 3D printing: an emerging tool for novel microfluidics and lab-on-a-chip applications. Microfluid Nanofluidics. 2016;20:94.
107. Sobrino A, *et al.* 3D microtumors in vitro supported by perfused vascular networks. Sci Rep. 2016;6:31589.
108. Homan KA, *et al.* Flow-enhanced vascularization and maturation of kidney organoids in vitro. Nat Methods. 2019;16:255–262.
109. Kim J, *et al.* Liver-on-a-chip platforms for drug screening and disease modeling. Micromachines (Basel). 2020;11:1.
110. Ronaldson-Bouchard K, Vunjak-Novakovic G. Organs-on-a-chip: A fast track for engineered human tissues in drug development. Cell Stem Cell. 2018;22:310–324.

https://doi.org/10.1142/9789819817597_0003

Chapter 3

# Automation in Organoid-Based Precision Medicine

Yanan Shi[1,*], Quanlin Xin[1], Wei Kang[2]

[1]*School of Pharmacy, Yantai University, Yantai 264005, Shandong Province, China*

[2]*MOE Key Laboratory of Bio-Intelligent Manufacturing, School of Bioengineering, Dalian University of Technology, Dalian 116024, China*

**Abstract:** *In vitro* disease research is usually performed by utilizing cultured 2D cells, and 2D cell lines suffer from the problem of not being able to restore certain biological properties of the original parental cells. As an alternative, the newly developed 3D organoid method allows for the cultivation of healthy human tissues, thus providing a new approach for *in vitro* studies of disease. Compared to simple 2D cells, organoid methods retain certain physiological properties of organs and can self-organize according to the same principles as organs. Organoid-based automation for precision medicine is a cutting-edge field that combines biotechnology and information technology, utilizing organoids to mimic real human physiological and pathological environments. These organoids can be cultured from a patient's stem cells, thus offering the possibility of personalized medicine. Through the application of automation technology, more efficient, accurate and reproducible experimental operations, as well as large-scale data analysis, can be achieved, which is crucial for the advancement of precision medicine.

**Keywords:** organoid, human tissue model, self-organization, precision medicine, automation

*Corresponding author. Email: shiyanan@ytu.edu.cn

## Key Points

1. Organoid technology simulates the physiological and pathological characteristics of human organs through 3D culture, overcoming the limitations of traditional 2D cell models and providing a more realistic experimental platform for precision medicine.
2. Precision medicine is the key to transforming the medical model from 'one-size-fits-all' to customized treatment based on individual genes, environment and lifestyle data, with the aim of improving efficacy and reducing healthcare costs.
3. The core advantages of organoids lie in their self-organizing ability, multi-cell type composition and genetic stability, which can be used in biomedical fields such as disease mechanism research, drug metabolism testing and regenerative medicine.
4. Organoid-based drug screening and biobanking combined with genomic analysis can identify sensitive drugs for specific tumor subtypes and provide functional predictive tools for personalized cancer therapy.
5. The integration of automation technology and artificial intelligence enables the standardization of organoid culture, high-throughput experiments and large-scale data analysis, accelerating the process of precision medicine from basic research to clinical translation.

## 3.1 Introduction

Precision medicine, also known as personalized medicine or customized medicine, is a medical approach that develops preventive and treatment strategies based on an individual patient's specific health condition, genetic make-up, living environment and habits. As shown in Figure 3.1, its core concept is to provide patients with more precise and effective diagnosis, treatment and prognosis plans by integrating various bioinformatic data, such as genomics, proteomics, metabolomics and other big data analysis. The importance of precision medicine is reflected in its ability to provide highly personalized diagnostic, therapeutic and preventive solutions based on information about an individual's genetic background, biomarkers, environmental factors and lifestyle habits [1]. This approach can significantly improve treatment outcomes and reduce side effects, while also helping to reduce unnecessary healthcare expenditures. Precision medicine is a revolution in medicine, enabling a shift from a one-size-fits-all model to a more refined, personalized approach to disease management [2].

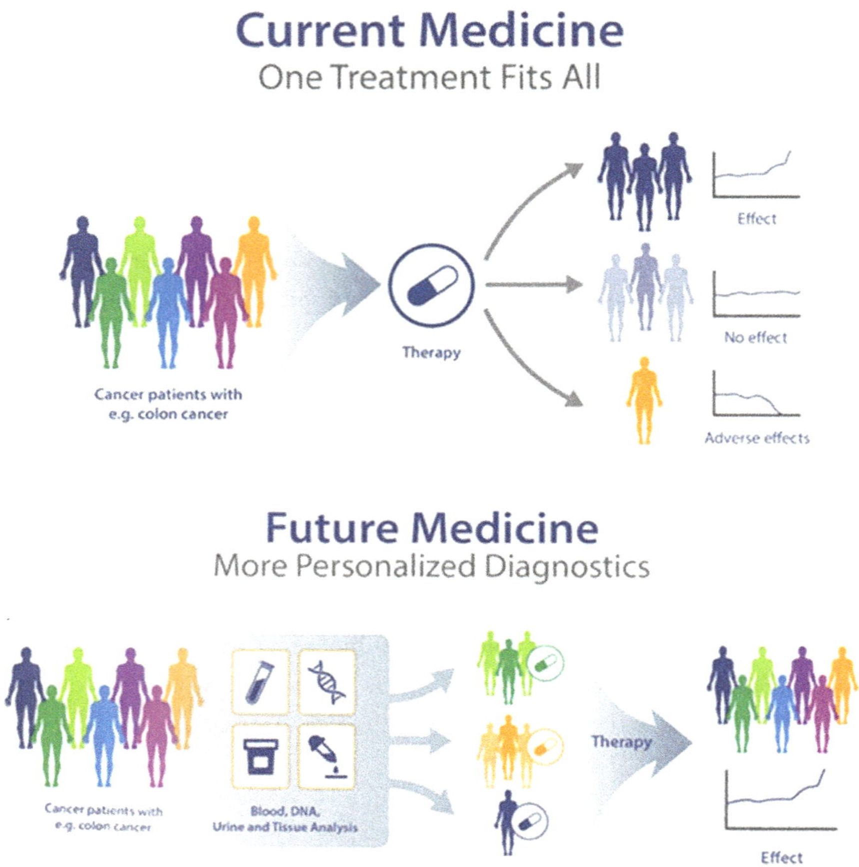


**Figure 3.1** Schematic diagram of precision medicine. Reproduced with permission from Barbeau J. PDX and personalized medicine — Crown Bioscience [Internet]. 2018. Available from: https://blog.crownbio.com/pdx-personalized-medicine.

Organoid technology is a cutting-edge biomedical research approach that uses stem or precursor cells to construct miniaturized, simplified versions of models with primitive tissue and organ structures and functions through *in vitro* 3D culture techniques. As shown in Figure 3.2, these organoids are able to self-organize and differentiate into complex structures containing multiple cell types and mimic to some extent the functions and microenvironmental characteristics of real organs [3].

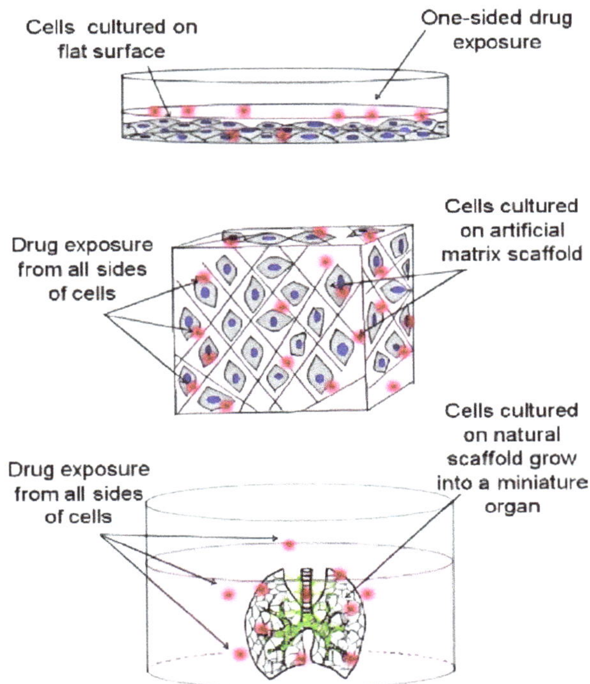


**Figure 3.2** A brief schematic of lung organoid construction. Reproduced with permission from Shete Y, Vavia P, Amiji M, *et al.* Pulmonary multifunctional nano-oncological modules for lung cancer treatment and prevention. J Biomed Nanotechnol. 2014 Oct;10(10):1–31.

Automation technology plays a crucial role in the biomedical field, covering drug discovery and development, biological sample processing and analysis, medical image processing and diagnosis, drug production and quality control, and medical services and rehabilitation. In drug research and development, automation of high-throughput screening and synthesis accelerates the process of drug discovery; biological sample processing achieves efficient and accurate pre-processing and analysis with the help of automated equipment; medical imaging assists diagnosis through automated acquisition, pre-processing and intelligent analysis; automated production lines and quality control in drug production ensure product quality and efficiency; and in medical services, automation technologies such as medical robots and telemedicine enhance the level and availability of medical services [4].

## 3.2 Basic Theory of Organoids

### 3.2.1 *The Concept of Organoids*

Organoids are tissue analogues with a certain spatial structure formed by *in vitro* 3D culture using adult stem cells or pluripotent stem cells. Although organoids are not human organs in the true sense of the word, they can mimic real organs in terms of structure and function, can simulate the structure and function of *in vivo* tissues to the greatest extent possible, and can be cultured in a long-term and stable way.

Functional organoid-based precision medicine is a therapeutic approach that seeks to exploit patient-specific personalized treatment strategies. Given their ease of handling and potential to capture the diversity of patients and tumor types, organoids are well suited to the development of personalized therapies.

### 3.2.2 *Biological Properties and Functional Modeling of Organoids*

Organoids are able to mimic the complex biological properties of the source organ, including self-organization, multicellular type composition, genetic stability, gene expression patterns, and microenvironmental reproduction. For example, intestinal organoids are capable of nutrient absorption and transport, and liver organoids can participate in drug metabolism [5]. At the same time, organoids can also simulate the development of diseases, providing an ideal model for studying disease mechanisms, drug screening and personalized medicine.

### 3.2.3 *Key Technologies for Organoid Culture*

The key technologies of organoid culture mainly include the following aspects: induction and differentiation of human embryonic stem cells or induced pluripotent stem cells, and inducing these stem cells to form embryoid bodies through specific culture medium and conditions, which contain three embryonic layers, namely, endoderm, mesoderm, and ectoderm; 3D culture system, in which organoids are cultured *in vitro* to simulate the 3D structure and physiological function of *in vivo* organs under normal or diseased conditions (Figure 3.3) [6, 7], providing a higher level of complexity compared to 2D cell cultures; and the use of extracellular matrix, where the self-renewal and differentiation of stem cells are influenced by growth factors and which provide scaffolds needed to support cell adhesion and growth during organoid formation. Hydrogels such as Corning Matrigel matrix and Corning® collagen are commonly used scaffolds to support cell expansion in organoid cultures [8]. Bio-orthogonal crosslinking

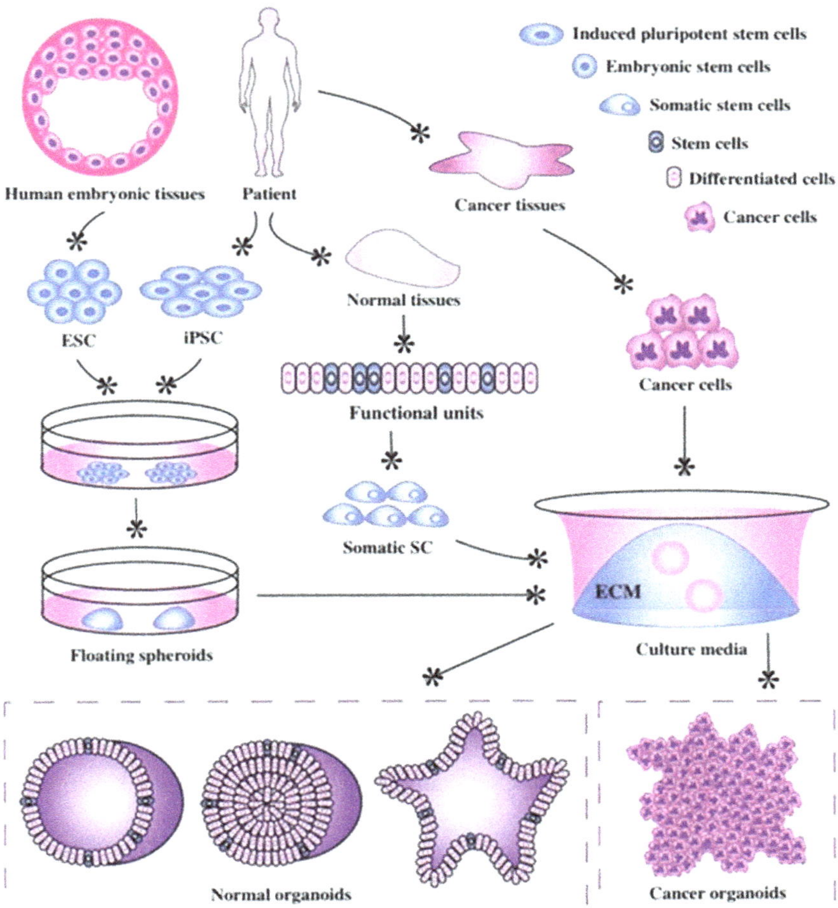


**Figure 3.3** A brief schematic of lung organoid construction. Reproduced with permission from Xu H, Lyu X, Yi M, Zhao W, Song Y, Wu K. Organoid technology and applications in cancer research. J Hematol Oncol. 2018;11(1):116.

hydrogel technology, where specific groups are introduced to gelatin precursors through chemical modification, forms hydrogels where the rheological, stability and mechanical properties can be regulated. By adjusting the gelatin concentration and stoichiometric ratio, the researchers effectively regulated the mechanical properties of the hydrogel, providing a suitable matrix environment for organoids. CRISPR-Cas9 genome editing technology, when used in conjunction with organoid technology, provides a better model for genetic and drug screening while opening new avenues for organ development research. Furthermore, personalized medical applications can be realized through organoids derived from individual stem cells, progenitor cells, or induced pluripotent stem cells. These organoids are valuable for disease modeling, efficacy and dosage testing, and regenerative medicine. In the realm of bioprinting, organoids serve as physiologically relevant models for the development of therapeutic drug candidates. Hydrogels can be used as bioinks for precise positioning and embedding of living cells/organoid in 3D bioprinting [9].

## 3.3 Organoid-Based Functional Precision Medicine

### 3.3.1 *Drug Screening Against Organoid Biobanks*

Organoid biobanks cover a wide range of cancer types and therefore have many applications in the screening of therapeutic agents. Sensitivity analyses for this class of drugs are particularly powerful when combined with genomic and/or transcriptomic characterization of organoids to identify specific drug response profiles for different tumor subtypes or to define sensitive and resistant patient-derived organoids (PDOs) [10]. PDOs can also be used to analyze synthetic lethality in order to identify drugs with selective efficacy against organoids with specific mutations [11]. Examples of such approaches abound, including the screening of a liver cancer organoid biobank with six liver PDOs against 29 anticancer drugs, with ERK inhibitors singled out as potential therapies to treat a subset of liver cancers [12]. Similarly, 27 hepatocellular carcinoma organoid cell lines from different tumor regions of five patients were exposed to 129 anticancer drugs approved by the U.S. Food and Drug Administration (FDA). This identified 13 drugs with a wide range of cytotoxicity, including inhibitors of histone deacetylase, proteasome, DNA topoisomerase II, protein translation and RNA synthesis, as well as several additional agents [13]. Comparison of the organisms' drug responses with data from publicly available drug response databases showed significant clustering of drug responses in organisms compared to conventional liver cancer cell lines, suggesting that primary pancreatic cancer may respond differently to drugs than conventional cultured 2D cells [14]. Systematic exposure of a genetically characterized biobank of 66 patients with pancreatic cancer to five clinically used chemotherapeutic drugs including gemcitabine showed that 33% of the pancreatic cancer tissue samples were sensitive to all drugs but half of the multidrug-resistant strains were sensitive to one of 21 such drugs for targeted therapy, suggesting that alternative therapeutic strategies may be used. In this context, correlation between RRG gene expression and drug sensitivity revealed a genetic signature of sensitivity to gemcitabine and in a cohort of 55 patients, gemcitabine was significantly associated with improved progression-free survival with adjuvant treatment after surgery [15]. As shown in Figure 3.4, large-scale screening for PDOs may also reveal unexpected treatments or combinations of treatments, such as the establishment and evaluation of a gastric cancer organoid repository. Further, the generation of matched tumor and normal organoids was exploited to reveal that gemcitabine can potentiate the EZH2 inhibitor UNC1999 in pancreatic ductal adenocarcinoma PDOs. Drug sensitivities between sibling pairs of PDOs and patient-derived xenografts (PDXs) have been compared in CRC models141. 'CRC models141' refers to an experimental model group used to compare the drug sensitivity of PDOs with PDXs in colorectal cancer studies. Specifically, this model set contained 19 pairs of matched PDOs and PDXs samples (46 PDOs and 59 PDXs in total), which were found to have high concordance in drug response by testing 16 anti-cancer drugs. This model set aims to validate the reliability of organoid and xenograft models in simulating patients' tumor characteristics and drug responses, and to provide an experimental basis for precision medicine. In a study group of 46 PDOs and 59 PDXs, 19 tumors detected by both systems responded fairly consistently to the 16 drugs tested [17]. However, different patterns were observed in terms of individual drug sensitivity and RNA profiles associated with hypoxia, epithelial-mesenchymal transition, G2/M checkpoint, proliferation, stemness and tumorigenicity. While PDOs and PDXs can mimic important genetic and phenotypic features of the primary tumor, both have inherent limitations.

Future studies will combine the strengths of both models and have the potential to provide actionable clinical information that will advance precision medicine [18]. The large number of organoid biobanks under development provides a unique opportunity for targeted drug development. Drug screening in large, well-defined organoid biobanks can identify drugs that are effective against tumor subpopulations with a specific genetic make-up. Although these screens are widely used for cells grown in 2D monolayers, recent evidence suggests that cells grown in 3D often respond differently to drugs, with differences that include increased resistance to chemotherapy [19]. For example, drug responses in 2D versus 3D for ovarian cancer show a correlation between cytotoxic and cytostatic drugs, but differences in cytostatic drugs. It is conceivable that 3D organoid biobanks could reduce false-positive results in large drug screens, and thus costly confirmatory preclinical studies with mice. In addition, organoids could be grown from corresponding healthy tissue, providing an early indication of substance toxicity as well as potential biological information [20]. Organoid-based models may never replace mouse experiments for drug discovery, but culturing organoids in block cultures with tumors, infiltrating immune cells, and multi-organoid systems integrated on microarrays can be used to study drug metabolism and toxicity. For the foreseeable future, xenograft experiments will still be required for positive compounds. In

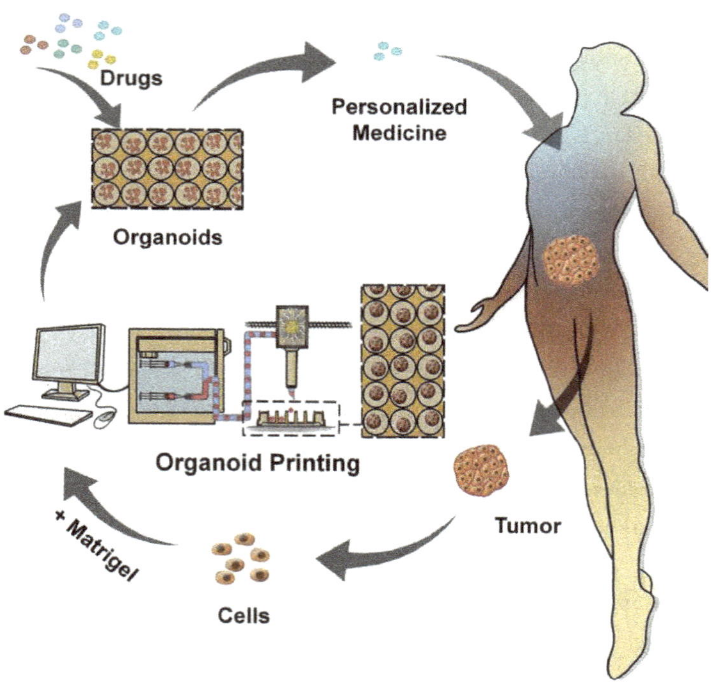


**Figure 3.4** PDO biobank established to screen therapies for molecular subtypes of different solid tumors. Reproduced with permission from Jiang S, Zhao H, Zhang W, *et al.* An automated organoid platform with inter-organoid homogeneity and inter-patient heterogeneity. Cell Rep Med. 2020;1(9):100161.

conclusion, the currently burgeoning PDO biobanks are a promising approach for screening therapies against different molecular subtypes within different solid tumors [21]. Rigorous genetic characterization of these PDOs in combination with small molecule screening could uncover new patient-relevant gene-drug interactions and synthetic fatalities, providing new insights compared to traditional cancer cell lines and PDX models. Furthermore, the biobanking paradigm has applications far beyond cancer, such as the recently established cystic fibrosis organoid resource [22].

### 3.3.2 *Precision Medicine and Personalized Therapy Design*

In precision oncology, predictive mutation biomarkers have traditionally been used for targeted therapy. However, such biomarkers are often lacking; for example, after whole-exome sequencing of a mixed group of tumors, only 3 out of 737 patients (0.4%) had actionable mutations found in the U.S. FDA-approved cognate. Even when targeted biomarkers are found, patients do not necessarily respond to targeted therapies, so there is an urgent need for predicting efficacy or identifying alternative regimens [23]. As shown in Figure 3.5, PDO technology offers an exciting opportunity to predict functional therapeutic responses in living cells. Several studies have reported that PDOs can predict patient response to anticancer drugs in a limited number of cases ($n < 5$). In general, published responses of tumor tissue cells to drugs have been correlated with patient prognosis. For example, in a biobank consisting of well-characterized PDO histiocytes from pancreatic cancer, eight out of nine histiocytes responded similarly to the corresponding patient's response to chemotherapy, with an 89% match rate [24]. In a study of patient responses to drugs and drug regimens for different types of gastrointestinal tumors, paired organ tissues correctly predicted whether or not they would respond to treatment in 20 out of 21 patients. Similarly, a comparison of in-patients with metastatic colorectal cancer with the PDO response in these patients found that irinotecan monotherapy (10 patients) and irinotecan in combination with 5-FU (12 patients) were relatively successful, but 5-FU in combination with oxaliplatin (10 patients) was unsuccessful [25]. The authors speculated that the inability of PDO to predict response to oxaliplatin may be due to the absence of the immune system and stroma in the organism. Two recently published papers concluded that organ tissue can accurately predict response to neoadjuvant chemotherapy in patients with rectal cancer. In a large study, 80 PDOs were measured in biopsy tissue from untreated patients with locally advanced rectal cancer from the phase 3 clinical trial of neoadjuvant radiotherapy combined with 5-FU with or without irinotecan [26]. Organ tissues were treated with radiotherapy, 5-FU or irinotecan instead of combination therapy. Defining the organoids as sensitive to neoadjuvant chemotherapy by response to at least one of the three treatments (radiation, 5-FU, irinotecan), the study correctly predicted outcomes in 85% of patients. Because many organoids were sensitive only to single or double agents, the authors hypothesized that not all three therapies are necessary in combination for every patient, and that organoid screening can identify ineffective treatments and thus avoid overtreatment. Another study, also of neoadjuvant chemotherapy in rectal cancer, found varying sensitivity of rectal PDOs to *ex vivo* radiation, which correlated with clinical response in a cohort of 19 patients [27]. Given these results, functional precision medicine, in which

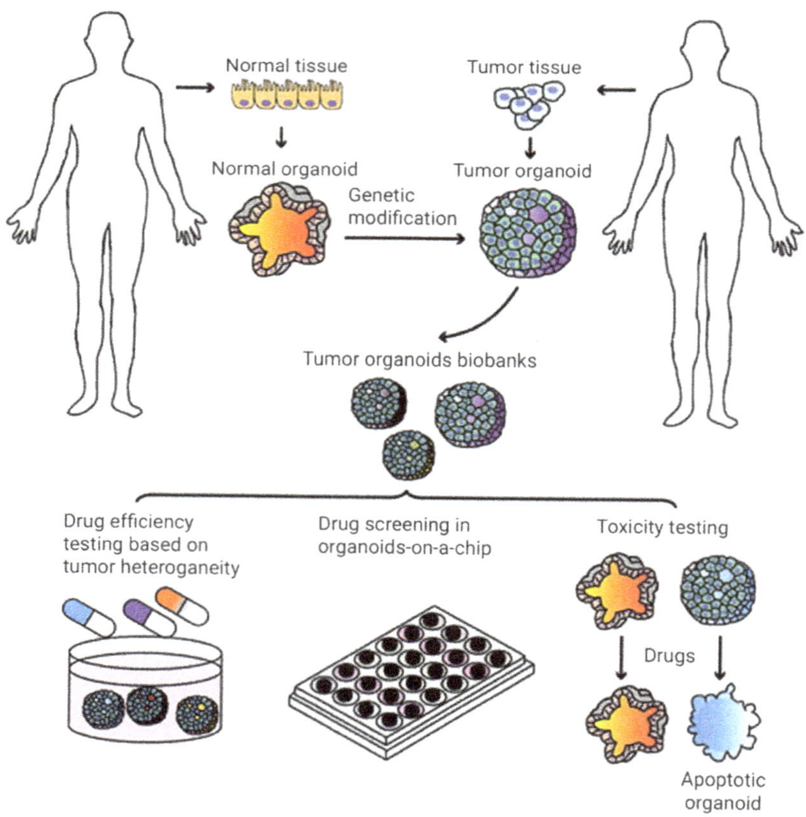


**Figure 3.5** Targeted therapy using predictive mutation biomarkers. Reproduced with permission from Kretzschmar K. Cancer research using organoid technology. J Mol Med (Berl). 2021;99(4):501–515.

individualized prediction is based on the testing of cellular responses to drugs rather than the identification of biomarkers, is an intriguing prospect for PDOs. In the current biobanking work, the success rate of establishing cultures varies greatly depending on tumor type, but is high (>80%), suggesting that functional precision medicine based on organ tissues may be feasible. Although tumor heterogeneity is an important potential confounding variable that militates against extrapolating treatment from a single biopsy region, functional prediction seems feasible, at least for specific tumor types and drug testing [28]. However, most current organoid-based treatment prediction systems lack stromal and immune regions, which may prevent their general application. Negative results are not characterized, which raises the issue of publication bias and, perhaps more importantly, the fact that studies to date have formed predictions based on prior knowledge of clinical outcomes. Although the current studies show high complication rates (80–95%), this does not mean that they are not applicable; it will be necessary to observe whether initial successes persist in larger prospective independent validation cohorts of patient–organoid pairs in which response metrics are fixed in advance.

### 3.3.3 *Organoid-Based Automation for Precision Medicine is a Cutting-Edge Field that Combines Biotechnology and Information Technology*

Organoid-based precision medicine automation is an innovative direction in the field of medicine that integrates biotechnology and information technology. Central to this approach is the utilization of organoids — 3D *in vitro* models that closely replicate the structural and functional complexity of human organs — integrated with high-throughput automated platforms and artificial intelligence (AI)-driven data analytics. By combining these technologies, this paradigm aims to enhance the precision, scalability, and efficiency of critical processes such as disease mechanism elucidation, drug discovery, and the development of personalized therapeutic strategies. Such integration holds promise for accelerating translational research and delivering tailored clinical interventions in precision medicine [29]. Derived from patients' pluripotent stem cells or tissue-specific stem cells, organoids are capable of self-assembling and reproducing the physiological and pathological characteristics of primary tissues under 3D culture conditions *in vitro*, providing a highly simulated experimental platform for disease modeling and drug response research (Figure 3.6). By leveraging automation

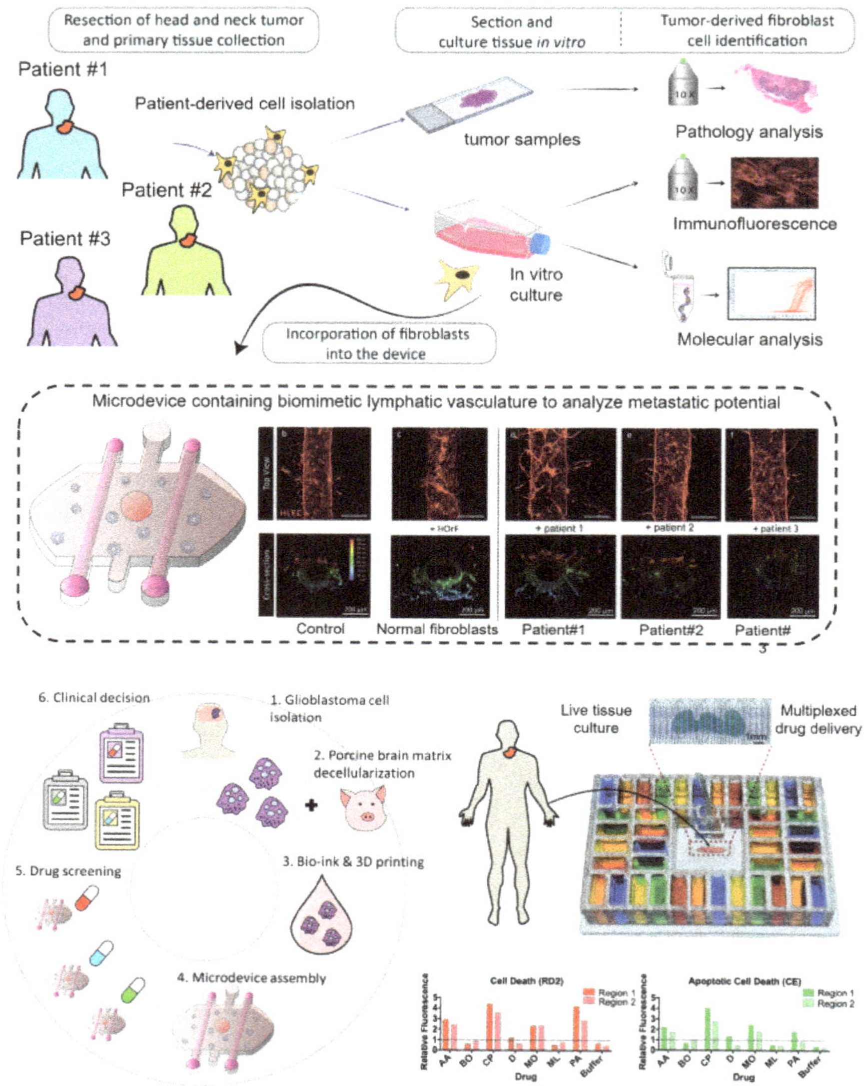


**Figure 3.6** Organoid derived from patient's pluripotent stem cells or tissue-specific stem cells. Reproduced with permission from Tuveson D, Clevers H. Cancer modeling meets human organoid technology. Science. 2019;364(6444):952–955.

technologies, researchers can streamline the cultivation, processing, and analysis of organoid samples at scale. When integrated with AI algorithms, these high-throughput approaches enable the extraction of actionable insights from vast experimental datasets. This synergy accelerates the identification of disease-specific biomarkers, novel therapeutic targets, and tailored treatment regimens, optimizing the discovery pipeline for precision medicine applications.

A specific example is in the precision treatment of colorectal cancer, where researchers can extract cells from a patient's tumor tissue and culture colorectal cancer organoids [30]. Subsequently, an automated drug-screening platform is used to test the organoid for a variety of chemotherapeutic and targeted drugs, recording its growth inhibition rate, apoptosis rate, and other key metrics. AI-driven algorithms synthesize and interpret these multidimensional datasets to predict patient-specific drug sensitivities, enabling data-guided recommendations for optimal therapeutic regimens. For instance, studies have demonstrated strong concordance between patient responses to EGFR inhibitors (e.g., cetuximab) and the corresponding organoid model's drug sensitivity profiles, validating the clinical utility of this strategy. By bridging experimental models with real-world patient outcomes, this organoid-based precision medicine automation strategy not only accelerates the drug development process, but also provides strong technical support to realize individualized treatment.

## 3.4 Challenges and Perspectives

Organoid culture technologies have rapidly exerted a transformative impact on cancer research, with widespread adoption for fundamental and translational applications. Despite promising studies to date, numerous challenges remain. Although PDOs often retain the genetic composition of the original tumor in early passages, the extent of genetic drift, clonal selection, and ongoing tumor evolution in later passages and after freeze-thaw cycles is not well documented and may be tumor-specific. Similar caveats also apply to oncogene engineering in normal tissues. Differences in apparently normal cells concerning telomere length, genetic, and epigenetic state could potentially influence phenotypic outcomes. Furthermore, variability can stem from multiple experimental factors: the sequence and timing of mutations introduced during multi-step genetic engineering protocols; the spatial precision, editing efficiency, and temporal persistence of CRISPR-mediated modifications; the artificial population bottlenecks imposed during clonal selection of rare genetically modified cells; and the inherent evolutionary dynamics of culture systems. This could explain differences in invasive behavior between two recent colorectal cancer organoid models introducing the same set of mutations. Another key limitation of conventional organoid methods is the demonstrated lack of endogenous tumor-associated stromal components, particularly immune cells and fibroblasts. Thus, the continued development of organoid systems that more holistically represent the tumor microenvironment is an urgent need. Ultimately, PDOs incorporating immune and stromal components could open new research directions such as immuno-oncology and realize the promise of precision cancer therapies.

While the essential culture components for growing organoids from different normal tissues and cancers have been extensively studied, the costs are substantial and reagents can vary between laboratories, facilitated by the use of conditioned medium containing factors such as Wnt3a, R-spondin, and Noggin. Additionally, the presence of serum in conditioned media may disadvantage long-term culture. Recently developed artificial water-soluble Wnt agonists or afamin-stabilized Wnt3a may facilitate the development of serum-free alternatives to conventional Wnt conditioned media and enable economical, fully defined, recombinant culture reagents. A practical challenge is reproducing the potency of organoid media across different batches and laboratories, which can exert selection pressure on a subset of cells that might not be representative of the original tumors. Simultaneously, evaluating many different culture conditions can improve PDO generation success rates. Oncogene engineering using CRISPR-Cas9 in primary human organoids is currently inefficient and largely restricted to selected genes. This limitation arises because activating mutational pathways in these genes enables custom, media-based functional selection strategies to enrich for gene knockouts. Future approaches might bypass such screening requirements, perhaps by enabling phenotypic screening, increasing efficiency, or using selectable knock-in cassettes. Opportunities also exist for large-scale genetic and chemical perturbation of organoids. Improved, highly efficient editing methods could facilitate screening of a broader range of target loci, extending to genome-wide high-throughput functional screens. Similarly, small molecule screening in organoids has been limited to modest panels of therapeutics, which could be expanded to larger compound libraries using ultra-high-throughput miniaturized cultures. The scale of genetic and small molecule screens could be significantly increased by methods to expand organoid biomass to degrees well beyond current practice. Among the potentially most beneficial applications of organoids in oncology lies therapeutic prediction. Numerous studies suggest the feasibility of PDO-based functional testing for patient drug responses, which now require prospective confirmation in validation cohorts. Optimally, organoid-based assays will require rapid turnaround within clinically actionable timeframes, evidence of an enhanced survival benefit and, presumably, extension to modalities such as immunotherapy.

Furthermore, the creation of ever-larger PDO biobanks, for example through the Human Cancer Models Initiative, can establish large collections representing diverse cancer subtypes and genotypes. Systematic drug screening of these could establish ready-to-use therapeutic response models, potentially relevant for patients with similar tumor genotypes. Such a transformation from previous descriptive metrics to predictive, organoid-based living-cell biological assays would be a culmination of the rapid progress made with cancer organoids to date, presaging further advances in both fundamental biology and clinical translation.

## Key Opinion Points

1. Construct a complete tumor microenvironmental organoid model containing immune and stromal components to enhance the physiological relevance of drug response prediction.
2. Develop chemically defined serum-free standardized culture medium to solve the problems of high culture cost and large batch variation.
3. Break through the bottleneck of CRISPR-Cas9 editing efficiency to achieve high-throughput gene editing and functional screening of organoids.
4. Establish a cross-center standardized organoid biosample library, and strengthen the foundation for translation through prospective clinical validation.
5. Deepen the integration of automation platform and AI algorithms to achieve the intelligent process of organoid culture, analysis and personalized treatment prediction.

## References

1. Wang Y, Zheng D. The importance of precision medicine in modern molecular oncology. Clin Genet. 2021 Sep;100(3):248–257.

2. Puccetti M, Pariano M, Schoubben A, Giovagnoli S, Ricci M. Biologics, theranostics, and personalized medicine in drug delivery systems. Pharmacol Res. 2024 Jan;201:107086.
3. Yang S, Hu H, Kung H, Zou R, Dai Y, Hu Y, Wang T, Lv T, Yu J, Li F. Organoids: The current status and biomedical applications. MedComm (2020). 2023 May 17;4(3):e274.
4. Peng J, Tang F, Zhou R, Xie X, Li S, Xie F, Yu P, Mu L. New techniques of on-line biological sample processing and their application in the field of biopharmaceutical analysis. Acta Pharm Sin B. 2016 Nov;6(6):540–551.
5. Yang S, Hu H, Kung H, Zou R, Dai Y, Hu Y, Wang T, Lv T, Yu J, Li F. Organoids: The current status and biomedical applications. MedComm (2020). 2023 May 17;4(3):e274.
6. Qu B, Mu Q, Bi H, Chen Y, Wang Q, Ma X, Lu L. Interpretation of the past, present, and future of organoid technology: an updated bibliometric analysis from 2009 to 2024. Front Cell Dev Biol. 2024 Aug 13;12:1433111.
7. Suarez-Martinez E, Suazo-Sanchez I, Celis-Romero M, *et al.* 3D and organoid culture in research: physiology, hereditary genetic diseases and cancer. Cell Biosci. 2022;12:39.
8. Li Y, Qin M, Liu N, Zhang C. Organoid development and applications in gynecological cancers: the new stage of tumor treatment. J Nanobiotechnol. 2025;23:20.
9. Karvinen J, Kellomäki M. Design aspects and characterization of hydrogel-based bioinks for extrusion-based bioprinting. Bioprinting. 2023;32:e00274.
10. Wang C, Zhang M, Zhao J, Li B, Xiao X, Zhang Y. The prediction of drug sensitivity by multi-omics fusion reveals the heterogeneity of drug response in pan-cancer. Comput Biol Med. 2023 Sep;163:107220.
11. Swain B, Maddi S. Patient-derived tumor organoids: generation and applications in disease modeling and personalized therapy. Nature Cell and Science. 2024;2(3):185–197.
12. Wang C, Cao Y, Yang C, Bernards R, Qin W. Exploring liver cancer biology through functional genetic screens. Nat Rev Gastroenterol Hepatol. 2021 Oct;18(10):690–704.
13. Rao J, Song C, Hao Y, Chen Z, Feng S, Xu S, Wu X, Xuan Z, Fan Y, Li W, Li J, Ren Y, Li J, Cheng F, Gu Z. Leveraging patient-derived organoids for personalized liver cancer treatment. Int J Biol Sci. 2024 Oct 7;20(13):5363–5374.
14. Kim S, Choung S, Sun RX, Ung N, Hashemi N, Fong EJ, Lau R, Spiller E, Gasho J, Foo J, Mumenthaler SM. Comparison of cell and organoid-level analysis of patient-derived 3D organoids to evaluate tumor cell growth dynamics and drug response. SLAS Discov. 2020 Aug;25(7):744–754.
15. Merrill NM, Kaffenberger SD, Bao L, Vandecan N, *et al.* Integrative drug screening and multiomic characterization of patient-derived bladder cancer organoids reveal novel molecular correlates of gemcitabine response. Eur Urol. 2024 Nov;86(5):434–444.
16. Smabers LP, Wensink E, Verissimo CS, *et al.* Organoids as a biomarker for personalized treatment in metastatic colorectal cancer: drug screen optimization and correlation with patient response. J Exp Clin Cancer Res. 2024 Feb 27;43(1):61.

17. Kim DW, Beato F, Kim Y, Tassielli AF, Dai R, Denbo JW, Hodul PJ, Malafa MP, Fleming JB. Real time ex vivo chemosensitivity assay for pancreatic adenocarcinoma. Oncotarget. 2023 Sep 15;14:811–818.
18. Wang X, Zhu J, Li L, Zhao Q, Huang Y, Wen C, *et al.* Utility of patient-derived xenografts to evaluate drug sensitivity and select optimal treatments for individual non-small-cell lung cancer patients. Mol Med. 2024 Nov 11;30:209.
19. Lo YH, Karlsson K, Kuo CJ. Applications of organoids for cancer biology and precision medicine. Nat Cancer. 2020 Aug;1(8):761–773.
20. Zhao Z, Chen X, Dowbaj AM, Sljukic A, Bratlie K, Lin L, Fong ELS, Balachander GM, Chen Z, Soragni A, Huch M, Zeng YA, Wang Q, Yu H. Organoids. Nat Rev Methods Primers. 2022;2:94.
21. Gao H, Korn JM, Ferretti S, *et al.* High-throughput screening using patient-derived tumor xenografts to predict clinical trial drug response. Nat Med. 2015 Nov;21(11):1318–25.
22. Ghandi M, Huang FW, Jané-Valbuena J, *et al.* Next-generation characterization of the Cancer Cell Line Encyclopedia. Nature. 2019 May;569(7757):503–508.
23. Choucair K, Morand S, Stanbery L, Edelman G, Dworkin L, Nemunaitis J. TMB: a promising immune-response biomarker, and potential spearhead in advancing targeted therapy trials. Cancer Gene Ther. 2020 Dec;27(12):841–853.
24. Yang R, Qi Y, Zhang X, Gao H, Yu Y. Living biobank: Standardization of organoid construction and challenges. Chin Med J (Engl). 2024 Dec 20;137(24):3050–3060.
25. Smabers LP, Wensink E, Verissimo CS, Koedoot E, Pitsa KC, Huismans MA, Higuera Barón C, Doorn M, Valkenburg-van Iersel LB, *et al.* Organoids as a biomarker for personalized treatment in metastatic colorectal cancer: drug screen optimization and correlation with patient response. J Exp Clin Cancer Res. 2024 Feb 27;43(1):61.
26. Wensink GE, Elias SG, Mullenders J, Koopman M, Boj SF, Kranenburg OW, Roodhart JML. Patient-derived organoids as a predictive biomarker for treatment response in cancer patients. NPJ Precis Oncol. 2021 Apr 12;5:30.
27. Chetty R, McCarthy AJ. Neoadjuvant chemoradiation and rectal cancer. J Clin Pathol. 2019 Feb;72(2):97–101.
28. Zhu L, Jiang M, Wang H, Sun H, *et al.* A narrative review of tumor heterogeneity and challenges to tumor drug therapy. Ann Transl Med. 2021 Aug;9(16):1351.
29. Gorshkov K, Chen CZ, Marshall RE, *et al.* Advancing precision medicine with personalized drug screening. Drug Discov Today. 2019 Jan;24(1):272–278.
30. Punt CJ, Koopman M, Vermeulen L. From tumour heterogeneity to advances in precision treatment of colorectal cancer. Nat Rev Clin Oncol. 2017 Apr;14(4):235–246.

https://doi.org/10.1142/9789819817597_0004

Chapter 4

# Organoid Engineering Techniques for Drug Discovery and Development

**George Michael Nicolas, Ut Fai Chao, Shaohua Ma***

*Institute of Biopharmaceutical and Health Engineering,*
*Tsinghua Shenzhen International Graduate School,*
*Tsinghua University, Shenzhen 518055, China*

**Abstract:** Organoids transform biomedical research by mimicking *in vivo* physiological and pathological characteristics — providing effective drug discovery and development platforms, enabling rapid assessment of drug efficacy and toxicity, and simulating patient responses *in vitro*. However, challenges in inadequate reproducibility, inter-laboratory variability, restricted culture durations, and suboptimal production efficiency limit their broader applications. Organoid-based screening also requires thorough characterization and improved cultivation procedures, yet current methodologies encounter limitations in organoid size variability, extended culture periods, and difficulty obtaining structural and functional data. Given the increased interest in organoid models for disease modelling and drug discovery, significant engineering technique developments have emerged to create physiologically suitable, high-throughput, and reproducible organoids, thus allowing improved microenvironment regulation, vascularization, and perfusion. At the same time, novel organoid characterization techniques provide rapid identification and accurate organoid structure, function, and composition deep evaluation. This chapter discusses the recent innovations in organoid engineering (bioprinting, well molding, and organ-on-a-chip models) and characterization (spatial transcriptomics and AI-assisted identification) for drug discovery and development.

**Keywords:** AI-assisted organoid identification, bio-ink, bioprinting, deep profiling, microfluidic systems, organoid engineering

*Corresponding author. Email: ma.shaohua@sz.tsinghua.edu.cn

## Key Points

- Traditional organoid culturing techniques encounter limitations in organoid size variability, inadequate reproducibility, restricted culture durations, suboptimal production efficiency, extended culture periods, and structural and functional data analysis.
- Engineering developments in 3D bioprinting, multi-cavity well molding, and organ-on-a-chip systems enabled the creation of physiologically suitable, high-throughput, reproducible organoids with improved microenvironment regulation, vascularization, and perfusion.
- Selecting suitable bio-inks that replicate *in vivo* the extracellular matrix and specific culture parameters (static vs. dynamic) greatly influence organoid development and differentiation.
- Organoid characterization employing enhanced imaging, AI-driven analysis, and novel omics approaches allows rapid, comprehensive confirmation of organoid integrity and increased reproducibility.

## 4.1 Introduction

Organoids are 3D *in vitro* cell culture systems that replicate *in vivo* physiological and pathological traits, exhibiting self-organization capabilities to create intricate organ-like structures via cell-to-cell interactions and differentiation processes [1]. This technology creates "mini-organs" from primary or patient-derived samples, including the brain, skeletal muscle, skin, liver, kidney, intestine, and other organs in their healthy or cancerous states [1]. In precision medicine, organoids enable researchers and clinicians to explore tissue-specific, disease, or drug mechanisms [2–4]. These provide viable drug discovery and development platforms that allow rapid evaluation of drug effectiveness and toxicity, simulating patient reactions *in vitro*, and identifying prospective therapeutic targets [2, 4]. However, limitations include decreased reproducibility and lab-to-lab variations, poor *in vitro* vascular network incorporation, limited culture maintenance period, and low organoid production efficiency [5].

Organoid modeling characterization techniques also show significance in precision medicine and drug development given the rising demand for organoid-based rapid screening approaches, underscoring the need for a rapid complete assessment of organoid cultures [6]. Detailed characterization of these complex structures is usually hindered due to increased cell count, size, culture period, and decreased homogeneity [6]. Inherent organoid sizes limit imaging and analysis to collect essential structural and functional information [6]. Despite having standard sequencing identification approaches, these procedures are often arduous and time-consuming, demanding numerous organoid samples and masking insubstantial variability within cell populations.

Developments in organoid engineering techniques have generated significant progress in addressing these limitations. These innovations enable more accurate microenvironment control, aiding the creation of physiologically suitable models with greater complexity [1, 7, 8]. Additionally, they offer precise cell and biomaterial spatial organization with adequate nourishment, oxygen, and signaling molecule distribution ratios to identify and produce vascularized and perfused organoid systems [1, 9]. This chapter presents current organoid culturing techniques, advances in organoid engineering research for drug discovery and development, and their rapid characterization processes.

## 4.2 Organoid Culturing Techniques

Unlike 2D cell lines, culturing organoids requires highly detailed procedures. This not only entails specific media compositions and incubation periods, but also specialized equipment used for organoid culture to ascertain proper growth conditions. Conventional organoid cultivation methods include scaffold-based and scaffold-free 3D cell cultures (Figure 4.1). Scaffold-based systems introduce cells into natural or synthetic substrates, supporting cell proliferation, aggregation, and 3D structure [10]. They enable the construction of cells into 3D models and scale to substantial quantities [10]. Scaffold-free culturing protocols are matrix-independent systems that facilitate the self-aggregation of certain cell types, comprised of growing organoids via suspensions or bioreactors [11]. Despite these advantages, conventional organoid culture protocols produce significant limitations on sample reproducibility, accuracy in replicating natural extracellular matrix (ECM), mechanical property heterogeneity, and potential human immunogenicity [12, 13]. Highlighting organoid production efficiency, reproducibility, and homogeneity requirements has led to numerous engineering advances in organoid culturing techniques, encompassing innovations in traditional non-engineered organoids and engineered organoids.

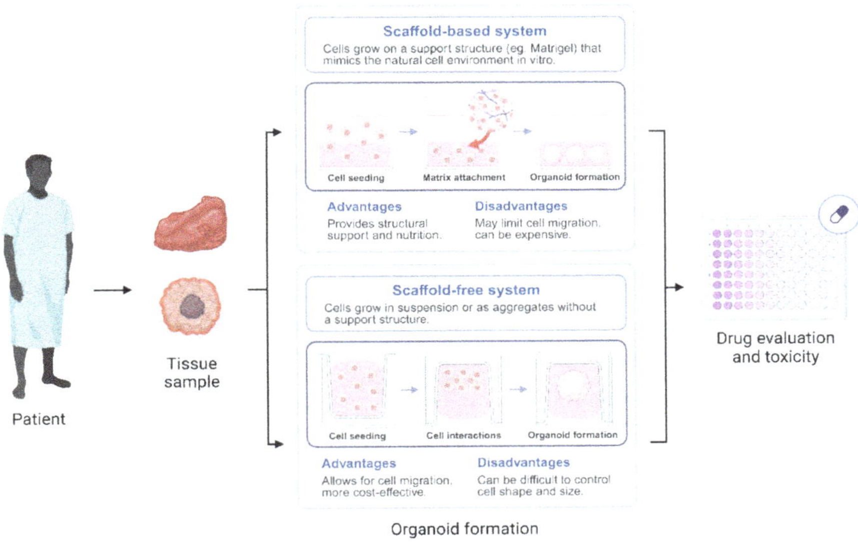


**Figure 4.1** Conventional methods used for organoid generation in precision medicine.

### 4.2.1 *Non-engineered Organoids*

Non-engineered organoids (NEOs) are 3D cell cultures typically used in primary or stem cell research. They are a fundamental platform for researching drug response and organ-specific cell activity for precision medicine applications. NEOs utilize traditional scaffold-based or scaffold-free systems, depending on the natural cell self-organizing capacities inside the organoid culture vessel.

#### 4.2.1.1 *Traditional Organoid Culture Vessels*

Traditional organoid culture vessels are specially designed containers for growing and maintaining these 3D structures. They are commonly manufactured using cell culture-compatible polystyrene materials, but some are made from polypropylene, polyethylene terephthalate, polyethylene, polyvinyl chloride, or borosilicate glass [14].

Polystyrene plastic materials are frequently used in culture vessels due to their great transparency, making them ideal for microscopic imaging and optical investigations [15, 16]. They are generally hydrophobic, allowing fast alterations with different physical surface treatments or coatings appropriate for cell culture, immunoassays, drug screening, and spectroscopic applications [15, 16]. Polypropylene, on the other hand, is resistant to most chemicals and possesses thermal stability [17]. Polar substances like DNA or proteins bind less to this material, making them ideal for screening and spectroscopic analyses. However, vessels made from polypropylene are commonly not surface-treated and show reduced transparency.

Traditional organoid culture vessels are also available in various shapes and sizes. These include T-flasks, cell-culture petri dishes, low-binding plates, transwells, hanging drop vessels, and custom cell culture vessels. Finding the appropriate vessel is essential in creating homogeneous structures for each specific organoid type (Figure 4.2).

Conventional T25 or T75 flasks are often used for cell-based assay research due to their cost-effectiveness for large-scale cell proliferation experiments. However, these vessels primarily facilitate 2D cell development, restricting intricate 3D organoid formations. T-flasks do not replicate *in vivo* architecture and microenvironments, leading to distinct characteristics of 2D-cultured cells and may provide inaccurate findings.

Cell culture petri dishes are shallow, covered cylindrical vessels that enable the observation and handling of organoids, but provide restricted environmental control. They are suitable for various analytical procedures, including immunofluorescence staining and high-content imaging tests, making them excellent for small-scale culture or control analysis research [18].

Low-binding 24- or 96-well plates, frequently covered with a covalently attached hydrogel layer, are commonly used to form spheroids or organoids, cell aggregates created by membrane protein 3D interactions. These simple and economical vessels are employed without specialized equipment and have been used for consistent spheroid formation from human-induced pluripotent stem cells (hiPSCs) or mesenchymal stem cells (MSCs) [19, 20]. Low-binding plates limit the attachment of semi-adherent and adherent cell lines via chemical surface modifications to prevent cell adhesion and promote cell aggregation, making them suitable substrates for 3D cell culture applications. They primarily feature U-bottom and V-bottom designs to address specific organoid requirements [21]. U-bottom wells facilitate gentle cell aggregation in rounded bases and are utilized for organoid or spheroid culture. V-bottom wells encourage

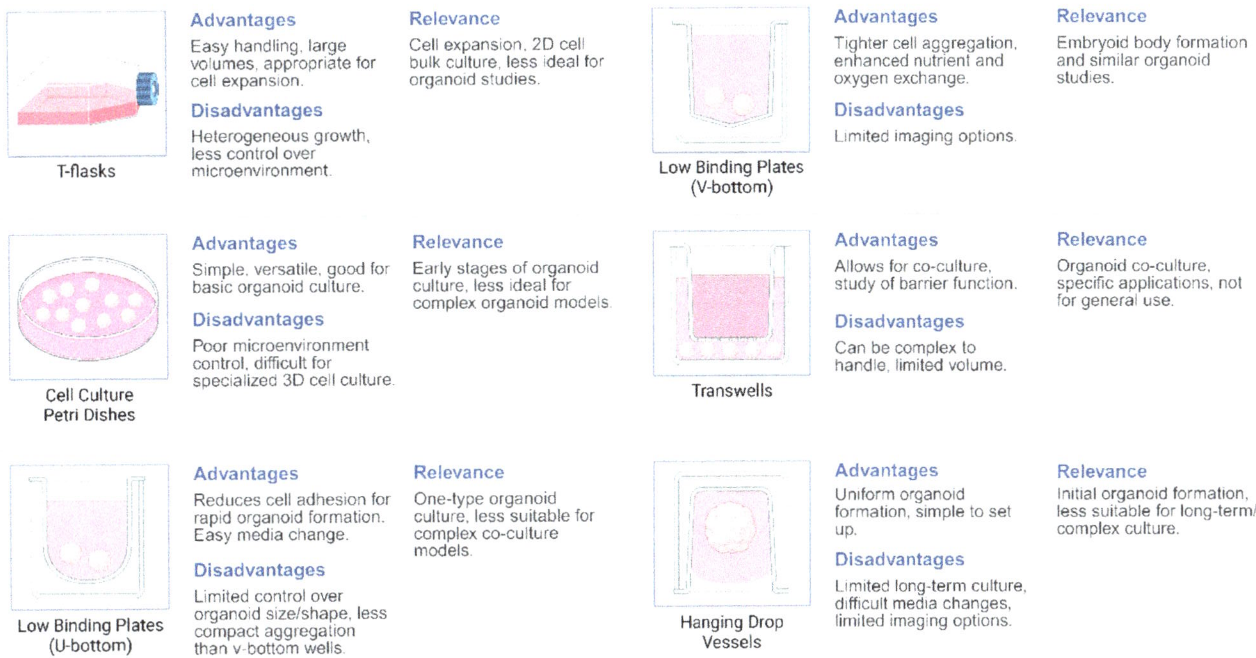


**Figure 4.2** Traditional organoid culture vessels, their advantages, disadvantages, and relevance.

tighter cell aggregation at the bottom due to their conical shape, making them well-suited for embryoid body formation.

Transwells are cell-culture vessels that enable cells to be cultivated in both chambers, the insert membrane and the well bottom. They are crucial for specialized organoid culture (e.g., epithelial tissue-derived organoids), establishing polarity necessary for understanding transport pathways, barrier function, and polarized gene expression [22]. Transwells also facilitate *in vitro* co-culture systems that mimic complex *in vivo* environments, allowing the investigation of cell-to-cell interactions between different organoid types.

Lastly, hanging drop vessels are specialized 3D cell culture vessels that form organoids or spheroids via single-cell suspension in droplets; they are inverted to maintain the droplets by liquid capillary tension forces [23, 24]. These vessels allow intercellular interactions without needing rigid support or hardened ECM scaffolding. Hanging drop vessels allow densely packed organoids to be created more often than loose cell aggregates, allowing the generation of organoids from diverse cell types and tissues like low-binding U-plates and V-plates.

#### 4.2.1.2 *Custom Organoid Culture Vessels*

Some NEO types require special growth conditions. However, current organoid culture approaches, which depend on embedding Matrigel in a dome shape, result in diverse sizes and morphological differences that hinder high-throughput analysis [7]. Although some researchers can administer growth factors every few hours to guide cell differentiation toward desired lineages, this technique is not economically practical due to concomitant pharmaceutical treatments and misleading reasons for size disparities [7], underscoring the need for custom cell culture vessels or inserts that provide convenience, efficiency, and high-resolution imaging.

Custom 3D-printed culture containers revolutionize organoid research by providing precise control over the cell microenvironment and vessel shape control. These vessels are utilized in tissue engineering, drug discovery, precision medicine, and disease modeling, providing high reproducibility, scalability, and customization. Jung *et al.* [25] designed a 96-well plate-compatible ECM plate to allow consistent culturing of tumor organoids. This plate is built similarly to a conventional 96-well plate, containing two types of central hole diameters appropriate for different applications. The D3 ECM plate (3-mm diameter central hole) is used for drug screening applications, whereas the D5 ECM plate (5-mm diameter central hole) is developed for organoid mass manufacturing. The central hole also contains an inverted pyramid structure on top to offer convenience in Matrigel placement, media change, or organoid washing.

Furthermore, most multi-well plates show inadequacies in high-resolution imaging of adult brain organoids, allowing constraints in studying neural spheroids and brain organoids. Mansilla *et al.* [26] developed 3D-printed microplate inserts to facilitate the development of brain organoids in conventional multi-well plates, increasing scalability in cerebral organoid culture. These inserts provide prolonged high-resolution imaging of adult brain organoids, permitting direct monitoring of individual cells inside intact living organoids, and enabling the evaluation of their growth, migration, and proliferation in a 3D milieu [26]. Organoid development, RNA sequencing, and immunofluorescence analyses also demonstrated similar results between organoids grown with plate-insert modifications and conventional methods, making 3D-printed inserts more appropriate for high-content studies to evaluate cellular responses [26].

## 4.2.2 *Engineered Organoids*

Although NEOs significantly contribute to *in vitro* organoid modeling, these models often encounter self-organization difficulties, slow growth, formation inconsistencies, and a lack of precise microenvironment control. With this, numerous researchers implemented modern bioprinting and microfluidic engineering technologies to exercise more control over organoid growth, formation, and differentiation, leading to the advancement of engineered organoids (EOs). This field of organoid research includes 3D bioprinting, multi-cavity well molding, microfluidic droplet-engineered organoids, and organ-on-a-chip models, enabling further advancements in developmental biology, drug discovery, and precision medicine [1, 27, 28].

### 4.2.2.1 *3D Bioprinting*

Bioprinting, a bio-additive manufacturing technique, has been widely used in tissue engineering and regenerative medicine due to its ability to control large-scale deposits of cells and biocompatible materials. It constructs intricate structures using a combination of living cells and support materials by accurately depositing and assembling cells and biomaterials in 3D [29, 30]. This fully customizable organoid engineering technique allows researchers to fully adjust bioprinting parameters and achieve precise spatial deposition of bio-inks, while programmed computer-aided automation facilitates repetitive operations and batch processing of many printed items.

In organoid culture, bioprinting enhances cell self-assembly and maturation, creating high-precision and high-throughput systems for organoid production [30]. It also assists in creating sophisticated ECM microenvironments around organoids, including spatial patterns of signaling molecules, or biochemical and biomechanical gradients to stimulate self-assembly [30–32]. Organoid bioprinting techniques can be divided into four groups. These include extrusion-based bioprinting, inkjet-based bioprinting, laser-assisted bioprinting, and bead-jet bioprinting (Figure 4.3).

#### 4.2.2.1.1 Extrusion-based Bioprinting

Extrusion-based bioprinting is a widely used approach in organoid engineering for producing large-scale tissue constructs with high cell density [33, 34]. This technique employs mechanical stress or air pressure to extrude bio-ink via a nozzle using various biocompatible materials such as hydrogels with fast cross-linking and shear-decreasing properties to create 3D-printed organoids or *in vitro* organ systems [33, 34]. Lawlor *et al.* [35] studied 3D cellular extrusion-based bioprinting techniques to automatically build self-organizing kidney organoids, dissociating a single cell suspension into a wet cell paste and fed into a syringe for automated deposition. This technology enabled the precise deposition of roughly one micromass every three seconds, creating approximately 200 organoids in 10 minutes with high diameter reproducibility. The extrusion bioprinting of hiPSC-derived kidney structures also effectively constructed large, homogeneously differentiated kidney organoids with functioning albumin absorption into proximal tubules, allowing a quality-controlled way of making transplantable kidney tissues utilizing cellular manufacturing methods [35].

Regardless, extrusion-based bioprinting presents issues on ensuring adequate cell nutrition and viability due to the increased mechanical pressure and shear stress from continuous squeezing. The size and variety of the printed organoids may also be

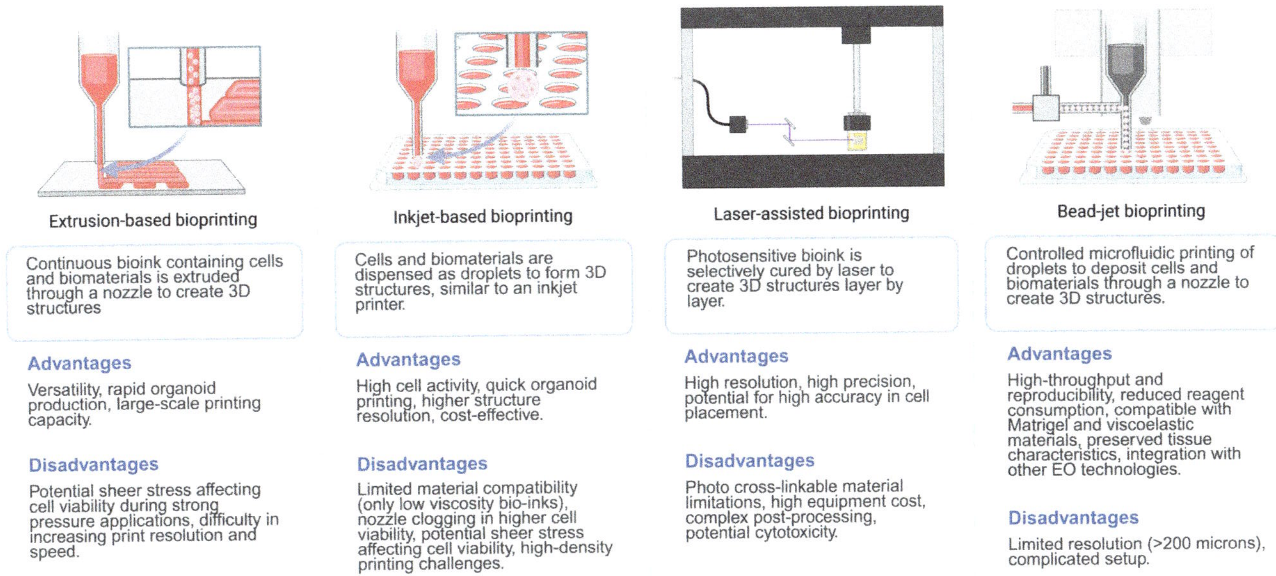


**Figure 4.3** Organoid 3D bioprinting technologies.

restricted by nozzle diameter and ink viscosity concerns. To address this, Brassard *et al.* [31] created bioprinting-assisted tissue emergence (BATE), a bioprinting system that employs a manually driven stage microscope and a syringe-based extrusion mechanism. This extrusion-based bioprinting technology provides real-time control and adjustment of the printing process, removing the need for an in-depth understanding of hydrogel rheology and bio-ink composition. Compared to existing bioprinting technologies, BATE provides various improvements, such as the capacity to organize fragile cells into complicated patterns in 3D culture matrices like Matrigel, coculture different organoid types, and decrease printing time and geometrical complexity, providing greater opportunities in stem cell biology and regenerative medicine research.

#### 4.2.2.1.2 Inkjet-based Bioprinting

Inkjet-based bioprinting is a contactless technology that generates liquid organoid droplets in a 3D biological ink structure by employing thermal or piezoelectric driving nozzles [34, 36]. Initially used due to their high cell activity, quick organoid printing, higher structure resolution, and affordability, this bioprinting method comprises several constraints in viscosity, shear stress, temperature, electric field, and stability [37]. Inkjet-based bioprinting also generates obstacles in cell viability and nozzle blockage, especially in high-density organoid synthesis [37]. Its low driving pressure disables printing materials with high viscosities or cell concentrations, making it challenging to produce complicated biomimetic tissues or organoids with high cell density. Low-viscosity biomaterials minimize mechanical characteristics but cannot supply a normal or similar physiological environment for cells, limiting *in vitro* and *in vivo* culturing efficiency [38].

#### 4.2.2.1.3 Laser-assisted Bioprinting

Laser-assisted bioprinting is a non-contact 3D bioprinting technology that employs laser direct-write and laser-induced transfer technologies to manufacture organoids with viscous biomaterials [34, 36]. The donor layer, comprised of a ribbon structure with an energy-absorbing layer and a bio-ink solution, responds to laser stimulation, activating a tiny piece of the absorbing layer and pushing the suspended bio-ink. Afterward, the organoid droplet is caught on the receiving substrate and cross-linked, providing better cell viability and enabling the printing of viscous bio-ink materials than droplet printing.

Stereolithography, a subset of laser-assisted bioprinting, employs photocurable materials to produce structures that simulate tissue and organs by pouring liquid photopolymer resin into a vat and exposing it to a computer-controlled laser beam during printing [36]. The light source is relocated further from the building platform, enabling the resin to be recoated at subsequent levels. This bioprinting method selectively hardens bio-inks layer-by-layer, providing enhanced spatial and temporal control and lowered heat output. Some digital light projectors can also cure bio-inks plane-by-plane, preserving excellent cell viability, and print in less than an hour with a 100 μm resolution.

Nevertheless, the deleterious consequences of laser exposure on cells are not well known, and laser diodes are more expensive than other nozzle-based printing methods. Further challenges include expensive machine costs, complex laser system management, requirement for photo-cross-linkable hydrogel materials, low printing efficiency, reproducibility concerns, and time-consuming production processes.

#### 4.2.2.1.4 Bead-jet Bioprinting

Novel bead-jet bioprinting approaches revolutionize EO research by combining controlled droplet production with microfluidics to manufacture homogeneous organoids by encasing primary or stem cells in bio-ink, addressing issues in traditional bioprinting methods. They encourage cell proliferation and self-organization, enabling fast production and differentiation of organoids. Unlike inkjet-based bioprinting, this method employs non-cytotoxic bio-inert oils or water instead of thermal or piezoelectric print heads to reduce cell shear stress. It also allows droplet modifications in cell type, growth factors, and signaling molecules to create organoids with specified features [39, 40]. In 2024, Yang *et al.* [37] designed OrgFab, an automated bioprinter that mitigates limitations in inkjet-based bioprinting, particularly the inability to process high cell densities with ultra-low volumes of viscous bio-inks, poor organoid scalability and throughput, and managing cell density and stability in organoid microenvironments. It offers highly compact sample processing capabilities, allowing 5 μL hydrogel volume processing compared to conventional 20 μL starting volumes. The system completely automates the process from sample loading, droplet generation, gel solidification, and accurate bioprinting onto 96 or 384-well plates. It also increases cell nutrient diffusion and permits high-density cell encapsulation into microdroplets, enabling intercellular interaction via paracrine signaling to develop organoids with exceedingly complicated biological systems and greater functional complexity.

Bead-jet bioprinting also enables fine-grain microenvironment control, high-throughput scalability, and homogeneity, potentially integrating with other EO technologies like multi-cavity well molding and organ-on-a-chip platforms to construct diverse organoid types from different cells and tissues, including patient-derived cells. This bioprinting method transforms organoid research and precision medicine, overcoming issues in organoid reproducibility, throughput, and long-term culture. According to Zhang *et al.* [41], droplet-engineered organoids from patient lung, esophageal, rectal, and colon tumor surgical samples revealed high similarities between the organoid and patient tissue morphology, as evidenced by histological staining. Immunohistochemistry staining of the organoids also showed preserved tumor purity by revealing negative tumor protein 63 and cytokeratin 5/6 with positive thyroid transcription factor-1 expression indicating non-small cell lung cancer adenocarcinoma, Kiel 67 antigen (Ki67), tumor protein p53, and caudal-type homeobox 2 (CDX2) expression indicating esophageal cancer, positive p53 and Ki67 with negative CDX2 indicating rectal cancer, and strong expression of Ki67, CDX2, and p53 indicating colon cancer. Subsequently, Liu *et al.* [40] devised a one-step bead-jet microfluidic system for creating cell-hydrogel capsules with high-throughput screening, reproducible 3D cell culture, and extended production of hiPSC organoids. This system utilizes pneumatic single-layer membrane valves to manage the formation of droplet templates and retain the constant size and shape of the capsules created, containing hollow-cored hybrid capsules to encase cells and shape them into homogenous spheres to display a unique core-shell structure with a thin shell. The properly permeable capsules safeguard against immunological rejection and mechanical damage while enabling the movement of gases, metabolites, and nutrients between cells and the external microenvironment.

Cao *et al.* [39] created a bead-jet printing system to improve cell retention in MSCs for rapid cell regeneration or wound healing therapy. Employing a specialized printing mechanism, monodispersed high-density MSC-laden Matrigel droplets exhibit remarkably superior proliferation and migration capabilities *in vitro*. These droplets markedly stimulated the production of functional extracellular vesicles, enhancing the regenerative potential of MSCs. Using a 3D bioprinter, ejection of the MSC-laden droplets onto injury sites in BALB/c mice via compressed air blasts formed sparse patterns, allowing effective coverage that maximizes MSC capacity and regeneration properties for large-scale injuries. It also rapidly accelerated skeletal muscle regeneration beneath the skin wounds, promoting deeper dermal layer formation. Lastly, Jiang *et al.* [42] developed an automated bead-jet bioprinting platform containing two modules (M1 and M2), utilizing microfluidic droplet engineering techniques followed by droplet bioprinting. M1 utilizes a continuous microfluidic tubing system to generate uniform cell-laden Matrigel droplets, minimizing mechanical interference, shear stress, and decreased organoid heterogeneity. M2 subsequently disperses these organoid precursors within the culture vessel chambers, achieving high throughput via spatial control over time. Rapid generation of numerous homogenous organoids using this dual-module platform revealed remarkably high accuracy, capturing patient-specific drug responses and predicting drug toxicity in healthy liver or kidney organoids.

#### 4.2.2.2 *Multi-cavity Well Molding*

Multi-cavity well molding (Figure 4.4) is another emerging EO technique that facilitates the fabrication of several identical microstructures in one well to enable consistent and reproducible platforms for organoid growth and testing. This innovation injects biocompatible micro-engineered hydrogel sheets into a cell culture vessel with well-designed chambers, allowing the simultaneous formation of numerous epithelial organoids from stem cell aggregates [7]. Multi-cavity well molding is excellent for scaling up organoid synthesis, enabling high-throughput applications in high-content phenotypic drug screening, disease modeling, precision medicine, and automated organoid production. It also permits the integration of varied competencies into a single device, such as electrodes for sensing organoid activity or optical windows for real-time imaging, presenting possibilities for standardizing organoid-based assays for diagnostics and drug research.

In 2020, Brandenberg *et al.* [7] designed the first micro-engineered platform for the rapid and uniform creation and characterization of gastrointestinal organoids, constructing a microcavity array system inside hydrogel substrates that enables simple access to individual organoids for downstream analysis and propagation. Evaluation of the cell aggregate size and microcavity diameters on organoid development and lifespan shows

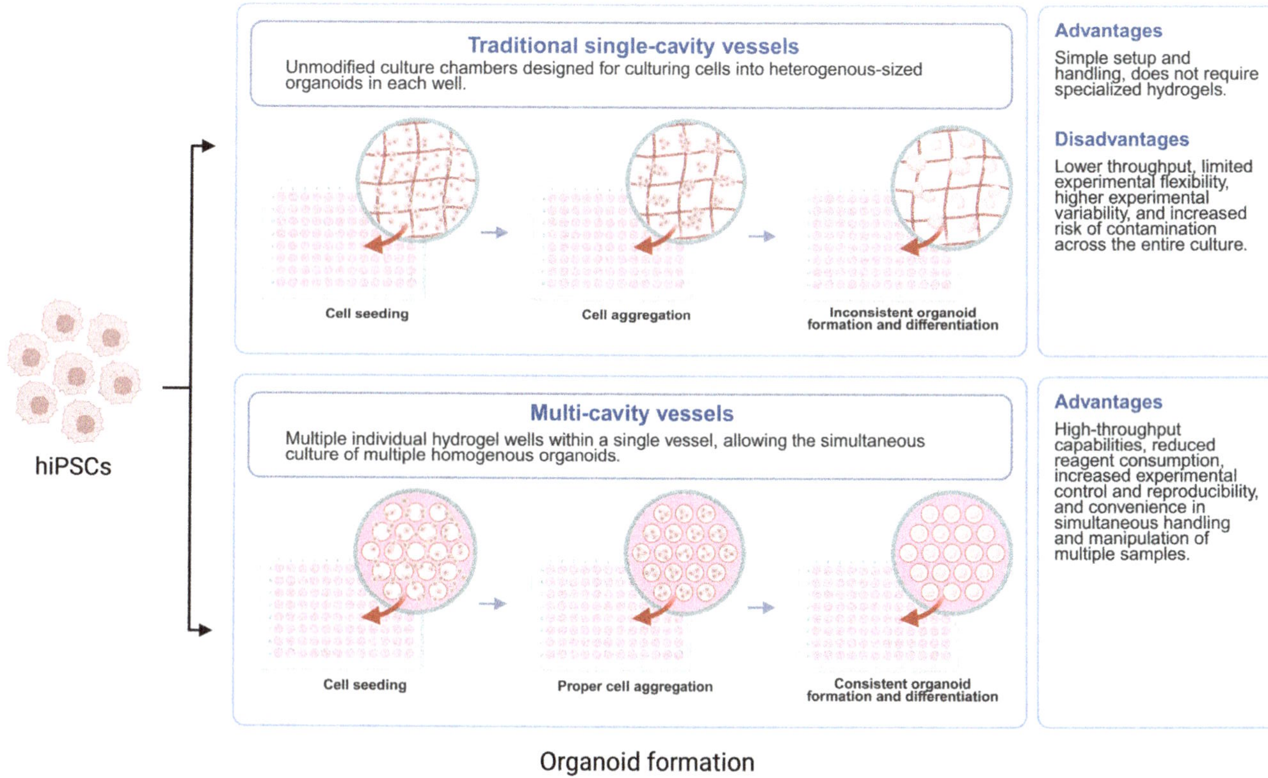


**Figure 4.4** Difference between traditional single-cavity vessels vs. multi-cavity wells for organoid engineering.

that optimal initial cell seeding density and microcavity size allow better organoid development in long-term culture. Subsequently, cells cultured in the micro-cavity platform with a more defined ECM formulation (containing laminin-111 and collagen IV) Matrigel alternative also increased organoid homogeneity and reproducibility, compared to standard Matrigel cultures, as they regulate the cell seeding process and avoid organoid fusion. Moreover, an automated high-content phenotypic drug screening assay of both mouse intestinal and human colorectal cancer organoids using this platform revealed the discovery of a unique phenotype linked with the protein kinase B (AKT) inhibitor drug afuresertib, further proving its application in high-throughput screening and thorough investigation of organoid growth and drug reactions.

At the same time, Harkin *et al.* [43] designed a similar vessel to construct homogenous retinal organoids, mitigating inherent differentiation diversity limitations of hiPSCs that lead to organoid size and shape heterogeneity via enzymatic lifting. They utilized single-cell suspensions with different amounts of cells per well, resulting in a controlled cellular aggregation size and consistent generation of uniformly sized aggregates following complete differentiation. Further genotypic analysis using this platform illustrated the importance of BMP4 signaling in cell development, acting as a developmental switch that promotes differentiation of retinal lineages.

#### 4.2.2.3 *Organ-on-a-chip*

Organ-on-a-chip models are miniature functional units that recreate human organs *in vitro* utilizing optically transparent materials like polydimethylsiloxane (PDMS) [44]. They are microfluidic cell culture systems with an irrigation-controlled micro-channel that assists the growth of primary cells, stem cells, and cell lines [1]. *In vitro*, these chips can reproduce organ microenvironments by coculturing two or more different cell types, such as stromal cells and organ-specific epithelial cells. Several organ chips have already been developed, accurately replicating *in vivo* organ structures *in vitro*. These include the lung alveoli [45, 46], bronchioles [46, 47], bone and bone marrow [48–50], kidney [51], heart [52], liver [53, 54], pancreas [55], and the blood-brain barrier [56, 57]. At the same time, certain orthotopic cancer organ chips are also constructed to simulate the anatomy and physiology of tumors [58–60]. Organ-on-chips are appropriate *in vitro* models for preclinical evaluation, showing human physiology and illness from a different aspect than single organoids. They regulate or combine complicated microenvironmental factors like dynamic fluids, mechanical signals, 3D topographical architecture, oxygen gradients, and partitioned space to drive the creation of functional organs and cell morphogenesis [1, 61]. This involves frequent replenishment of nutrients and waste discharge made possible by microfluidic flow in channels and reducing physiological shear stress, promoting physiological activity that allows systematic interaction across numerous organoids in the same chip system.

In 2024, Xue *et al.* [62] introduced a neural tube-like structure (μNTLS) and forebrain-like structure (μFBLS) human organ-on-a-chip microfluidic gradient systems for simulating human neurodevelopment. These hiPSC-derived neural patterning systems mimic important characteristics of neural patterning along the rostral-caudal and dorsal-ventral axes inside a 3D tubular shape to replicate *in vivo* neural tube formation. The device provides spatial and temporal control of morphogens and other signaling molecules, enabling microenvironments that simulate dynamic signaling gradients critical for brain development. It comprises a lumen, offering a regulated environment for sensitive real-time cell activity monitoring. Results showed that the μNTLS microfluidic system replicated patterned expression of regional markers (e.g., HOX family) along the rostral-caudal axis and dynamic development of neuromesodermal progenitors and neural crest cells, exhibiting an axial position-dependent induction into various cell types similar to *in vivo* neural crest development. Conversely, the μFBLS microfluidic system recapitulated spatially segregated dorsal and ventral regions with distinct apicobasal cellular structures in a layered morphology characteristic of human forebrain pallial and subpallial development.

### 4.2.3 *Bio-ink Design*

Bio-inks are essential in scaffold-based organoid modeling to establish a specialized cell microenvironment, enabling physiological cell growth, differentiation, and maturation activities. These biomaterials must be bioactive, biodegradable, and cytocompatible, containing adequate viscosity, surface tension, and elastic modulus mechanical properties, ultimately tied to the organoid type and printing procedure [36]. Common bioinks in organoid bioprinting comprise natural materials like alginate, agarose, hyaluronic acid, collagen, fibrin, gelatin, chitosan, and Matrigel. Synthetic materials include hyaluronic acid methacryloyl, polyethylene glycol, polyethylene glycol diacrylate, and gelatin methacrylic (GelMA), as shown in Table 4.1.

With the increased limitations of Matrigel and natural hydrogels, the discovery of novel bio-inks with high similarities to the natural ECM or moldable bio-inks to create differently shaped organoids that replicate *in vivo* organ structures revolutionizes 3D cell culture technology. Although widely used in 3D culture, the Engelbreth-Holm-Swarm mouse sarcoma cells-derived bio-ink Matrigel has several limitations. These include mechanical property heterogeneity and non-modifiability, batch variability due to its composition, nutrient and growth factor insufficiency, and decreased affordability — affecting organoid efficiency, reproducibility, and differentiation properties [83, 84]. In contrast, other natural hydrogels (e.g., collagen, hyaluronic acid) provide biocompatibility yet typically lack cues and mechanical qualities essential for organoid growth [83]. These materials also frequently display batch variability and are relatively prone to enzymatic breakdown, limiting long-term culture stability. Lastly, synthetic hydrogels (e.g., polyethylene glycol, GelMA) present promising solutions in modifiability, reproducibility, affordability, and long-term culture stability [8, 85]. However, they encounter difficulty in biodegradation due to complex polymer structures, duplication of biological signal and structural support like Matrigel, and potential cytotoxicity.

Jamaluddin *et al.* [86] developed unique hydrogels from decellularized bovine endometrium, successfully promoting endometrial organoid development in *in vitro* culture conditions. As decellularization process optimization considerably affects hydrogel quality and function, they tested decellularization techniques with drastically varying sodium dodecyl sulfate (SDS) and sodium deoxycholate (SDC) ionic detergent concentrations on endometrial tissue, discovering a 4% SDC-based approach that notably decellularizes organoid cell membranes and exhibits greater preservation of critical ECM proteins (laminins and collagen). This natural ECM biomechanical property preservation plays a key significance in the biocompatibility of rapid tissue regeneration *in vivo*. Further mechanical tests also demonstrated that the viscoelastic characteristics (loss modulus and storage) of SDC were higher than those of SDS-derived hydrogels. This hydrogel also efficiently supported human and animal endometrial organoid

**Table 4.1** Bio-inks used in organoid culture.

| Bio-ink | Cell Type | Method | Description | Reference(s) |
|---|---|---|---|---|
| Alginate (natural) | Human adipose-derived stem cells (hADSCs) and immortalized hepatic cells (HepaRG™) | Extrusion-based bioprinting, droplet-based bioprinting, and laser-assisted bioprinting (when functionalized with photo-cross-linkable properties) | Natural polysaccharide. Inexpensive, biocompatible, and quick ionic gelation.<br>Degrades slowly, has poor cell adhesion, does not boost cell growth rates, and brief duration of mechanical stability. | [63, 64] |
| Agarose (natural) | hiPSC-derived liver cells, human umbilical vein smooth muscle cells, and human skin fibroblast cells | Extrusion-based bioprinting | Excellent gel-forming ability, strong mechanical qualities, and biological tolerance.<br>Limited potential to maintain cell development. | [65, 66] |
| Hyaluronic acid (natural) | Patient-derived brain tumor cells and primary liver cells | Extrusion-based bioprinting and laser-assisted bioprinting (when functionalized with photo-cross-linkable properties) | Natural ECM component.<br>Boosts cell proliferation, can be readily changed, improves stability and viability, and has greater biocompatibility.<br>Slower gelation and inferior mechanical characteristics. | [67, 68] |
| Collagen (natural) | Human cardiomyocyte cells and breast cancer cells (21PT and MDA-MB-231) | Extrusion-based bioprinting and droplet-based bioprinting | Natural ECM component.<br>Outstanding cell transporters with great cell adhesion qualities.<br>Poor gelation rate and unstable structure. | [69, 70] |
| Fibrin (natural) | Mouse fibroblast cells (L929), endothelial colony-forming cells, and hADSCs | Droplet-based bioprinting and laser-assisted bioprinting (when functionalized with photo-cross-linkable properties) | Possesses intrinsic cell adhesion signaling molecules.<br>Low mechanical qualities, low infectious transmission, and non-shear-thinning behavior. | [71, 72] |
| Gelatin (natural) | Patient-derived liver cells and liver cancer cells (HepG2) | Extrusion-based bioprinting | Derived from collagen polymers. Water-soluble and low immunogenicity, with improved biodegradability and cell remodeling.<br>Thermally sensitive, need toxic cross-linking agents to address low mechanical qualities. | [73, 74] |

| | | | | |
|---|---|---|---|---|
| Chitosan (natural) | Pre-osteoblast cells (MC3T3-E1) and human umbilical vein endothelial cells | Extrusion-based bioprinting and laser-assisted bioprinting (when functionalized with photo-cross-linkable properties) | Natural ECM material.<br>Mechanically stable and mixable with other hydrogel components.<br>Acidic and damaging to cell pH, needing pH neutralization and combination with other materials. | [75, 76] |
| Matrigel (natural) | hiPSC-derived foregut cells | Extrusion-based bioprinting | Widely used in organoid culture.<br>Mechanically stable.<br>Increased cost and may induce potential immunogenicity to human samples. | [77] |
| Hyaluronic acid methacryloyl (synthetic) | Bone marrow-derived MSCs | Laser-assisted bioprinting (when functionalized with photo-cross-linkable properties) | Increased mechanical stiffness and long-term stability.<br>Low immunogenicity with high cytocompatibility.<br>May induce spontaneous differentiation. | [78] |
| Polyethylene glycol (synthetic) | Human chondrocyte cells | Extrusion-based bioprinting and droplet-based bioprinting | Produced by photopolymerization, are hydrophilic, biocompatible, and immunocompatible. Non-biodegradable, needing biodegradable segments for a higher decomposition rate. | [79] |
| GelMA (synthetic) | Cardiac myocyte and fibroblast cells, bone marrow-derived primary MSCs, human embryonic kidney cells (HEK293T), human colon myofibroblasts (CCD18Co), and human skeletal myoblasts | Extrusion-based bioprinting, droplet-based bioprinting, and laser-assisted bioprinting (when functionalized with photo-cross-linkable properties) | Possesses natural cell adhesion signaling molecules.<br>Thermoresponsive, supports excellent cellular proliferation and has minimal immunogenicity.<br>Mechanically weak during physiological temperatures. | [80–82] |

formation equivalent to Matrigel substrates, mirroring natural endometrial tissue via advantages in proteomic content signaling, and developing tubular structures comparable to the decellularized mouse uterus.

Conventional Matrigel cultures also typically limit deep tissue development due to the limitations in dynamic stress-relaxing matrices that are essential for organoid growth *in vitro*. Using reversible hydrogen bonding methods, Chrisnandy *et al.* [8] developed synthetic hydrogels (Hybrid50) with distinctive characteristics that enable extensive organoid development. Unlike conventional ineffective covalent gels, this custom hydrogel reduces stress in activities like crypt sprouting, exhibiting significant stress relaxation akin to Matrigel. The dynamic nature facilitates the matrix's stress absorption produced during rapid organoid development via intricate morphological interactions, providing great control over matrix stiffness and stress relaxation. It also profoundly influences mechanosensing pathways via increased nuclear yes-associated protein 1 localization to enhance early symmetry breaking, promote organoid formation, and improve Paneth cell proliferation. This synthetic hydrogel enables researchers to customize matrices for diverse organoid kinds in precision medicine, enhancing the prolonged growth of human organoids via complex mechanisms, including degradation facilitated by the enzyme sortase-A for cell adhesion and nutrient uptake.

Despite these promising advances, engineering perfect bio-inks that meet physiological demands poses significant difficulties due to mechanical property degradation, cell compatibility constraints, and *in vivo* environment recapitulation. Further bioink development must prioritize crafting fully defined hydrogels with similar *in vivo* ECM properties, promoting crucial biological functions with greater physical and biochemical property control. This includes controlling hydrogel stiffness, porosity, modifiability, and degradability while promoting a homeostatic microenvironment composition of growth factors and signaling molecules to improve cell proliferation and aggregation, organoid uniformity, and tissue differentiation containing complex *in vivo*-like structures.

### 4.2.4 *Static vs. Dynamic Organoid Culture*

In addition to replicating the natural cell microenvironment, organoids require specific growth circumstances to promote proper cell aggregation, nutrition supply delivery, and waste removal. This led to diverse organoid culture approaches, which can be

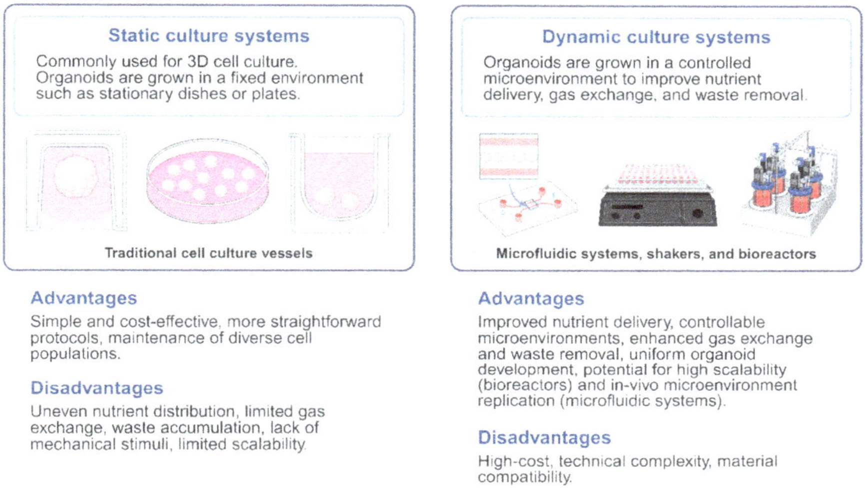


**Figure 4.5** Comparison of static vs. dynamic organoid culture conditions.

separated into static or dynamic systems. Static culture provides stationary environments within traditional vessels, while dynamic culture employs equipment such as microfluidic systems, shakers, and bioreactors, providing agitation and flow that simulate *in vivo* dynamic conditions (Figure 4.5).

Both organoid culture systems offer unique advantages and disadvantages. Static systems are simple and cost-effective when maintaining diverse cell populations. It is fully accessible in most laboratories, requiring simple traditional culture vessels and equipment without specialized training. However, these systems promote uneven nutrient distribution, limited gas exchange, and potential accumulation of metabolic waste, leading to significant variations in organoid growth, viability, development, and differentiation. In contrast, dynamic systems provide numerous advantages with improved nutrient delivery in a controlled microenvironment. Nevertheless, it necessitates specialized equipment, intricate laboratory configurations, and tremendous amounts of culture media, making it extremely expensive. These systems also pose sterility and sheer stress challenges due to their material composition, mechanical properties, and convoluted mechanisms, underscoring the importance of inventing new culture systems with diverse applications.

#### 4.2.4.1 *Microfluidic Systems*

Advancements in fluidic systems generate significant interest in organoid research, enabling the creation of novel culture systems. Microfluidic systems are vital in organoid engineering and precision medicine, allowing the production of vascularized organoids that promote differentiation, development, maturity, and function. They offer a steady supply of nutrients and oxygen while eliminating metabolic waste, creating synthetic *in vivo* environments for organoid development. Microfluidic chips generally involve carefully constructed channels, one for housing the organoids and another for nutrition exchange, typically made using microfabrication. The organoids are implanted inside a hydrogel framework to provide structural support, imitating the natural ECM. This technology offers easy, versatile, and robust formation of vascularized organoids with precise control over fluxes produced during both short- and long-term perfusion.

Yue *et al.* [87] devised a modular technique for microfabricating multilayer fluidic chips to generate large-scale perfusable microvascular networks by developing a multilayered architecture that splits tissue chambers and culture media tubes into multiple layers, allowing for individual manufacturing and customization that facilitates dense tissue packing and vertical flow of culture media into numerous tissues. They employed fast microfluidic manufacturing methods to microfabricate 43 flow-focusing droplet producers and built a droplet generator tool based on user requirements. The vertical anastomosis structure also allows direct connectivity across tissue rows, creating more complicated systems for researching organ interactions or confirming circulatory functions. At the same time, a PDMS plastic mold manufacturing process was designed to create a vertical two-layer platform, providing microchannels with narrow widths and trapezoidal cross-sectional forms.

Furthermore, Fonseca *et al.* [88] also developed a novel 96-well fluidic system to carry out image-based high-throughput organoid screenings under laminar high sheer stress flow rates. This vessel is suited to traditional and robotic platforms for organoid culture and transfection operations, facilitating cell seeding and transfection. Using cell culture and microscopic imaging techniques, this system's compatibility with automated systems was validated, while immunofluorescence and RT-qPCR showed efficiency in siRNA transfection, inhibiting the expression of two endothelial cell adherens junction proteins. The endothelial cell flow response was also verified using eight different channels with independent shear stress conditions, showing greater expression levels of two stress-sensitive transcription factors, Krüppel-like factor 2 and Krüppel-like factor. This validates the device's ability to generate controlled shear stress, allowing high-throughput studies of flow effects in organoids. It also promotes the creation of complex vascular systems in disease modeling by significantly improving vascularization, organoid maturation, and nutrient uptake.

#### 4.2.4.2 *Shakers and Bioreactors*

Shakers and bioreactors are also crucial for organoid development, providing controlled conditions for 3D cell growth. Shakers guarantee uniformly distributed nutrients and growth factors, avoiding cell settling and promoting cell aggregation. Bioreactors precisely control over various culture parameters (e.g., fluid flow, temperature, pH, and oxygen levels). Both shakers and bioreactors exert control over organoid growth via mechanical forces and nutrient distribution. These include simple shaker agitations or highly regulated bioreactor flows, which greatly affect organoid structure, cell differentiation, and tissue development by mixing cells with culture material. Despite these advantages, shakers provide limited control over certain parameters (e.g., oxygen, pH, temperature, shear stress, and organoid uniformity). Bioreactors address these limitations by providing superior oversight of these parameters. However, they are not cost-effective and require specialized equipment and expertise.

Recent breakthroughs in organoid engineering introduced spinning bioreactors that promote enhanced cell nutrition and oxygen absorption, permitting the production of epithelial zones and facilitating the growth of sophisticated organoids that closely mimic human structures. Despite this, spinning bioreactors incur significant limitations given the high amount of culture medium (75 to 100 mL) and incubator space required, preventing consistency, scalability, growth agent usage, and drug screening. To address these limitations, Qian *et al.* [89] designed a miniature heat-resistant 12-well tissue culture plate-sized spinning bioreactor Spin Omega (Spin$\Omega$) that utilizes hiPSCs to generate unique brain organoid parts. The Spin$\Omega$ spinning mechanism contains three fins with a single electric motor, working similarly to a bioreactor flask required for enhanced organoid oxygen supply. This mechanism only requires 2 to 3 mL of media and growth factors in each flask, with organoid treatments that can be conducted for up to 200 days. Further analysis resulted in the creation and proliferation of massive neuroepithelial structures that eventually evolved into ventricular zones in forebrain organoids following the implantation of embryoid bodies in Matrigel.

However, it has been recently found that the hardware composition of SpinΩ is not applicable for longer-term culturing as it may induce potential experimental variabilities due to contamination and mechanical failure. Romero-Morales *et al.* [90] redesigned SpinΩ into Spin Infinity (Spin∞), an easily maintained compact spinning bioreactor for long-term organoid culture. Manufactured from 3D-printed ULTEM™ 1010 resin, this heat- and humidity-resistant bioreactor can withstand multiple autoclaving and months-long incubation sessions after assembly. The Spin∞ system contains a separate acrylic sheet, hex standoffs, and a sturdy motor to avoid oscillation. A lid was also firmly placed on the 12-well plate to prevent leakage and contamination. Like the SpinΩ bioreactor, the Spin∞ brain organoids also showed growth and laminar structure potentials, with organoids reaching above 3 mm in diameter and demonstrating a distinct neural progenitor zone. At the same time, no contamination was discovered following long-term culture.

Although Spin∞ addresses SpinΩ's hardware, contamination, and long-term culture problems, their scalability remains in a 12-well plate format, limiting organoid high-throughput screening. The specific shear stress distribution may also not be uniform, potentially causing variations in organoid development within the same well. Moreover, their applications in different organoid types and co-culture setups possibly reduce their function due to specific requirements for media composition, oxygenation, shear stress, and matrix support. Future bioreactor developments should prioritize creating user-friendly scalable systems, allowing precise control over multiple parameters (shear stress oxygen levels and nutrient gradients) with real-time monitoring capabilities. These next-generation bioreactors must accommodate various cell types and tissue constructs, effectively enabling optimized culture conditions that yield accurate results for organoid studies in precision medicine.

## 4.3 Rapid Organoid Characterization

In addition to culturing procedures, the characterization of organoids is crucial for model fidelity validation, standardization, and reproducibility in disease modeling, drug discovery, and precision medicine. However, cellular heterogeneity and dynamic behavior pose significant challenges to accurate characterization. Rapid characterization is a multifaceted analytical approach that combines advanced imaging technologies, artificial intelligence (AI)-driven computational tools, and new transcriptomics techniques, invented to advance the comprehensive understanding of organoids.

Microscopy remains a cornerstone in organoid characterization, enabling researchers to observe morphological features, track developmental processes, and assess functional properties. Yet, these characterization tools show accuracy, scalability, and depth penetration limitations. Beyond visual assessment, AI-assisted identification appeared as a transformative tool in studies of organoids. Integrating deep learning algorithms with imaging platforms enables automated segmentation, classification, and phenotypic analysis of organoids with high precision. Large dataset training allows AI models to detect subtle variations of organoids in morphology, cellular composition, and functional responses that might be easily overlooked by human observation. At the same time, deeper genomic examination provides valuable information about the organoids' profile, leading to the development of data acquisition techniques such as genome sequencing, spatial transcriptomics, and electrophysiological signal detection.

This section elaborates on the evolving landscape of organoid characterization, and expatiates the recent advancements in imaging modalities, AI-powered analytical tools, innovative omics techniques, and other depth data acquisition methods in organoid research (Figure 4.6). These cutting-edge technologies not only refine the capacity to

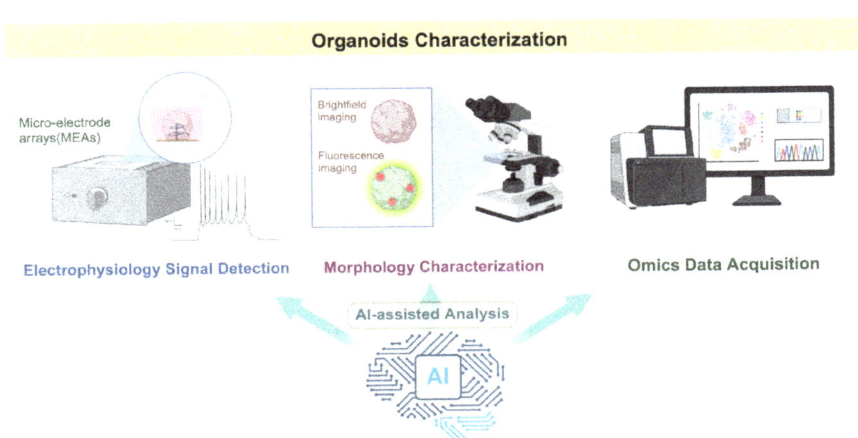


**Figure 4.6** Overview of organoid characterization methods.

evaluate the organoid structure and functions, but also expand their utility in precision medicine, drug design, and regenerative therapies. By strengthening the reliability and reproducibility of organoid-based studies, these superiorities pave the way for future innovations in biopharmaceutical research, enabling us to discover a more effective way of disease modeling and therapeutic development.

### 4.3.1 *Acquisition of Morphological Information*

Various imaging methods are utilized to capture *in vitro* organoid morphological information. These include non-specific microscopic techniques designed for integral shape capturing and specific marker detection associated with lower cost and technical requirements. Traditional brightfield microscopy offers a straightforward approach to observing the culture environment and monitoring the morphological development of organoids. This technique is useful for rapid, simple meso- and macro-scale observations, including assessment of individual organoids and overall organoid culture for their growth and general health. However, its utility is limited to deeper, more detailed observation. In particular, for 3D samples such as organoids, the central regions of the structure are often difficult to analyze effectively using only brightfield microscopy. The light scattering and absorption in thicker areas hinder resolution, making it challenging to visualize internal cellular structures or study complex developmental processes.

Apart from brightfield imaging, fluorescence imaging is also commonly used in organoid characterization. Confocal fluorescence microscopy (CFM) is a widely used imaging technique, especially for imaging cellular structures and analyzing the localization of proteins or other molecular markers. CFM employs laser light to excite fluorescent molecules in a sample with native or pre-labeled fluorophores. A key feature of confocal microscopy is its ability to optically section thick samples, allowing for high-resolution imaging of structures at various depths. This is achieved using a pinhole to exclude out-of-focus light, ensuring that only light from the focal plane is detected. The image is then captured by a detector, and a 3D representation of the sample is reconstructed by the computer. However, in thick organoids, this labeling method may not allow fluorophores to uniformly penetrate sample central regions. In such cases, physically sectioning the organoid into slices before labeling ensures that the fluorophores reach all areas of the sample, thereby maintaining the validity of the detection. This approach is particularly beneficial for subsequent quantitative analysis. Multiphoton Fluorescence Microscopy (MPM) is an extension of confocal microscopy that uses two or more photons of lower energy to excite a fluorophore. The longer-wavelength photons allow for deeper tissue penetration. Unlike single-photon excitation, which is used in CFM, multiphoton excitation occurs only at the focal point where the photons converge, minimizing scattering and photo-toxicity to surrounding tissue — making MPM useful for imaging thick tissues and viable organoids at greater depths without causing significant cell damage [91]. Meanwhile, MPM systems are more complex and costly than CFM.

Additionally, fluorescence micro-optical sectioning tomography (fMOST) is a 3D imaging technique that utilizes semi-ultrathin sectioning tomography to generate high-resolution 3D datasets of the entire organoid. fMOST favored large-scale samples that required real-time staining because the samples could be immersed in a fluorescent dye solution. Numerous studies utilize fMOST to analyze cerebral organoids at a multiscale level. Ma and colleagues [92] successfully performed whole-volume 3D imaging of large cerebral organoids at single-cell resolution. This enabled the reconstruction of individual neurons and GFAP+ cells and the visualization of cortical layer marker distribution, serving as powerful tools for analyzing cellular composition, structural organization, pathological alterations, and even the developmental processes of other organoids. However, fMOST involves the process of embedding samples in resin, which may affect cell viability and organoid morphology.

Another 3D imaging technique is light-sheet fluorescence microscopy (LSFM). LSFM generates a thin light sheet to selectively excite samples at a specific plane, while the emitted fluorescence is detected orthogonally. This enables 3D imaging with higher acquisition efficiency and reduced photobleaching and phototoxicity compared to other techniques [93]. It has been extensively used for 3D imaging of various tissues, organs, and organoids. However, LSFM systems with conventional orthogonal setups require special sample mounting methods and are unsuitable for imaging samples in flat microchips. In traditional microfluidic chips using materials (e.g., PDMS), the refractive index difference is unfavorable for light-sheet imaging systems. Therefore, some developments have been made, such as open-top optical systems combined with novel chip materials.

Existing imaging approaches show limitations in performing large numbers of 3D organotypic culture multi-scale characterization, hindered by the low imaging throughput, with subcellular resolution, complex sample mounting requirements, and inability to permit long-term sterile culture. In 2022, Beghin *et al.* [94] developed an automated imaging platform to overcome these problems. This platform rapidly synergizes high-density organoid cultures with live 3D single-objective light-sheet imaging. It incorporates disposable micro-fabricated organoid culture chips (JeWells) embedded with optical components and a laser beam-steering device linked to a commercial inverted microscope [94], allowing streamlined organoid culture and high-content 3D imaging with few interventions and an output of 300 organoids per hour. JeWells are designed with a specific geometry and coating that allow optimal cell seeding and growth. The light-sheet imaging is performed using 45° gold-coated micro-mirrors to reflect laser beams, creating a light-sheet perpendicular to the objective's optical axis for 3D optical sectioning [94]. Moreover, it enables the training of deep learning-based algorithms for the multi-scale quantification of organoid morphogenesis. However, the JeWell architecture creates several organoid restrictions, including physical confinements that may affect its development. The JeWell dimensions are also limited, restricting the utility for smaller organoids or cell aggregates.

## 4.3.2 *Deep Profiling of Organoids*

### 4.3.2.1 *Omics Data Acquisition*

Omics data provides comprehensive insights into their molecular landscape, enabling a deeper understanding of cellular heterogeneity, developmental processes, and disease modeling. Researchers can analyze the biological regulation of organoids through genomics, transcriptomics, epigenomics, proteomics, and metabolomics. Transcriptomics, particularly single-cell RNA sequencing, is the most common technique utilized to assist in mapping gene expression patterns within organoids, revealing cellular diversity and lineage trajectories.

### 4.3.2.2 *Lamination Methods for Spatial Transcriptomics*

The characterization of primary tissue-derived organoids using traditional spatial transcriptomics methods has been hindered by several challenges, primarily due to the small size of the organoids and the limited number of cells available in cross-sections. Existing tissue sectioning techniques are often labor-intensive and unsuitable for these delicate 3D structures, restricting the advancement of organoid technology. Ma *et al.* [95] developed a lamination-based organoid spatially resolved transcriptomics (LOSRT) technique to address these issues, streamlining the spatial transcriptomics workflow while preserving organoid integrity (Figure 4.7). In this approach, organoids are first produced using the Matrigel droplet encapsulation and templating method [96], ensuring uniform and structurally stable samples. A homemade lamination device with weight compression is then used to gently flatten the organoids, which is more accessible for spatial transcriptomics analysis (Figure 4.2). The Stereo-seq technique from Beijing Genomics Institute is employed to capture spatial and molecular information, providing a high-resolution transcriptomics map. Compared to traditional methods, LOSRT significantly reduces processing complexity, enhances cell retention, and preserves spatial relationships between cells, making it highly compatible with various organoid types. This innovation overcomes the limitations of conventional sectioning techniques, holding great potential for standardizing and accelerating organoid application in precision medicine and drug development.

#### 4.3.2.3 *Electrophysiological Signal Detection*

Signal conduction monitoring within organoids is vital to further understand *in vivo* physiological activities. The study of electrophysiology is a common way to discover the cell-cell interaction mechanisms and to detect the specific activities for function determination, particularly in neural-related organoids, such as brain organoids. Electrophysiological studies of brain organoids have advanced significantly with the development of micro-electrode arrays (MEAs) and bioelectronic interfaces, enabling researchers to probe neural activity in a minimally invasive manner. 2D MEAs establish long-term bioelectronic interfaces with brain organoids [97]. These arrays, composed of micro-electrodes embedded in a silicon org glass substrate, record action potentials and field potentials from neurons at the bottom of the organoid. 2D MEAs are non-invasive, allowing for long-term monitoring of neuronal activity without causing structural damage. However, 2D MEAs are limited by restricted spatial access; only neural signals from the bottom layer can be detected. Moreover, the resolution is relatively low, representing multi-unit activity rather than a single-neuron action potential.

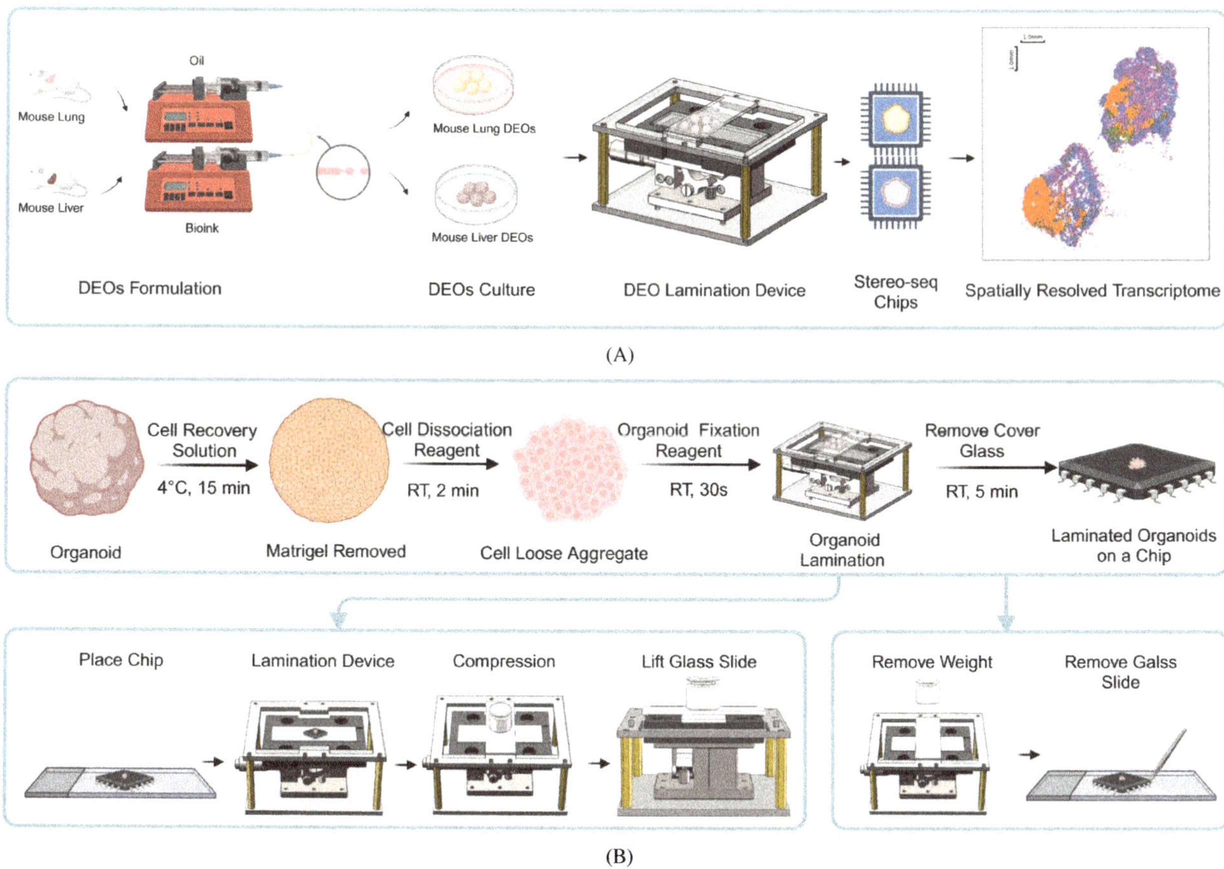


**Figure 4.7** Lamination-based organoid spatially resolved transcriptomics technique (LOSRT). Reproduced with permission from [95]. (A) Schematic illustration of LOSRT. DEO: droplet-engineered organoid. (B) Stepwise description of organoid lamination.

To overcome this, 3D MEAs have been developed, offering deeper penetration into the brain organoid's structure, enabling the detection of electrical activity throughout its entire volume [98]. These MEAs employ probes such as Michigan [99] and Neuropixel [100], which are fabricated with flexible encapsulating materials, to provide a more comprehensive view of neuronal networks that allow researchers to study neural synchronization and activity mapping at higher spatial resolutions. However, insertion can damage neural networks and disrupt normal physiological functions. A promising alternative is the use of 3D flexible bioelectronics, which are designed to conform to the morphology of brain organoids, creating a seamless and non-invasive electrical interface. It comprises gold micro-electrodes encapsulated in polyimide, recording complex neural dynamics, including field potentials, wave propagation, and bursting events across cortical spheroids. Their soft and shape-matched design minimizes mechanical stress on the organoid, preserving its structural integrity. These bioelectronics support multimodal interrogation by integrating advanced semiconductor-based electronic and optoelectronic components. Despite the advantages, challenges remain in achieving long-term stable single-cell electrophysiological recordings, as these flexible electronics must adapt to the rapid volumetric changes that occur during organoid growth and maturation [101].

### 4.3.3 *Artificial Intelligence-assisted Identification*

As 3D *in vitro* models, organoids offer a closer representation of human organs than traditional 2D cultures and a more precise perspective of cellular interaction than animal models. Although there is remarkable progress in the characterization techniques of organoids, some challenges are still hindering the efficient analysis of organoids. In addition to limitations on continuous monitoring and analysis of the organoids' growth status mentioned above, another significant challenge is the examination of a large volume of microscopy images and thus the necessity of a set of highly robust automatic analysis algorithms. Presently, several studies have provided diverse data sets of organoid microscopic images to establish AI-derived analysis tools. AI-enabled organoids are an interdisciplinary field that integrates AI with organoid research to enhance various aspects of their development, analysis, and applications [102]. Some of the organoid morphology analysis AI tools, such as OrganoidID [103], OrgaQuant [104], OrganoSeg [105], and ilastik [106], employed a large set of brightfield organoid image data for machine learning based on various models. By quantifying the segmentation result of the organoid external structure using different metrics, they can assess the current physiological state of the living organoids. These tools can assist in tracing identical organoids temporally, detecting their size, or predicting fluorescence staining phenotypes with a simple optical microscope. AI tools reduce the cost and time associated with high-throughput screening, facilitating the process of monitoring and analyzing organoid growth.

Beyond image analysis, AI significantly contributes to optimizing organoid construction strategies. In the organoids' construction strategy, selecting appropriate ECM materials is the first and most critical step [107]. Machine learning offers a powerful solution to the complex challenges inherent in designing hydrogels as biomaterials for specific applications like personalized customization matrix gel, including organoid research. The machine learning algorithms process large datasets related to matrix gel synthesis, cell culture conditions, growth factors, and external stimuli. This allows for a more precise and reproducible approach to organoid development, reducing variability and improving efficiency. AI also assists in analyzing multi-omics data including genomics, transcriptomics, proteomics, and single-cell omics. The complexity and volume of the omics data bring challenges for deep understanding of cellular development. Therefore, AI tools like UnitedNet and devCellPy [108] have been developed to handle this complexity, offering automated data analysis and meaningful biological insights. For instance, UnitedNet merges various tasks and helps evaluate single-cell multi-modality data using an interpretable multi-task deep neural network. Moreover, this interpretable machine learning technique to analyze the trained UnitedNet can discover the direct correlation between gene expression and cell types-specific modalities [109]. This is especially useful in disease modeling and drug screening of organoids, identifying key biomarkers, predicting disease progression, and even assessing drug responses. These technologies lead to more effective organoid research in discovering new personalized therapeutic strategies.

Furthermore, AI has shown promise in enabling rapid and personalized drug response prediction through digital markers. Traditional precision drug administration methods, such as genomic sequencing and tumor organoid evaluation, often require extended processing time, which delays immediate chemotherapy decisions for hospitalized patients. Fan *et al.* [110] proposed an AI-based approach using multiplex gene-based digital markers. By screening transcriptional profiles and constructing small gene libraries, digital markers are developed for drug sensitivity prediction. This method incorporates k-nearest neighbors models for classification and regression, along with qRT-PCR quantification to measure transcription levels within a short time frame. Training datasets from Genomics of Drug Sensitivity in Cancer v1 and v2 (GDSC), Cancer Cell Line Encyclopedia (CCLE), and The Cancer Genome Atlas (TCGA) sources enable model validation and cross-verification. This AI-driven framework offers an efficient and rapid evaluation system for personalized drug response, potentially integrating with clinical workflows to streamline chemotherapy decision-making. Despite challenges such as limited and inconsistent training datasets, the study highlights AI's potential to enhance precision medicine through accelerated and data-driven drug sensitivity assessment.

Despite the potential benefits, AI integration with organoid research offers challenges. Variations in organoid structure and function arise from different culture conditions or protocols, resulting in difficulty collecting consistent data for AI analysis. Additionally, AI requires substantial computational resources, especially when dealing with large datasets from organoid imaging or multi-omics analysis. These computational capacities are essential for deep learning techniques and can be costly and limit accessibility for some researchers. The "black box" nature of AI algorithms, particularly deep learning models, also poses transparency and trust challenges among healthcare professionals [111].

## Key Opinion Points

- Organoid bioprinting and microfluidic engineering advancements significantly improved high-throughput automated organoid production by providing spatial control over cell and bio-ink deposition. Given the early stages in organoid engineering research, emerging AI-assisted robotic culture platforms may contribute to full organoid generation automation, enabling real-time culture parameter optimization and organoid assessment to increase efficiency and consistency while reducing human error.
- Reproducibility and standardization remain a significant challenge in organoid research despite optimized bio-ink formulations and culture protocols. Establishing standardized experimental designs aided by organoid engineering techniques allows universal culture guidelines and standard reference models to

ensure reproducibility and replicability for organoid-based therapeutics and drug discovery research.

- High-throughput organoid scaling is critical for meeting drug screening and therapeutic application demands. Despite the availability of numerous suspension culture bioreactors, this limits microenvironmental fidelity, resulting in reduced cell viability or incorrect differentiation. Recent bioprinting innovations allow high-throughput organoid production. Future modular culture systems and bioreactors should focus on facilitating organoid system expansion to create consistent and physiologically relevant organoids.
- Accurate tissue-specific microenvironment recapitulation is essential to developing functional organoid models. Although recent ECM scaffold designs have improved organoid physiological relevance, research in vascularization, immune components, and dynamic flow remains in the earlier stages. Integrating bioengineered vascular systems and advanced perfusion models allows the creation of highly functional and physiologically accurate organoids for studying complex diseases *in vitro* and creating novel drugs that target specific disease mechanisms.
- Integrating high-resolution imaging techniques and advanced analytical workflows greatly enhances organoid structure and function characterization. The discovery of new AI-assisted imaging and analysis tools and cloud-based data platforms allows increased data acquisition efficiency, seamlessly integrating multi-modality datasets that facilitate high-throughput organoid comprehensive evaluation to ensure accurate, scalable, and reproducible analyses.

## References

1. Hofer M, Lutolf MP. Engineering organoids. Nat Rev Mater. 2021;6(5):402–420.
2. Kim J, Koo B-K, Knoblich JA. Human organoids: model systems for human biology and medicine. Nat Rev Mol Cell Biol. 2020;21(10):571–584.
3. Drost J, Clevers H. Organoids in cancer research. Nat Rev Cancer. 2018;18(7):407–418.
4. Verstegen MMA, *et al.* Clinical applications of human organoids. Nat Med. 2025.
5. Zhao Z, *et al.* Organoids. Nat Rev Methods Primers. 2022;2(1):94.
6. Ma S, *et al.* Lamination-based organoid spatially resolved transcriptomics technique for primary lung and liver organoid characterization. Proc Natl Acad Sci U S A. 2024;121(46):e2408939121.
7. Brandenberg N, *et al.* High-throughput automated organoid culture via stem-cell aggregation in microcavity arrays. Nat Biomed Eng. 2020;4(9):863–874.

8. Chrisnandy A, *et al.* Synthetic dynamic hydrogels promote degradation-independent in vitro organogenesis. Nat Mater. 2022;21(4):479–487.
9. Nwokoye PN, Abilez OJ. Bioengineering methods for vascularizing organoids. Cell Rep Methods. 2024;4(6).
10. Abuwatfa WH, Pitt WG, Husseini GA. Scaffold-based 3D cell culture models in cancer research. J Biomed Sci. 2024;31(1):7.
11. Kronemberger GS, *et al.* Spheroids and organoids as humanized 3D scaffold-free engineered tissues for SARS-CoV-2 viral infection and drug screening. Artif Organs. 2021;45(6):548–558.
12. Shao Y, *et al.* Biomaterial-assisted organoid technology for disease modeling and drug screening. Mater Today Bio. 2025;30:101438.
13. Tong L, *et al.* Patient-derived organoids in precision cancer medicine. Med. 2024;5(11): 1351–1377.
14. ThermoFisher Scientific. Culture plastics. Technical Reference Library. 2023 [cited 2025 Feb 16]; Available from: https://www.thermofisher.com/au/en/home/references/gibco-cell-culture-basics/cell-culture-environment/culture-media/culture-plastics.html.
15. Zeiger A, Hinton B, Van Vliet K. Why the dish makes a difference: Quantitative comparison of polystyrene culture surfaces. Acta Biomater. 2013;9.
16. Lerman MJ, *et al.* The evolution of polystyrene as a cell culture material. Tissue Eng Part B Rev. 2018;24(5):359–372.
17. Hossain MT, *et al.* Research and application of polypropylene: a review. Discov Nano. 2024;19(1):2.
18. Nebuloni F, *et al.* A platform for modular assembly and feeding of micro-organoids on standard Petri dishes. Biol Open. 2023;12.
19. Acharya P, *et al.* Uniform cerebral organoid culture on a pillar plate by simple and reproducible spheroid transfer from an ultralow attachment well plate. bioRxiv. 2023.
20. Redondo-Castro E, *et al.* Generation of human mesenchymal stem cell 3D spheroids using low-binding plates. Bio-protocol. 2018;8(16).
21. Buentello D, *et al.* Use of standard U-bottom and V-bottom well plates to generate neuroepithelial embryoid bodies. PLoS One. 2021;17.
22. Ubertini V, *et al.* Abstract 2754: Transwell-grown monolayers derived from small intestinal organoids to study the effects of tight junction modulators that may improve the absorption of orally-administered, anti-neoplastic drugs. Cancer Res. 2023.
23. Foty R. A simple hanging drop cell culture protocol for generation of 3D spheroids. J Vis Exp. 2011;(51).
24. Eder T, Eder I. 3D Hanging drop culture to establish prostate cancer organoids. Methods Mol Biol. 2017;1612:167–175.

25. Jung YH, *et al.* Development of an extracellular matrix plate for drug screening using patient-derived tumor organoids. BioChip J. 2023;17(2):284–292.
26. Oksdath Mansilla M, *et al.* 3D-printed microplate inserts for long term high-resolution imaging of live brain organoids. BMC Biomed Eng. 2021;3(1):6.
27. Yu F, Choudhury D. Microfluidic bioprinting for organ-on-a-chip models. Drug Discov Today. 2019;24(6):1248–1257.
28. Miri A, *et al.* Bioprinters for organs-on-chips. Biofabrication. 2019;11.
29. Saini G, *et al.* Applications of 3D bioprinting in tissue engineering and regenerative medicine. J Clin Med. 2021;10.
30. Huang MS, *et al.* Organoid bioprinting: from cells to functional tissues. Nat Rev Bioeng. 2025;3(2):126–142.
31. Brassard JA, *et al.* Recapitulating macro-scale tissue self-organization through organoid bioprinting. Nat Mater. 2021;20(1):22–29.
32. Xu J, *et al.* 3D bioprinting of colon organoids in ultrashort self-assembling and decorated peptide matrices. Int J Bioprint. 2024.
33. Jiang T, *et al.* Extrusion bioprinting of soft materials: An emerging technique for biological model fabrication. Appl Phys Rev. 2019.
34. Ren Y, *et al.* Developments and opportunities for 3D bioprinted organoids. Int J Bioprint. 2021;7(3):364.
35. Lawlor KT, *et al.* Cellular extrusion bioprinting improves kidney organoid reproducibility and conformation. Nat Mater. 2021;20(2):260–271.
36. Mandrycky C, *et al.* 3D bioprinting for engineering complex tissues. Biotechnol Adv. 2016;34(4):422–434.
37. Yang H, *et al.* Ultra-small tissue-compatible organoid printer for rapid and controllable modeling of respiratory organoids. Device. 2024;2(8).
38. Carvalho E, Kumar S. Lose the stress: Viscoelastic materials for cell engineering. Acta Biomater. 2022.
39. Cao Y, *et al.* Bead-jet printing enabled sparse mesenchymal stem cell patterning augments skeletal muscle and hair follicle regeneration. Nat Commun. 2022;13(1):7463.
40. Liu H, *et al.* A droplet microfluidic system to fabricate hybrid capsules enabling stem cell organoid engineering. Adv Sci (Weinh). 2020;7(11):1903739.
41. Zhang W, *et al.* Microfluidic droplet encapsulation-guided organoid growth promotes parental tumor phenotype recapitulation. Int J Cancer. 2024;154(1):145–154.
42. Jiang S, *et al.* An automated organoid platform with inter-organoid homogeneity and inter-patient heterogeneity. Cell Rep Med. 2020;1(9):100161.
43. Harkin J, *et al.* A highly reproducible and efficient method for retinal organoid differentiation from human pluripotent stem cells. Proc Natl Acad Sci U S A. 2024; 121(25):e2317285121.

44. Campbell S, *et al.* Beyond polydimethylsiloxane: alternative materials for fabrication of organ-on-a-chip devices and microphysiological systems. ACS Biomater Sci Eng. 2020;7(7):2880–2899.
45. Kim SK, Sung E, Lim K. Recent advances and applications of human lung alveolar organoids. Mol Cells. 2024;47(12):100140.
46. Kim HJ, *et al.* Lung organoid on a chip: a new ensemble model for preclinical studies. Int J Stem Cells. 2024;17(1):30–37.
47. Sun C-H, *et al.* A bronchiole-on-a-chip and a stretching system for studying human disease model of asthma attack. Sens Actuators B Chem. 2024;416:136031.
48. Khan AO, *et al.* Human bone marrow organoids for disease modeling, discovery, and validation of therapeutic targets in hematologic malignancies. Cancer Discov. 2023;13(2):364–385.
49. Glaser DE, *et al.* Organ-on-a-chip model of vascularized human bone marrow niches. Biomaterials. 2022;280:121245.
50. Frenz-Wiessner S, *et al.* Generation of complex bone marrow organoids from human induced pluripotent stem cells. Nat Methods. 2024;21(5):868–881.
51. Kroll KT, *et al.* Immune-infiltrated kidney organoid-on-chip model for assessing T cell bispecific antibodies. Proc Natl Acad Sci U S A. 2023;120(35):e2305322120.
52. Xia X, *et al.* Engineering cardiology with miniature hearts. Mater Today Bio. 2025; 31:101505.
53. Yang J, *et al.* Integrated-gut-liver-on-a-chip platform as an in vitro human model of non-alcoholic fatty liver disease. Commun Biol. 2023;6(1):310.
54. Deguchi S, Takayama K. State-of-the-art liver disease research using liver-on-a-chip. Inflamm Regen. 2022;42(1):62.
55. Shik Mun K, *et al.* Patient-derived pancreas-on-a-chip to model cystic fibrosis-related disorders. Nat Commun. 2019;10(1):3124.
56. Hajal C, *et al.* Engineered human blood–brain barrier microfluidic model for vascular permeability analyses. Nat Protoc. 2022;17(1):95–128.
57. Koh I, Hagiwara M. Modular tissue-in-a-CUBE platform to model blood-brain barrier (BBB) and brain interaction. Commun Biol. 2024;7(1):177.
58. Haque MR, *et al.* Patient-derived pancreatic cancer-on-a-chip recapitulates the tumor microenvironment. Microsystems Nanoeng. 2022;8(1):36.
59. Liu X, *et al.* Tumor-on-a-chip: from bioinspired design to biomedical application. Microsystems Nanoeng. 2021;7(1):50.
60. Zhu J, *et al.* Organoids and organs-on-chips: insights into predicting the efficacy of systemic treatment in colorectal cancer. Cell Death Discov. 2023;9(1):72.
61. Urciuolo F, Imparato G, Netti P. Engineering cell instructive microenvironments for in vitro replication of functional barrier organs. Adv Healthc Mater. 2024.

62. Xue X, *et al.* A patterned human neural tube model using microfluidic gradients. Nature. 2024;628(8007):391–399.
63. Jia J, *et al.* Engineering alginate as bioink for bioprinting. Acta Biomater. 2014;10(10): 4323–4331.
64. Yang H, *et al.* 3D bioprinted hepatorganoids prolong survival of mice with liver failure. Gut. 2021;70(3):567–574.
65. Jiang S, *et al.* Development of a high-throughput micropatterned agarose scaffold for consistent and reproducible hPSC-derived liver organoids. Biofabrication. 2022;15(1).
66. Norotte C, *et al.* Scaffold-free vascular tissue engineering using bioprinting. Biomaterials. 2009;30(30):5910–5917.
67. Clark CC, *et al.* Immersion bioprinting of hyaluronan and collagen bioink-supported 3D patient-derived brain tumor organoids. Biomed Mater. 2022;18(1).
68. Skardal A, *et al.* Bioprinting cellularized constructs using a tissue-specific hydrogel bioink. J Vis Exp. 2016;(110):e53606.
69. Bergmann O, *et al.* Dynamics of cell generation and turnover in the human heart. Cell. 2015;161(7):1566–1575.
70. Shi W, *et al.* Embedded bioprinting of breast tumor cells and organoids using low-concentration collagen-based bioinks. Adv Healthc Mater. 2023;12(26):e2300905.
71. Gamboa-Martínez TC, *et al.* Crosslinked fibrin gels for tissue engineering: two approaches to improve their properties. J Biomed Mater Res A. 2015;103(2):614–621.
72. Gruene M, *et al.* Laser printing of three-dimensional multicellular arrays for studies of cell–cell and cell–environment interactions. Tissue Eng Part C Methods. 2011;17(10): 973–982.
73. Bernal PN, *et al.* Volumetric bioprinting of organoids and optically tuned hydrogels to build liver-like metabolic biofactories. Adv Mater. 2022;34(15):e2110054.
74. Flores-Torres S, *et al.* Alginate-gelatin-Matrigel hydrogels enable the development and multigenerational passaging of patient-derived 3D bioprinted cancer spheroid models. Biofabrication. 2021;13(2).
75. Demirtaş TT, Irmak G, Gümüşderelioğlu M. A bioprintable form of chitosan hydrogel for bone tissue engineering. Biofabrication. 2017;9(3):035003.
76. He Y, *et al.* A photocurable hybrid chitosan/acrylamide bioink for DLP-based 3D bioprinting. Mater Des. 2021;202:109588.
77. Shrestha S, *et al.* Reproducible generation of human liver organoids (HLOs) on a pillar plate for high-throughput drug screening. SLAS Technol. 2024.
78. Skylar-Scott MA, *et al.* Biomanufacturing of organ-specific tissues with high cellular density and embedded vascular channels. Sci Adv. 2019;5(9):eaaw2459.

79. Nguyen D, *et al.* Vascularized liver tumor model engineered from a tri-cell co-culture and its application in drug screening. Sci Rep. 2016;6:26750.
80. Amodio S, *et al.* A three-dimensional system to model tumor-stroma interactions in pancreatic cancer. Theranostics. 2022;12(15):6521–6537.
81. Kornaszewska A, *et al.* Bioprinting of 3D breast cancer models for radiobiology applications. Front Bioeng Biotechnol. 2021;9:734940.
82. Brancato V, *et al.* 3D tumor microenvironment models: drug screening, biomarkers, immuno-oncology and patient-tailored therapy. Biotechnol Adv. 2024;66:108219.
83. Zang X, *et al.* 3D bioprinting in tissue engineering for cancer therapy. Bioact Mater. 2023;22:133–154.
84. Langer EM, *et al.* Heterotypic 3D culture models for precision medicine. Nat Rev Cancer. 2024;24(5):295–312.
85. Davidson MD, *et al.* Engineered 3D vascular and neuronal networks in a microfluidic platform: applications for modeling neural-vascular interactions. Nat Commun. 2022;13(1):4086.
86. Jiang Z, *et al.* Organotypic 3D culture models of human pancreatic cancer. Biomaterials. 2020;232:119673.
87. Kolesky DB, *et al.* 3D bioprinting of vascularized, heterogeneous cell-laden tissue constructs. Adv Mater. 2014;26(19):3124–3130.
88. Zhang B, *et al.* Bioprinting the cancer microenvironment for cancer models and therapy. Nat Rev Cancer. 2023;23(4):240–256.
89. Liu R, *et al.* Engineering multiscale vascular networks for tissue regeneration. Trends Biotechnol. 2023;41(3):281–297.
90. Xie X, *et al.* Tumor organoid-on-a-chip for personalized oncology. Biomaterials. 2020; 254:120858.
91. Yi HG, *et al.* A bioprinted human-glioblastoma-on-a-chip for the identification of patient-specific responses to chemoradiotherapy. Nat Biomed Eng. 2019;3(7):509–519.
92. Bracher MG, *et al.* Tumor-on-chip models for the development of personalized cancer treatment: the role of bioengineering and biomaterials. Biomaterials. 2022;280:121274.
93. Liu L, *et al.* Personalized cancer-on-a-chip design using advanced 3D bioprinting technology. Micromachines (Basel). 2023;14(1):55.
94. Dijkstra KK, *et al.* Generation of tumor-reactive T cells by co-culture of peripheral blood lymphocytes and tumor organoids. Cell. 2018;174(6):1586–1598.e12.
95. Neal JT, *et al.* Organoid modeling of the tumor immune microenvironment. Cell. 2018;175(7):1972–1988.e16.
96. Hofer M, Lutolf MP. Engineering organoids. Nat Rev Mater. 2021;6(5):402–420.

97. Puca L, *et al.* Patient-derived organoids to model rare prostate cancer phenotypes. Nat Commun. 2018;9(1):2404.
98. Yuki K, *et al.* Organoid models of human gastrointestinal development and disease. Gastroenterology. 2020;159(4):1090–1105.
99. Li R, *et al.* Patient-derived organoids (PDOs) as a novel in vitro model for radiobiology. Clin Transl Radiat Oncol. 2022;33:1–7.
100. Sato T, *et al.* Long-term expansion of epithelial organoids from human colon, adenoma, adenocarcinoma, and Barrett's epithelium. Gastroenterology. 2011;141(5):1762–1772.
101. van de Wetering M, *et al.* Prospective derivation of a living organoid biobank of colorectal cancer patients. Cell. 2015;161(4):933–945.
102. Sachs N, *et al.* A living biobank of breast cancer organoids captures disease heterogeneity. Cell. 2018;172(1–2):373–386.e10.
103. Calandrini C, *et al.* An organoid biobank for childhood kidney cancers that captures disease and tissue heterogeneity. Nat Commun. 2020;11(1):1310.
104. Maenhoudt N, *et al.* Organoid culture of epithelial ovarian cancer captures the genomic landscape of primary patient tumors. J Pathol. 2020;250(3): 445–460.
105. Ganesh K, *et al.* A rectal cancer organoid platform to study individual responses to chemoradiation. Nat Med. 2019;25(10):1607–1614.
106. Vlachogiannis G, *et al.* Patient-derived organoids model treatment response of metastatic gastrointestinal cancers. Science. 2018;359(6378):920–926.
107. Kim M, *et al.* Patient-derived lung cancer organoids as in vitro cancer models for therapeutic screening. Nat Commun. 2019;10(1):3991.
108. Driehuis E, *et al.* Oral mucosal organoids as a potential platform for personalized cancer therapy. Cancer Discov. 2019;9(7):852–871.
109. Lin M, *et al.* 3D organoid model for studying early-stage lung cancer and drug screening. Cancer Lett. 2023;563:216181.
110. Hill SJ, *et al.* Prediction of DNA repair inhibitor response in short-term patient-derived ovarian cancer organoids. Cancer Discov. 2018;8(11):1404–1421.
111. Phan N, *et al.* A simple high-throughput approach identifies actionable drug sensitivities in patient-derived tumor organoids. Commun Biol. 2019;2:78.

https://doi.org/10.1142/9789819817597_0005

Chapter 5

# Organoid-Driven Drug Discovery: Precision Screening and Target Validation

Yunqi Man[1,†], Yanfei Liu[2,†], Qiwen Chen[2], Zhenbao Liu[1,*]

[1]*Department of Pharmaceutics, Xiangya School of Pharmaceutical Sciences, Central South University, Changsha 410013, Hunan Province, China*

[2]*Department of Pharmaceutical Engineering, College of Chemistry and Chemical Engineering, Central South University, Changsha 410083, Hunan Province, China*

**Abstract:** Organoids, 3D cultures derived from individual stem cells or progenitor cells that exhibit differentiated structures, have been rapidly advancing in the field of biomedicine. These organoids can closely mimic the biological characteristics of the donor, reconstruct the microenvironment of tissues or organs, and exhibit a high degree of consistency with the donor in terms of drug target expression and responses to drugs. In this chapter, we explore the critical applications and advancements of organoid technology in drug screening and development. We discuss how organoid technology can be leveraged for high-throughput drug screening to identify potential therapeutic compounds. Additionally, we highlight its role in the screening and identification of drug therapy targets. Finally, we summarize the progress achieved and the challenges faced in applying organoid technology to drug development. We anticipate that the integration of organoid technology will revolutionize traditional drug development paradigms, bringing us closer to the vision of intelligent precision medicine and shaping the future of healthcare and societal advancement.

**Keywords:** organoids, drug screening, target identification, target validation

---

*Corresponding author. Email: zhenbaoliu@csu.edu.cn
†These authors contributed equally to this work.

## Key Points

1. Patient-derived organoids retain donor-specific genetic and phenotypic features and provide a physiologically relevant preclinical model that more accurately simulates human tissue architecture and function, enabling improved prediction of drug efficacy and safety.
2. Their compatibility with high-throughput screening platforms allows for efficient evaluation of large compound libraries under near-physiological conditions.
3. Organoid systems support the identification and validation of therapeutic targets by preserving *in vivo*-like molecular expression and cellular interactions.
4. Integration with microfluidic platforms gives rise to organoid-on-a-chip systems, which allow fine control of the microenvironment, dynamic perfusion, and real-time monitoring of drug responses.
5. Integration of organoid technology into early drug development pipelines enhances lead optimization and informs translational decision-making with higher clinical relevance.

## 5.1 Introduction

Traditional approaches in early-stage drug development face significant limitations. 2D cell culture systems fail to replicate the complexity of native tissue architecture and microenvironmental cues, resulting in a lack of predictive accuracy for evaluating drug efficacy and safety. Similarly, animal models, while providing systemic context, may lack translatability to human physiology due to species-specific differences in genetics, metabolism, and immune responses. These discrepancies contribute to high failure rates in clinical trials, particularly in the search for treatments for complex diseases. Additionally, constructing robust animal disease models is challenging. Of the more than 7,000 rare diseases recognized globally, fewer than 400 are actively studied using animal models, highlighting a significant gap in preclinical research [1].

In 2009, Toshiro Sato and colleagues made a groundbreaking discovery by demonstrating that adult intestinal stem cells could proliferate and self-organize *in vitro* [2]. Stem cells marked by the expression of LGR5, a gene encoding the receptor for the Wnt agonist R-spondin, depend on a defined set of signaling cues, notably Wnt, epidermal growth factor, and Noggin, to preserve their proliferative potential and functional integrity. Leveraging on these findings, researchers established a 3D culture system that emulates the intestinal stem cell niche with high fidelity. This system facilitated the derivation of intestinal organoids from either isolated $Lgr5^+$ stem cells or differentiated intestinal epithelial cells. The resulting organoids exhibited a crypt-villus architecture analogous to the native intestinal epithelium and demonstrated long-term self-renewal capability. The ability to culture these organoids for up to three months while maintaining genomic stability provided a robust model for large-scale production. This breakthrough laid the foundation for modern organoid culture systems, revolutionizing research in stem cell biology and tissue engineering.

Organoids are 3D cellular structures derived from stem or progenitor cells under carefully controlled culture conditions. These systems recapitulate the structural, cellular, and functional complexity of primary tissues or organs on a miniature scale. Unlike 2D cell lines or biopsied tissues, organoids replicate the 3D architecture, cellular heterogeneity, and physiological state of their tissue of origin. For instance, organoids can reproduce key functional attributes of organs such as intestinal peristalsis [3], neurotransmission [4] and neurodevelopment [5] in brain models, and metabolic processes in liver models. This makes organoids a highly accurate platform for studying both physiological and pathological processes, particularly in preclinical drug testing. By faithfully simulating the *in vivo* environment, organoids improve the predictive power of drug response studies, offering insights into drug sensitivity, selectivity, and mechanisms of action that are often unattainable with traditional models.

Organoid technology offers a promising solution to the limitations of conventional *in vitro* and *in vivo* models by providing a physiologically relevant intermediate that more accurately reflects human tissue architecture and function. This approach has been effectively applied across a broad spectrum of disease models, including malignancies, neurodegenerative conditions, infectious diseases, and inherited disorders. By recapitulating key aspects of disease pathology, organoid systems enable detailed analysis of the molecular and cellular events driving disease progression. Moreover, they serve as a powerful platform for the discovery of therapeutic targets and the development of early diagnostic and prognostic biomarkers, thereby advancing both mechanistic research and translational applications. Furthermore, patient-derived organoids (PDOs) offer an unprecedented opportunity to study the heterogeneity of human diseases at the individual level. PDOs retain the genetic, phenotypic, and functional characteristics of the donor tissue, including tumor architecture, cellular diversity, and interactions within the microenvironment. This level of fidelity enables personalized drug testing, where therapeutic strategies can be tailored to the unique characteristics of each patient's disease.

In cancer research, PDOs have been particularly transformative. Traditional cancer cell lines often fail to capture the complexity of tumor microenvironments, limiting their utility in studying drug resistance or metastasis. In contrast, PDOs preserve key features such as intratumoral heterogeneity, tumor-stroma interactions, and genetic stability over extended culture periods. This allows researchers to track tumor progression, metastasis, and therapeutic resistance with unprecedented accuracy. PDOs have also facilitated the creation of biobanks, where organoid models representing diverse cancer subtypes are stored and made available for high-throughput drug screening and biomarker discovery. These biobanks are cost-effective and scalable, making precision oncology more accessible and efficient.

Moreover, organoids align with the ethical principles of the 3Rs (Replacement, Reduction, and Refinement) by offering an alternative to animal models in preclinical research. The ability to simulate human physiological processes *in vitro* reduces the need for animal experiments, minimizing ethical concerns and improving experimental reproducibility. For instance, organoid models have been used to study drug toxicity in liver tissues [6] and barrier integrity in intestinal tissues [7], all without relying on animal testing. This shift toward human-relevant models not only accelerates drug discovery but also enhances the reliability of preclinical findings.

Organoid technology represents a paradigm shift in biomedical research and drug development. By combining the structural complexity of *in vivo* systems with the experimental control of *in vitro* models, organoids provide an unparalleled platform for studying human biology and disease. From early-stage drug discovery to personalized medicine, organoids are transforming how researchers approach scientific challenges, ultimately paving the way for more effective, efficient, and ethical healthcare solutions.

## 5.2 High-throughput Screening and Automation

Currently, over 90% of new drugs fail during clinical trials or the subsequent drug approval process after entering clinical research [8]. On average, drug development takes more than 10 to 15 years and costs billions of dollars. This high failure rate leads to significant losses in time, financial resources, and clinical opportunities, underscoring the urgent need for innovative technologies in the early stages of drug screening. These technologies are crucial for reducing costs, improving efficiency, and accelerating drug discovery. Such technologies must combine large-scale screening capabilities with a high degree of automation, low liquid volume, consistent results between samples, highly simulated *in vivo* physiological conditions, and precise, controllable interventions.

High-throughput screening (HTS) has emerged as a critical tool in this effort, enabling the rapid and systematic evaluation of large numbers of chemical compounds, biological molecules, or genetic material. HTS utilizes microplate formats of various densities (e.g., 96-well, 384-well, or 1536-well plates) as experimental platforms. It integrates automated robotic systems, highly sensitive detection methods like fluorescence and luminescence assays, and advanced data analysis software to ensure efficient and accurate operation. Compared to traditional drug screening methods, HTS significantly accelerates testing, allowing researchers to screen multiple compounds simultaneously on the same biological sample. This capability greatly enhances the identification of potential active compounds and their subsequent application in clinical treatments [9]. However, as an *in vitro* 2D culture approach, HTS cannot fully replicate the complex physiological and biochemical conditions of living organisms. HTS models often lack critical microenvironmental cues, such as extracellular matrix interactions and signaling gradients, and are limited in their ability to simulate the dynamic interconnectivity among organs. As a result, discrepancies between HTS findings and clinical outcomes are common.

The advent of organoid technology has addressed many of these limitations, transforming HTS and revitalizing its potential in drug discovery. Organoids are 3D structures derived from stem cells or primary tissues that self-organize into models resembling their *in vivo* counterparts. Unlike traditional human- or animal-derived cell lines, PDOs retain the genetic, epigenetic, and histopathological features of the original tissues, allowing them to closely mimic physiological and pathological conditions. Organoids can undergo cell sorting and lineage differentiation to create niche environments that simulate the biochemical and biophysical dynamics of living tissues. These features enhance the translational relevance of organoid-based experiments and help bridge the gap between preclinical findings and clinical applications. In cancer research, for example, PDOs have demonstrated the ability to classify malignancies more precisely based on histopathology and molecular profiles [10]. Organoids also enable the development of biobanks that represent diverse models of the same disease, capturing the genetic and phenotypic heterogeneity of tumor tissues. Such biobanks facilitate the correlation of drug sensitivity with specific tumor subtypes, enabling more accurate personalized drug screening. Moreover, organoids provide a dynamic platform for studying tumor biology and drug responses. By incorporating immune cells, fibroblasts, or endothelial cells into co-culture systems, researchers can reconstruct the tumor microenvironment and investigate complex interactions, such as immune evasion and stromal regulation of therapy. These models have been used to evaluate immunotherapies, such as immune checkpoint inhibitors, and to identify novel therapeutic targets within the tumor microenvironment [11].

The process of organoid-based HTS involves several key steps: organoid culture, construction of screening components, drug dosing and data collection, and result analysis. Each of these steps is outlined in the following sections. Organoids are derived from either pluripotent stem cells (PSCs), including embryonic stem cells and induced pluripotent stem cells, or adult stem cells (ASCs) sourced from tissue-specific progenitor cells. These stem cells undergo self-organization in a controlled environment, guided by critical developmental signaling pathways, such as Wnt, Notch, Hedgehog, and TGF-β/BMP, each with distinct roles:

- Wnt/β-catenin Signaling: Regulates stem cell proliferation and differentiation, playing a pivotal role in the development of intestinal and neural organoids.
- Notch Signaling: Regulates cell fate determination and tissue homeostasis, influencing the development of liver, pancreas, and neural organoids.
- Hedgehog Signaling: Directs organ patterning and is crucial for the formation of brain, kidney, and lung organoids.

- TGF-β/BMP Signaling: Modulates epithelial-mesenchymal interactions, contributing to the differentiation of gastric, hepatic, and lung organoids, etc.

In contrast to conventional cell cultures, organoids exhibit self-organizing properties. Cells differentiate and spatially arrange themselves according to intrinsic developmental programs rather than relying on external scaffolds. For example, intestinal organoids closely mimic the architecture of the intestinal epithelium, forming crypt-villus structures that contain absorptive enterocytes, goblet cells, Paneth cells, and enteroendocrine cells, which are key elements for intestinal function. Similarly, cerebral organoids develop distinct regions resembling the forebrain, midbrain, and hindbrain, demonstrating cellular diversity and neuronal functionality, making them invaluable models for neurodegenerative disease research and drug screening. The ability to generate tumor organoids from patient-derived biopsies further enables precision oncology, allowing for the evaluation of patient-specific drug responses *in vitro* before clinical trials.

For PSC-derived cells, maintain them in a feeder-free system using Essential 8 or mTeSR1 medium on vitronectin- or laminin-coated plates. Ensure that PSC colonies exhibit compact morphology, a high nuclear-to-cytoplasmic ratio, and minimal spontaneous differentiation. Pass cells using EDTA-based dissociation methods to preserve genomic stability. Detach PSCs and plate them in ultra-low attachment 96-well plates to form embryoid bodies. Culture the embryoid bodies in neural induction medium containing dual-SMAD inhibitors (SB431542 and LDN193189) to suppress mesodermal and endodermal differentiation. Transition the embryoid bodies into Matrigel droplets to promote 3D self-organization. Supplement differentiation media with region-specific growth factors (e.g., Wnt activators for intestinal organoids, Sonic Hedgehog for neural organoids). For long-term cultures, maintain dynamic shaking conditions (for cerebral organoids) or microfluidic perfusion (for liver/kidney organoids) to enhance nutrient exchange.

For ASC-derived cells, obtain tissue samples via biopsy (e.g., intestinal crypts from colon samples, liver progenitors from hepatocytes). Digest the tissue with collagenase IV and mechanically dissociate it to release epithelial stem cells. Filter and centrifuge to isolate the stem/progenitor populations. Embed these isolated cells in dome-shaped

Matrigel structures to promote 3D self-organization. Use chemically defined growth factor media containing R-spondin, Noggin, and Wnt3a for intestinal organoids, or FGF and HGF for liver organoids. Allow the organoids to grow for 7–14 days, monitoring morphology and proliferation rates. Passage organoids through mechanical disruption or enzymatic digestion with TrypLE. Freeze organoids in CryoStor CS10 or similar cryopreservation medium for long-term storage and experimental reproducibility.

Next, construct the HTS components. The design of the system may vary depending on specific needs, but it generally incorporates the following characteristics:

- Miniaturization of Assays: HTS requires thousands of replicates, making microscale culture systems, such as 96-, 384-, and 1536-well plates, essential. Organoids must be adapted to these miniaturized platforms while maintaining physiological relevance.
- Automated Drug Dispensing and Handling: Robotic liquid handling systems are crucial to ensure precise and uniform drug application across all wells, reducing errors associated with manual pipetting.
- Multiparametric Readouts: Unlike conventional endpoint assays, organoid-based HTS utilizes live-cell imaging, functional assays (e.g., ATP-based viability assays), high-content microscopy, and omics-based readouts (transcriptomics, proteomics) to capture comprehensive data on drug effects.
- Computational Data Analysis: Due to the complexity and volume of HTS data, artificial intelligence (AI)-driven image analysis and machine learning algorithms are used to identify hit compounds, analyze changes in organoid morphology, and classify drug response patterns.

For binding to organoids, controlling organoid size and density is critical, as variations can significantly affect drug diffusion and response. Several strategies are used to achieve uniformity:

- Microwell Arrays: Pre-patterned microwells (e.g., AggreWell™ plates) enable the formation of uniformly sized organoids by restricting cell aggregation.
- Droplet-based Microfluidics: Encapsulating organoid-forming cells in controlled droplet systems ensures consistent spheroid size.

Organoids are embedded in low-viscosity extracellular matrix (e.g., 2% Matrigel or synthetic hydrogels) to preserve their 3D architecture while facilitating automated pipetting.

A suitable liquid flow system and dosing setup are essential for HTS. A highly automated dosing system not only reduces manual labor but also minimizes inter-well errors, ensuring stable and reliable screening results. Automated pipetting systems (e.g., Tecan Fluid, Hamilton STAR) enable precise medium exchange, drug dispensing, and organoid passaging. Perfusion-based bioreactors enhance organ viability by continuously supplying fresh nutrients and removing metabolic waste. The main dosing modes include:

- Static Diffusion: Drugs are added to the culture medium and passively diffuse into organoids. This is suitable for small, permeable compounds.
- Microfluidic Perfusion Systems: Continuous drug flow enhances penetration into large organoids, reducing concentration gradients between surface and core.
- Hydrogel-Embedded Drug Release: Slow-release drug encapsulation within synthetic hydrogels allows for long-term exposure studies.
- Droplet-Based Single-Organoid Drug Delivery: Microdroplet technology enables precise drug titration onto individual organoids, ensuring controlled exposure.

Following drug dosing, high-throughput reads and analysis of organoid responses are essential. Automated fluorescence microscopy systems (e.g., Opera Phenix, ImageXpress Micro Confocal) or high-content imaging, coupled with AI-based image analysis, enable real-time monitoring of organoid morphology and drug response. High-content imaging is a powerful tool for multiplexed analysis in organoid-based HTS. By combining advanced microscopy with automated image acquisition and analysis, it allows for quantifying a wide range of phenotypic changes at single-cell resolution within organoids. In cancer organoids, for example, high-content imaging can assess changes in cell proliferation, apoptosis, invasion, and differentiation, providing insights into how drug candidates influence tumor growth and behavior. Furthermore, advanced image analysis algorithms can extract spatial and temporal patterns from organoid data, enabling researchers to monitor dynamic processes like drug-induced cell death or tissue remodeling in real time [12, 13].

Imaging observations typically include determining organoid size, morphology, and growth rate under visible light. Fluorescent staining with Calcein AM/Propidium Iodide can assess organoid viability and survival post-treatment. Additionally, Caspase 3/7 staining can reveal drug-induced apoptosis. Nuclear chromatin staining with Hoechst or DAPI dyes aids in localizing cells for fluorescence imaging. Molecular assays are equally essential. Biochemical and genetic assays provide deeper insights into drug efficacy and mechanisms of action. For instance, ATP-based luminescence assays quantitatively detect cellular activity by measuring intracellular ATP levels (Table 5.1).

Transcriptomic and proteomic approaches are indispensable tools for multiplexed analysis in organoid-based research, as they generate comprehensive molecular profiles that elucidate treatment-induced responses. Transcriptomics, encompassing methods such as single-cell RNA sequencing and spatial transcriptomics, enable high-resolution mapping of gene expression dynamics at both the single-cell and tissue architecture levels. In the context of cancer organoids, spatial transcriptomics are particularly informative for detecting localized transcriptional changes within distinct cellular compartments, such as cancer stem cells, immune infiltrates, or stromal elements, thereby shedding light on therapeutic mechanisms and resistance pathways. Complementing these insights, proteomics — including mass spectrometry and innovative techniques like proximity labeling and single-cell proteomics — facilitate the

**Table 5.1** Detection methods for organoid-based drug screening.

| Detection | Technical Methods | Purposes |
|---|---|---|
| Viability assay | MTT, CCK-8, ATP and other assays to assess organoid vitality | Cell inhibition rate, dose-response curve |
| Cell viability staining | Use of Calcein AM-PI or Caspase-3/7 staining with fluorescence microscopy to visually assess organoid cell viability | Organoid viability and intra-organoid cell apoptosis rate |
| Bright-field imaging | Bright field image analysis of organoids captured via microscope | Organoid number, morphology, and average size |
| Immunofluorescence/ Immunohistochemistry | Immunohistochemical or immunofluorescent staining to target specific molecules in organoids | Viability/quantity of target cells, changes in target expression |
| Live cell imaging | Dynamic monitoring of organoids after drug treatment using live cell dyes or cell tracer dyes | Cell behavior and interactions |

direct assessment of protein abundance, post-translational modifications, and signaling cascades. This layer of analysis bridges the gap between transcriptional alterations and phenotypic outcomes. For instance, proteomic interrogation of drug-treated organoids can uncover perturbations in key regulatory networks involved in cell cycle control, programmed cell death, and cellular stress responses, offering a more integrative and functional perspective on drug efficacy and mechanism of action.

Functional assays further enhance multiplexed analysis by measuring key physiological responses in organoids, such as metabolic activity, barrier integrity, and electrophysiological properties. For example, in organoids derived from intestinal or lung tissues, barrier function assays can evaluate how drugs impact epithelial tight junctions and permeability. Similarly, in cardiac or neural organoids, electrophysiological assays can assess the effects of compounds on tissue excitability and conductivity. These functional readouts are particularly valuable for assessing the safety and efficacy of drugs targeting specialized tissues or systems [14]. Figure 5.1 depicts the main processes of individual source cells to construct organoids and organoids-on-chips (OoCs) and use them for HTS of drugs.

Various methods are currently available for cultivating organoids, each offering distinct advantages and challenges. Traditional approaches often rely on micro-engineered systems composed of natural hydrogels, animal-derived extracellular matrices such as Matrigel, or synthetic matrices. These materials provide the biochemical environment

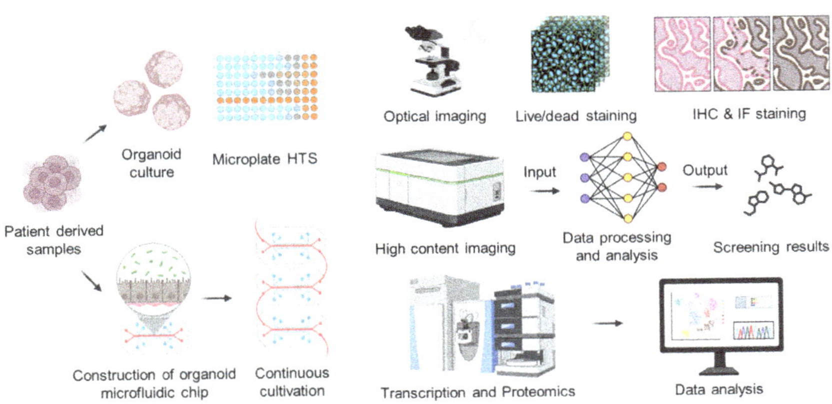


**Figure 5.1** Schematic diagram of organoids and organoid chips for HTS.

and nutrients necessary to support organoid growth [15, 16]. However, in drug screening applications, achieving high uniformity and minimizing batch-to-batch variability are critical requirements. While natural matrix materials are rich in biochemical complexity and can mimic native tissue environments, they often suffer from significant batch-to-batch variability. This inconsistency can affect the reproducibility and stability of organoid cultivation, limiting their applicability in HTS workflows.

Engineered synthetic materials, particularly hydrogels, have gained attention as viable alternatives to natural extracellular matrices in organoid culture due to their customizable physical and biochemical properties. These synthetic scaffolds offer precise modulation of key parameters, such as stiffness, porosity, and ligand presentation, enabling the fine-tuning of microenvironmental cues critical for organoid development and function. Moreover, their adaptability allows for integration with cutting-edge platforms such as 3D bioprinting, thereby promoting the generation of highly reproducible and standardized organoid models suitable for high-throughput applications. Despite these advantages, synthetic matrices often fall short in recapitulating the complex biochemical milieu found in native tissues, as they may lack essential bioactive components like growth factors and native extracellular matrix proteins required for optimal organoid growth, differentiation, and maturation. Consequently, a major challenge in organoid engineering lies in achieving a balance between the controllability and uniformity of synthetic systems and the biological relevance of natural microenvironments. To overcome these limitations, microfluidic technology has emerged as a next-generation platform for organoid cultivation, particularly in HTS applications [17]. Microfluidics involves the precise manipulation and control of fluids at microscopic scales, typically within channels smaller than 1 mm in diameter. At these scales, fluid behavior is governed by forces such as surface tension and capillary action rather than gravity, enabling precise control over fluid dynamics. Microfluidic devices, often referred to as "lab-on-a-chip" systems, integrate various components such as valves, pumps, actuators, sensors, mixers, and heaters. This integration allows for complex analyses and reactions to occur with minimal fluid volumes, making microfluidics an ideal platform for high-precision applications like organoid culture.

In organoid research, microfluidic systems enable the creation of OoCs. These devices consist of microscale chambers where live cells are cultured under continuously perfused conditions, mimicking the physiological functions of tissues and organs. Constructed from biocompatible materials like polydimethylsiloxane or polymethyl methacrylate, these chips are fabricated using advanced techniques such as soft lithography, sacrificial molding, or micropatterning [18]. Microfluidic chips offer unparalleled control over the organoid microenvironment, allowing for precise regulation of nutrient delivery, oxygenation, carbon dioxide levels, and waste removal. This level of control enhances the reproducibility of organoid cultures and facilitates their scalability for high-throughput applications [19].

Furthermore, microfluidic platforms enable seamless integration with biosensors, addressing a significant limitation of traditional organoid cultivation methods. In conventional systems, organoid monitoring, whether through imaging, viability assays, or other analytical techniques, is conducted as a separate step from cultivation. This separation can introduce delays, reduce accuracy, and increase workflow complexity. By incorporating biosensors directly into microfluidic systems, real-time monitoring of organoid responses to various stimuli, such as drug treatments, becomes possible. These integrated systems allow for continuous collection of high-resolution data on organoid growth, viability, metabolism, and other key parameters, thereby expanding the range of organoid applications in both basic research and translational medicine.

One of the most transformative aspects of microfluidic organoid systems is their ability to simulate multi-organ interactions. Many physiological and pathological processes in the human body are driven by crosstalk between multiple organs. Traditional single-organ models often fail to capture these complex interactions, limiting their predictive value in drug screening and disease modeling. Microfluidic technology allows for the integration of multiple organoid models onto a single chip, creating "body-on-a-chip" platforms that replicate inter-organ communication and systemic effects. For example, Skardal and colleagues successfully developed an OoC system that integrated six bioengineered tissue models, representing the liver, heart, vascular system, lungs, testes, and colon, to test drugs previously withdrawn from the market due to adverse reactions. Their studies demonstrated how body-on-a-chip platforms could simulate the interdependent metabolic and downstream effects of drugs across multiple tissues in a single experimental setup [20].

These multi-organ systems offer unprecedented insights into the systemic effects of drugs, enabling researchers to evaluate not only the efficacy but also the potential toxicity of therapeutic compounds. By simulating organ-to-organ communication, they provide a more comprehensive understanding of drug mechanisms and adverse reactions, reducing the reliance on animal models and increasing the translational relevance of preclinical findings. As microfluidic and organoid technologies continue to advance, their integration is set to revolutionize drug discovery and development, paving the way for more accurate, efficient, and ethical approaches to precision medicine.

The integration of organoids with HTS has significantly improved the predictive accuracy and efficiency of drug screening. Organoids' ability to replicate *in vivo* micro-environments enhances the reliability of predictions related to drug efficacy and toxicity. Furthermore, their 3D structure enables the study of dynamic biological processes, such as feedback loops, compensatory signaling, and drug resistance mechanisms, which are often overlooked in traditional 2D systems. For example, studies using colorectal cancer organoids have shown how targeted therapies against the Wnt signaling pathway interact with other pathways, such as PI3K/AKT, leading to drug resistance. This insight has informed the development of combination therapies targeting multiple pathways to improve treatment outcomes [21].

Despite these advancements, organoid-based HTS still faces several challenges that must be addressed to unlock its full potential in drug discovery and precision medicine. These challenges are primarily related to the standardization of organoid culture protocols, the integration of automation, and the improvement of data acquisition and analysis systems.

A major hurdle lies in the complexity and intricacy of organoid culture processes, which pose significant obstacles to large-scale drug screening. The time-consuming nature of constructing organoids, coupled with variability introduced during manual handling, makes it difficult to achieve consistent and reproducible results. Uniform protocols for organoid generation, maintenance, and experimentation are essential. Current methods often require precise control over cell seeding, media composition, and differentiation cues to produce organoids that closely mimic *in vivo* conditions. However, this complexity inherently limits throughput and scalability. Reducing manual interventions and increasing automation could help address these issues.

Automation has become crucial in overcoming these limitations and is now foundational for scaling organoid-based HTS. Robotic platforms enable precise execution of tasks such as cell plating, media exchange, compound distribution, and endpoint analysis, reducing the burden of manual labor and ensuring consistency across experiments. For example, liquid-handling robots with multi-channel pipettes can process hundreds of wells simultaneously, delivering reagents with exceptional uniformity and precision. Innovations in microfluidics, bioprinting, and bioreactor technologies further enhance automation by enabling the generation of standardized organoids compatible with HTS formats. Microfluidic systems, in particular, streamline organoid workflows by offering precise control over fluid delivery, timing, and reagent concentration, thereby improving reproducibility and scalability [22].

Integrated automated platforms designed specifically for organoid-based HTS represent the next step in advancing this technology. These platforms combine liquid handlers, automated incubators, centrifuges, and high-content imaging systems into a fully automated workflow. Such systems not only automate organoid construction but also facilitate downstream processes such as drug treatment, imaging, and data collection, enabling seamless translation from laboratory research to high-throughput applications. By ensuring consistency in organoid size, morphology, and cellular composition across experimental replicates, these platforms enhance the reliability of drug screening data and reduce inter-experimental variability.

Another critical challenge in organoid-based HTS lies in acquiring and analyzing the complex datasets generated. Unlike traditional 2D cell cultures, organoids present unique imaging challenges due to their 3D structure and dynamic nature. Conventional imaging techniques, such as Live/Dead staining, are often inadequate for capturing the intricate physiological and morphological features of organoids. Advanced imaging technologies that combine 3D imaging with high-speed data collection are essential to overcome these limitations. These systems must be capable of capturing detailed information on organoid architecture, growth patterns, viability, and microenvironmental composition during drug treatment. Additionally, they should provide insights into spontaneous cellular behaviors, such as antagonistic interactions, regulatory feedback mechanisms, and physical responses to environmental stimuli.

For instance, high-resolution imaging platforms integrated with real-time analysis tools can reveal structural changes, gene expression profiles, metabolic states, and phenotypic differentiation within organoids. In cancer research, such technologies enable the monitoring of tumor invasion, metastasis, and drug-induced cell death at a cellular level. These detailed assessments not only improve our understanding of drug mechanisms but also help identify resistance pathways and potential therapeutic targets.

The high-resolution and high-throughput imaging technologies employed in organoid research generate large-scale, multidimensional datasets that pose considerable computational demands. Traditional image analysis tools, which are predominantly optimized for 2D data, often fall short when applied to the intricate 3D structures of organoids. To overcome these limitations, the integration of machine learning and deep learning methodologies into image analysis workflows has become increasingly vital. These advanced computational approaches are particularly well-suited to managing and interpreting complex, high-dimensional data, enabling robust and scalable analysis of 3D organoid imaging. Deep learning algorithms, for instance, can accurately classify organoid morphologies, quantify treatment responses, and detect nuanced alterations in cellular dynamics, thereby enhancing the precision and efficiency of phenotypic profiling in drug screening and disease modeling applications [23].

By combining traditional imaging techniques with advanced computational tools, researchers can analyze organoid-based HTS data with greater precision and efficiency. This integration not only streamlines the drug discovery process but also enhances the predictive power of organoid models, accelerating the development of personalized therapies and novel treatment strategies. As these technologies evolve, organoid-based HTS holds immense promise for revolutionizing preclinical drug screening and advancing precision medicine.

Multiplexed analysis is a cornerstone of organoid-based HTS, allowing researchers to leverage the multidimensional data that organoids inherently provide. Unlike traditional screening methods, which often rely on single endpoints such as viability or cytotoxicity, organoid-based HTS captures a broader spectrum of biological responses, encompassing molecular, cellular, and functional parameters. This comprehensive approach is crucial for understanding the complex and nuanced effects of drug candidates, especially in disease models where cellular heterogeneity and microenvironmental factors are key [24]. By integrating these diverse analytical methods, organoid-based HTS goes beyond simple endpoints, capturing the full complexity of drug responses. This integration enables researchers to link molecular changes, such as shifts in gene expression or protein activity, with phenotypic outcomes like tissue remodeling or tumor regression. For example, in cancer research, combining high-content imaging with transcriptomics and functional assays can help identify novel biomarkers associated with drug sensitivity or resistance. Such biomarkers can guide the development of personalized therapies, tailoring treatments to the unique molecular and phenotypic characteristics of individual tumors. Moreover, multiplexed analysis facilitates the study of combination therapies, which are increasingly being explored to overcome drug resistance and enhance treatment efficacy. By evaluating the effects of multiple drugs on various molecular and functional parameters within organoids, researchers can identify synergistic interactions and optimize dosing regimens. This approach is particularly valuable for complex diseases, such as cancer or neurodegenerative disorders, where targeting multiple pathways is often necessary to achieve therapeutic success.

The integration of organoids into HTS has revolutionized drug discovery, providing unparalleled physiological relevance while maintaining scalability. Although challenges such as batch-to-batch variability, drug penetration limitations, and high costs remain, advancements in automation, microfluidics, AI-driven data analysis, and synthetic biology continue to propel the field forward. With ongoing technological innovations, organoid-based HTS is poised to play a central role in personalized medicine, oncology drug screening, and toxicology testing, bridging the gap between preclinical models and human clinical trials.

## 5.3 Target Identification and Validation

The development of disease models with clinical relevance is a cornerstone for target identification and validation. By accurately replicating the genetic, molecular, and cellular characteristics of patient tissues, these models provide essential tools for identifying and validating therapeutic targets. This is particularly crucial for addressing rare subtypes of common diseases and rare diseases that lack standardized treatment protocols. Creating tissue substitutes that authentically mimic the organ-specific microenvironment is key to enhancing the predictive power of preclinical studies. The closer a model replicates the niche of the target tissue, the more reliable its predictions of drug responses, bridging the gap between laboratory research and clinical applications.

Organoids, derived from patient-specific tissues, are uniquely positioned to replicate the genetic features and drug target profiles of their sources. They retain key characteristics, such as specific mutations, chromosomal rearrangements, and epigenetic landscapes, which are essential for understanding the mechanisms of disease initiation and progression. These organoids allow researchers to investigate how genetic alterations influence molecular pathways, cellular behavior, and responses to pharmacological interventions. For instance, organoids derived from colorectal cancer patients preserve the oncogenic Wnt signaling pathways that drive tumor growth while interacting with secondary pathways like PI3K/AKT or Notch. By targeting these interconnected pathways using genetic tools like CRISPR-Cas9 or pharmacological inhibitors, researchers can identify critical nodes and potential therapeutic targets necessary for tumor survival and progression.

The principles and methods for identifying and validating organoids as therapeutic targets are outlined below. These approaches can be based on genetic perturbation-based screening (such as CRISPR and RNA interference, or RNAi) to identify potential targets. Genetic perturbation-based screening utilizes tools like CRISPR-Cas9, RNAi, or transposon-based mutagenesis to systematically modify gene expression within organoids, enabling the identification of essential genes involved in disease progression. This method is particularly valuable for uncovering oncogenic dependencies, synthetic lethal interactions, and essential survival pathways in tumor organoids.

The underlying principle of genetic perturbation-based screening is that disrupting key regulatory genes will reveal their functional roles in maintaining disease. By introducing gene knockouts (via CRISPR), knockdowns (via RNAi), or overexpression constructs, researchers can identify genes essential for organoid survival, proliferation, or drug resistance. The general procedure involves the following steps: first, organoids are cultured in Matrigel or other defined extracellular matrix substrates to maintain stem cell niches. Organoids are pre-treated with ROCK inhibitors to enhance single-cell survival during the genetic perturbation process. Next, lentiviral or electroporation-based methods are used to deliver whole-genome or targeted single-guide RNA libraries. Successfully transduced organoids are selected using antibiotic resistance markers (such as puromycin or hygromycin) or fluorescence sorting. Finally, organoid viability and growth dynamics post-gene knockout are assessed using live-cell imaging and metabolic assays. RNA sequencing and proteomics are then performed on the treated organoids to determine transcriptional and post-translational changes associated with gene perturbations.

In addition to genetic perturbation, multi-omics-based screening for organoid targets has proven highly effective. Multi-omics profiling integrates genomic, transcriptomic, proteomic, and metabolomic analyses to systematically map molecular pathways altered in disease states. This approach is particularly powerful for identifying biomarkers, metabolic dependencies, and novel signaling pathways that can be targeted therapeutically (Figure 5.2A). The principle behind multi-omics is that by simultaneously analyzing multiple molecular layers, this approach provides a comprehensive view of disease pathophysiology, helping researchers prioritize targets that are consistently dysregulated across various molecular dimensions. To conduct multi-omics profiling, organoid samples are collected under optimized conditions to preserve RNA, proteins, and metabolites. Organoids are snap-frozen or preserved in stabilizing buffers (e.g., RNAlater for RNA and protease inhibitors for proteins). RNA sequencing captures gene expression changes in response to perturbations, while mass spectrometry is used for proteomic and metabolomic profiling to detect alterations in protein abundance and metabolic shifts, especially with the advancement of high-resolution accurate mass. Computational tools are employed to integrate multi-omics data and construct disease-specific molecular networks, and machine learning algorithms are applied to predict druggable nodes within these networks.

Additionally, direct screening of organoids for drug sensitivity and resistance is a straightforward and intuitive approach. This method involves exposing organoids to drug libraries and analyzing the differential responses. The core principle of drug

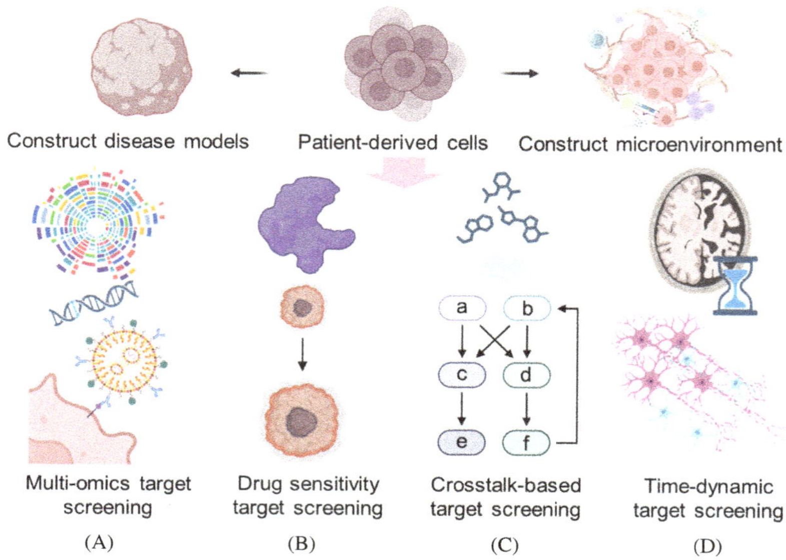


**Figure 5.2** Schematic diagram of organoids and organoid chips for target identification and validation. (A) Multi-omics testing based on simulating complex environments *in vivo* using organoids, which is more closely related to the situation *in vivo*. (B) Using organoids for drug sensitivity testing is more closely related to patients' reactions to drug sensitivity. (C) Compared to single cell lines and 2D culture, organoids can provide a more comprehensive cross-talk. (D) Organoids can introduce temporal observation and intervention, providing a foundation for model construction and research on development and degenerative diseases.

sensitivity screening is to evaluate how different compounds affect organoid viability, morphology, and functional outputs, which helps identify targetable vulnerabilities in specific disease contexts. The workflow begins by treating organoids with a drug library consisting of clinically relevant agents, including chemotherapy drugs, targeted inhibitors, and immunotherapies. High-throughput viability assays, such as ATP-based luminescence measurements and live-cell imaging, are used to assess treatment responses in real time. Generation of dose-response curves allows the calculation of $IC_{50}$ values, which quantify the potency of each drug in inhibiting organoid growth.

To better understand resistance mechanisms, drug-resistant organoid subpopulations are isolated and subjected to transcriptomic and proteomic analyses to identify compensatory pathways that allow survival. This process reveals secondary targets that may be co-inhibited to overcome resistance, facilitating the development of combination therapies. The integration of drug sensitivity data with genetic and multi-omics insights ensures that the identified targets are not only functionally relevant but also clinically actionable (Figure 5.2B). The ultimate aim of this approach is to refine therapeutic strategies by aligning drug target identification with precision medicine principles, thereby tailoring treatment regimens to the molecular characteristics of individual patients [25].

The temporal versatility of organoid models also makes them ideal for studying diseases with dynamic progression, such as neurodegenerative disorders. Brain organoids, derived from human pluripotent stem cells, can recapitulate both early and late pathological events [26]. In the early stages, they allow researchers to investigate key processes such as protein misfolding, aggregation, and synaptic dysfunction, while in the later stages, they provide insights into neuronal death and glial activation. This longitudinal perspective is crucial for identifying drug targets that not only prevent disease onset but also slow or reverse disease progression, offering new therapeutic opportunities for conditions like Alzheimer's, Parkinson's, and Huntington's diseases [27].

In cancer research, PDOs have emerged as powerful tools for precision oncology. PDOs faithfully preserve the driver mutations, chromosomal abnormalities, and clonal diversity of the original tumor, providing a robust platform for high-throughput functional genomics and drug screening. Combining organoid models with transcriptomics and proteomics enables researchers to explore the molecular underpinnings of tumor biology at a systems level. For instance, transcriptomic analyses can identify subpopulations of cancer cells within an organoid that are inherently resistant to treatment, guiding the development of more effective combination therapies.

Moreover, co-culture systems that incorporate additional cell types, such as immune cells, fibroblasts, and endothelial cells, recreate the tumor microenvironment, providing valuable insights into how stromal or immune components influence treatment outcomes. These models facilitate the study of tumor-immune interactions, such as immune evasion or resistance to checkpoint blockade therapies. For example, immune checkpoint inhibitors can be tested in tumor organoids co-cultured with T cells or NK cells to assess their efficacy in restoring anti-tumor immunity. By integrating these co-culture systems with PDOs, researchers can identify novel immunotherapy targets, optimize drug combinations, and gain a deeper understanding of the mechanisms driving resistance to immunotherapy.

The utility of organoid models extends well beyond oncology, offering transformative potential in the field of infectious disease research. Organoids provide a physiologically relevant platform for investigating host-pathogen interactions with a level of fidelity unattainable in traditional cell lines or animal models. For example, intestinal organoids have been instrumental in modeling viral infections such as norovirus and SARS-CoV-2, while hepatocyte-derived organoids are used to explore the replication and pathogenesis of hepatotropic viruses, including hepatitis B and C. These systems support the evaluation of antiviral therapeutics and vaccine candidates by accurately capturing the dynamic interplay between human host cells and invading pathogens. Organoids derived from patient-specific tissues such as the intestine, lung, and liver further enhance this approach by enabling individualized assessments of susceptibility and immune responses.

Moreover, organoid-based models have significantly advanced our understanding of bacterial pathogenesis. Studies employing intestinal organoids infected with pathogens like *Salmonella enterica* or *Escherichia coli* have elucidated key mechanisms of bacterial adhesion, epithelial invasion, and toxin-mediated disruption. These insights have unveiled novel molecular targets involved in early infection processes. Targeting bacterial effectors critical for host cell attachment or entry represents a promising therapeutic avenue, offering a targeted alternative to conventional broad-spectrum antibiotics. This strategy holds particular promise in the context of rising antimicrobial resistance, as it aims to disarm pathogens without exerting widespread selective pressure on microbial communities.

Additionally, organoids provide a platform to study viral infections, enabling researchers to explore viral entry, replication, and host immune responses. Lung organoids, for example, have been instrumental in uncovering the mechanisms of SARS-CoV-2 infection, identifying viral entry points such as ACE2 and TMPRSS2 receptors, and testing antiviral compounds. Similarly, liver organoids have been used to model the life cycles of hepatitis B and C viruses, providing a valuable means for screening antiviral drugs and investigating host genetic factors that influence infection outcomes [28].

One of the most significant advantages of organoids over traditional *in vitro* cell culture models is their ability to replicate the complex feedback loops and pathway crosstalk inherent to biological systems. Unlike monolayer cell cultures, which simplify cellular interactions and signaling, organoids preserve the spatial and functional complexity required to study dynamic processes. Signaling pathways such as PI3K/AKT/mTOR, MAPK, and JAK/STAT are not isolated networks but are interconnected, regulated by both feedback and feedforward mechanisms. These pathways play critical roles in disease progression and therapeutic response. Organoids provide a platform for observing these processes in real time, under conditions that closely mimic both physiological and pathological states. For instance, studies using organoid models have shown how the inhibition of one pathway can lead to compensatory activation of alternative signaling cascades, contributing to therapeutic resistance. In melanoma organoids, for example, inhibition of the oncogenic BRAF pathway often triggers compensatory activation of the ERK or MEK pathways, enabling tumor cell survival despite targeted therapy. These insights have driven the development of combination therapies targeting multiple nodes within interconnected pathways. By simultaneously inhibiting both primary and compensatory survival mechanisms, such therapies achieve more durable treatment responses, reducing the likelihood of resistance and relapse (Figure 5.2C). Organoids also allow researchers to explore the role of the microenvironment in shaping disease progression and treatment responses. Tumor organoids co-cultured with immune cells, fibroblasts, or endothelial cells replicate the interactions between cancer cells and their surrounding stroma. These models provide valuable insights into how the tumor microenvironment influences immune evasion, drug resistance, and metastatic behavior. For example, organoid-immune co-culture systems have revealed mechanisms of immune checkpoint blockade resistance, guiding the development of novel immunotherapies aimed at restoring anti-tumor immunity.

In addition, organoids also add temporal simulation to the scope of research. For example, organoids with more complex shapes can better mimic the development of the human fetal brain *in vivo*, reflecting the abnormal temporal progression of organoids with disrupted tissue structures. Moreover, organoids can provide physiological models for neurodegenerative diseases, providing a good foundation for the screening and identification of drug targets [29, 30] (Figure 5.2D).

As organoid technology continues to advance, its integration with cutting-edge tools such as single-cell genomics, high-content imaging, and computational modeling is expanding its potential. Single-cell sequencing of organoids enables the study of heterogeneity within complex tissues, shedding light on how distinct cell populations respond to therapeutic interventions. High-content imaging captures both the spatial and temporal dynamics of organoid models, providing visual insights into structural changes, cellular behavior, and drug-induced effects. Meanwhile, computational tools powered by AI and machine learning facilitate the analysis of vast datasets generated from organoid studies, identifying patterns and relationships that would otherwise go unnoticed. Overall, as shown in Figure 5.2, organoids allow for the construction of disease models that highly mimic the biological characteristics of the source individual and allow for the formation of microenvironments in the vicinity of the organ or tumor, which allows for more accurate and reliable screening and identification of drug targets. This approach allows the construction of dynamic models in the temporal dimension and the reproduction of *in vivo* pathway crosstalk and interactions, which can be used for drug target screening through either multi-omics identification or direct drug sensitivity experiments.

For example, in COVID-19 caused by SARS-CoV-2, the development of anti-SARS-CoV-2 drugs may change the epidemic situation and control the scope of the epidemic. At this point, it is crucial to use human disease-related cells to create novel models for studying the biology of SARS-CoV-2 and promoting drug screening. Studies have shown that the lung organ-like model induced by human pluripotent stem cells (hPSC LOs) can infect COVID-19 and show strong chemokine induction of SARS CoV-2 infection. Research has found that the alveolar type II-like cell (AT2) marker can be highly expressed in stem cells, and the AT2-like cell population in lung organoids is highly similar to human lung AT2 cells. In addition, key factors involved in the entry of SARS-CoV-2, such as ACE2, SARS-CoV-2 receptor, TMPRSS2 (protease involved in virus entry), and FURIN (pre-activated SARS-CoV-2 protein-converting enzyme), were enriched in AT2-like cells. Next, SARS-CoV-2 infects hPSC LOs. The results confirmed that hPSC LOs have robust SARS-CoV-2 infection. The hPSC LOs infected with SARS-CoV-2 exhibit strong induction of chemokines, which is consistent with the findings detected in lung autopsy tissues of COVID-19 patients. Due to the association between gastrointestinal complications and poorer outcomes in COVID-19 patients, researchers tested whether SARS-CoV-2 could infect colon cells. Research has confirmed that ACE2 is expressed in human colon tissue keratin 20 $(KRT20)^+$ intestinal cells, and pathological analysis of colonoscopy samples from COVID-19 patients detected significant damage to the colon mucosa, manifested as intestinal luminal epithelial cell damage and goblet cell depletion. SARS-CoV-2 infection was confirmed by *in situ* hybridization of viral RNA and electron microscopy examination. This study identified five cell clusters of hPSC colonic organoids (CO), including $KRT20^+$ intestinal cells, $MUC2^+$ goblet cells, $EPHB2^+$ transient expansion cells, $CHGA^+$ intestinal endocrine cells, and $LGR5^+$ or $BMI1^+$ stem cells. ACE2, TMPRSS2, and FURIN are also expressed in all five cell clusters, but highly enriched and correlated in $KRT20^+$ intestinal cells. This study validated the expression of ACE2 in $KRT20^+$ intestinal cells. Using organoids for HTS of the U.S. Food and Drug Administration (FDA)-approved drugs, it was found that three drugs, including imatinib, mycophenolic acid, and quinacrine hydrochloride, can significantly inhibit SARS-CoV-2 infection in hPSC LOs and hPSC COs under physiological treatment. Research shows that lung- and colon-like organs can be used as disease models to study COVID-19 infection and identify potential COVID-19 therapies, so as to achieve HTS of drugs [31].

Organoids are revolutionizing our ability to study disease mechanisms and identify therapeutic targets. Their capacity to model the molecular, cellular, and microenvironmental complexities of human tissues offers unparalleled insights into drug action, resistance, and host-pathogen interactions. As technological advancements continue to enhance organoid systems, their role in drug discovery and personalized medicine will only expand, bridging the gap between laboratory research and clinical application. This progress not only accelerates the development of effective treatments but also ensures that therapeutic strategies are tailored to the unique needs of individual patients.

Organoid technology is transforming drug discovery by accelerating the development of personalized therapies tailored to individual patients. Patient-specific organoids enable HTS, allowing researchers to test thousands of compounds simultaneously while maintaining the biological relevance of the models. When integrated with microfluidic chips, this approach not only improves the evaluation of drug efficacy and toxicity but also facilitates the rapid identification of active compounds for specific patients. These advancements bridge the gap between preclinical research and clinical applications, providing a faster and more reliable path for drug development.

A groundbreaking milestone was achieved in August 2022 when the FDA approved the world's first drug developed entirely based on OoC research (NCT04658472). Supported by robust preclinical data generated through OoC models, this drug bypassed traditional animal testing and directly entered clinical trials. This achievement marked a historic shift in the drug development paradigm, demonstrating the potential of OoCs to replace animal models and gain regulatory recognition.

The growing recognition of organoid and OoC technologies has prompted international regulatory bodies to establish guidelines and policies to support their adoption. The International Council for Harmonisation (ICH) of Technical Requirements for Pharmaceuticals for Human Use has incorporated organoids and OoCs into its regulatory framework. For example, the ICH guidelines reference these alternative models in documents such as E14 (clinical and non-clinical evaluation of QT/QTc prolongation and potential arrhythmogenic effects) and S12 (consideration of non-clinical biodistribution of gene therapy products). These guidelines affirm the scientific validity of organoids and OoCs as reliable alternatives for evaluating drug safety and efficacy.

In China, regulatory advancements have similarly highlighted the importance of innovative models in drug development. In 2021, the National Medical Products Administration issued groundbreaking guidelines, including the "Guiding Principles for Non-clinical Research and Evaluation Technology of Gene Therapy Products (Trial)" and the "Guiding Principles for Non-clinical Research Technology of Gene-modified Cell Therapy Products (Trial)." For the first time, these guidelines explicitly encouraged the use of 2D and 3D tissue models, organoids, and microfluidic models as substitutes for animal experiments. These models were recognized as valuable tools for proof-of-concept research and supplementing drug efficacy and safety data in preclinical studies.

The United States has also taken significant steps to modernize its drug development regulations. In September 2022, the FDA Modernization Act 2.0 redefined non-clinical trial requirements by eliminating the mandatory use of animal testing in drug research and development. This legislative change underscores the FDA's support for scientifically validated alternatives, including OoCs, bioprinting, and computer modeling, to demonstrate the safety and efficacy of new drugs. This shift not only accelerates the drug approval process but also aligns with ethical principles by reducing reliance on animal testing.

These breakthrough advances highlight the enormous potential of organoid technology in the development of biomedicine in the new era. The application of organoid technology in pharmaceutical research makes drug development more efficient and cost-effective, enabling faster and more effective entry into clinical research.

## 5.4 Conclusion

Organoid technology, alongside OoC systems, is rapidly reshaping the landscape of drug discovery and development. By faithfully replicating the complexities of human tissues and organs, organoids provide a more accurate platform for drug screening and target identification, offering a closer approximation of clinical outcomes compared to traditional 2D cell cultures. This technology enables HTS of drug candidates, the discovery of novel therapeutic targets, and a deeper understanding of disease mechanisms. Furthermore, the integration of patient-specific organoids and microfluidic technologies has the potential to significantly enhance drug efficacy and safety evaluations, accelerating the transition from preclinical to clinical stages. In addition to its scientific and technological advances, regulatory frameworks are evolving to incorporate organoid models into drug development pipelines. The FDA's approval of a drug based on OoC research and the global push toward reducing animal testing are critical milestones that validate the therapeutic and ethical value of organoid technologies. As regulations continue to adapt, the widespread adoption of organoid-based drug screening will streamline drug discovery, reduce costs, and foster personalized medicine strategies that are more aligned with individual patient profiles. These advancements position organoid technologies as a cornerstone for the future of drug development, healthcare, and ethical scientific progress, marking a significant step toward more efficient, reliable, and humane medical innovations.

## Key Opinion Points

1. Organoid models are expected to become standard tools in early-phase drug discovery, particularly for diseases where conventional models fail to capture human-specific pathophysiology, such as neurological disorders and rare cancers.
2. The development of automated, high-throughput-compatible organoid culture systems will be essential to meet industrial scalability requirements, enabling their integration into pharmaceutical screening pipelines and regulatory toxicology studies.
3. OoC technologies are anticipated to evolve into multi-tissue or body-on-a-chip platforms, allowing simultaneous assessment of drug efficacy, metabolism, and systemic toxicity within interconnected organoid systems.
4. Advances in single-cell sequencing, spatial transcriptomics, and AI-powered image analytics will significantly enhance the resolution and interpretability of organoid-based assays, transforming them into data-rich platforms for mechanism-driven drug discovery.
5. In the future, regulatory agencies may adopt organoid-based models as part of accepted preclinical testing frameworks, especially when combined with patient-derived data, to support clinical trial design, drug repurposing, and adaptive therapeutic strategies.

## Acknowledgments

This research was funded by the National Natural Science Foundation of China (32271464), the Hunan Provincial Natural Science Foundation for Distinguished Young Scholars (2022JJ10086), the Innovation-Driven Project of Central South University (2020CX048), Hunan Provincial High-Level Health Talents (20240304088), the Joint Fund of the Hunan Provincial Natural Science Foundation and the Hunan Medical Products Administration (2023JJ60501).

## References

1. Moutinho S. Researchers and regulators plan for a future without lab animals. Nat Med. 2023;29(9):2151-4.
2. Sato T, Vries RG, Snippert HJ, van de Wetering M, Barker N, Stange DE, *et al.* Single Lgr5 stem cells build crypt–villus structures in vitro without a mesenchymal niche. Nature. 2009;459(7244):262–5.
3. Lee KK, McCauley HA, Broda TR, Kessler SP, Mangold KA, Wells JM, *et al.* Human stomach-on-a-chip with luminal flow and peristaltic-like motility. Lab Chip. 2018;18(20):3079–85.
4. Dixon TA, Muotri AR. Advancing preclinical models of psychiatric disorders with human brain organoid cultures. Mol Psychiatry. 2023;28(1):83–95.
5. Lancaster MA, Renner M, Martin C-A, Wenzel D, Bicknell LS, Hurles ME, *et al.* Cerebral organoids model human brain development and microcephaly. Nature. 2013; 501(7467):373–9.
6. Jin Y, Liu Y, Li Z, Santostefano KE, Shi J, Zhang D, *et al.* Vascularized liver organoids generated using induced hepatic tissue and dynamic liver-specific microenvironment as a drug testing platform. Adv Funct Mater. 2018;28(37):1801954.
7. Xu P, Becker H, Elizondo DM, Zhang Y, Wu J, Yong M, *et al.* Intestinal organoid culture model is a valuable system to study epithelial barrier function in IBD. Gut. 2018;67(10):1905.
8. Sun D, Li X, He Y, Ren Y, Zhang X. Why 90% of clinical drug development fails and how to improve it? Acta Pharm Sin B. 2022;12(7):3049–62.
9. Errico A. High-throughput screen identifies a roadmap for combination drug trials. Nat Rev Clin Oncol. 2014;11(3):124.
10. Kratochvil MJ, Seymour AJ, Li TL, Paşca SP, Kuo CJ, Heilshorn SC. Engineered materials for organoid systems. Nat Rev Mater. 2019;4(9):606–22.
11. Organoids. Nat Rev Methods Primers. 2022;2(1):95.
12. Herpers B, van der Wiel B, Span PN, van den Heuvel M, Verhaegh G, van der Burgt C, *et al.* Functional patient-derived organoid screenings identify MCLA-158 as a therapeutic EGFR × LGR5 bispecific antibody with efficacy in epithelial tumors. Nat Cancer. 2022;3(4):418–36.
13. Patel ZH, Berrios DI, Yu X, Xu Z, Mahalingam G, Yuan J, *et al.* Evaluating anticancer agents on 3D bioprinted organoid tumors (BOT) to reduce cost and accelerate therapeutic discovery. J Clin Oncol. 2022;40(16):e13500.
14. Tao M, Wu X. The role of patient-derived ovarian cancer organoids in the study of PARP inhibitors sensitivity and resistance: from genomic analysis to functional testing. J Exp Clin Cancer Res. 2021;40(1):338.

15. Bernal PN, Bouwmeester M, Madrid-Wolff J, van der Sloot T, Schleider Y, Wei K, *et al.* Volumetric bioprinting of organoids and optically tuned hydrogels to build liver-like metabolic biofactories. Adv Mater. 2022;34(15):e2110054.
16. Hernandez-Gordillo V, Kassis T, Lampejo A, Gamboa ME, Khazal F, Jensen J, *et al.* Fully synthetic matrices for in vitro culture of primary human intestinal enteroids and endometrial organoids. Biomaterials. 2020;254:120125.
17. Mullard A. Microfluidics platform lowers barrier to drug combination screening. Nat Rev Drug Discov. 2018;17(10):691–2.
18. McDonald JC, Duffy DC, Anderson JR, Chiu DT, Wu H, Schueller OJA, *et al.* Fabrication of microfluidic systems in poly(dimethylsiloxane). Electrophoresis. 2000;21(1):27–30.
19. Man Y, Li S, Zhou L, Zheng J, Liu L, Li J, *et al.* Organoids-on-a-chip for personalized precision medicine. Adv Healthc Mater. 2024;13(30):e2401843.
20. Sackmann EK, Fulton AL, Beebe DJ. The present and future role of microfluidics in biomedical research. Nature. 2014;507(7491):181–9.
21. Sachs N, de Ligt J, Kopper O, Gogola E, Bounova G, Weeber F, *et al.* A living biobank of breast cancer organoids captures disease heterogeneity. Cell. 2018;172(1–2):373–86.e10.
22. Czerniecki SM, Cruz NM, Harder JL, Menon R, Annis J, Otto EA, *et al.* High-throughput screening enhances kidney organoid differentiation from human pluripotent stem cells and enables automated multidimensional phenotyping. Cell Stem Cell. 2018;22(6):929–40.e4.
23. Kong J, Cooper LA, Wang F, Yin X, Moses N, Chapuy B, *et al.* Network-based machine learning in colorectal and bladder organoid models predicts anti-cancer drug efficacy in patients. Nat Commun. 2020;11(1):5485.
24. Sufi J, Poulain S, Mulas C, Attar M, Li M, Rognan D, *et al.* Multiplexed single-cell analysis of organoid signaling networks. Nat Protoc. 2021;16(10):4897–918.
25. Lane SW, Williams DA, Watt FM. Modulating the stem cell niche for tissue regeneration. Nat Biotechnol. 2014;32(8):795–803.
26. Ao Z, Tao M, Huang Y, Wu L, Wang S, Zhang Y, *et al.* Understanding immune-driven brain aging by human brain organoid microphysiological analysis platform. Adv Sci. 2022;9(27):2200475.
27. Amartumur S, Liu Y, Zhang X, Lin Y, Xu Y, Li H, *et al.* Neuropathogenesis-on-chips for neurodegenerative diseases. Nat Commun. 2024;15(1):2219.
28. Wang P, Song Y, Li Y, Chen L, Li D, Sun Y, *et al.* Blood–brain barrier injury and neuroinflammation induced by SARS-CoV-2 in a lung–brain microphysiological system. Nat Biomed Eng. 2024;8(8):1053–68.

29. Chiaradia I, Lancaster MA. Tissue morphology influences the temporal program of human brain organoid development. Cell Stem Cell. 2023;30(10):1351–67.
30. Pellegrini L, Bonfio C, Chadwick J, Lancaster MA. Modeling neurodegeneration with mutant-tau organoids. Cell. 2021;184(17):4377–9.
31. Han Y, Duan X, Yang L, Nilsson-Payant BE, Wang P, Duan F, *et al.* Identification of SARS-CoV-2 inhibitors using lung and colonic organoids. Nature. 2021;589(7841):270–5.

https://doi.org/10.1142/9789819817597_0006

Chapter 6

# Perspectives from a High-throughput Screening and Target Identification Laboratory

Valentina Gonzalez-Pecchi[1], Elizabeth L. Zoeller[2,3], Matías I. Hepp[1], Sebastián Vera[1], Xiulei Mo[2], Kecheng Lei[4], Yuhong Du[2,3,*]

[1]*Laboratorio de Investigación en Ciencias Biomédicas, Universidad Católica de la Santísima Concepción, Concepción, Chile*

[2]*Emory Chemical Biology Discovery Center, Emory University School of Medicine, Atlanta, USA*

[3]*Department of Pharmacology and Chemical Biology, Emory University School of Medicine, Atlanta, USA*

[4]*Department of Neurosurgery, Emory University School of Medicine, Atlanta, GA, USA*

**Abstract:** 3D organoids have emerged as a revolutionary tool in drug discovery, bridging the gap between traditional 2D cell cultures and complex *in vivo* systems with applications in the drug discovery field. This chapter explores the development and applications of organoids in drug discovery, highlighting their use in high-throughput screening assays and target identification and validation. We discuss key advancements in the establishment of organoids as a model system for high-throughput screening, and their implications for personalized medicine. Additionally, we examine the utility of organoids in cancer, to be used as a physiological relevant screening platform to model tumors for primary high-throughput screening campaign for drug discovery. By integrating organoids in the early drug development pipeline, researchers can reduce the reliance on using 2D transformed cell lines as screening tool and improve the efficiency and translational potential of new therapies. Ultimately, this chapter aims to illustrate the transformative role of 3D organoids in modern pharmacology and accelerating the discovery of novel therapeutics.

**Keywords:** organoids, high-throughput screening (HTS), ultra-HTS (uHTS), target identification

[*]Corresponding author. Email: dyuhong@emory.edu

## Key Points

1. Introduction to high-throughput screening
2. Miniaturization of organoids culture into 384-well HTS and 1536-well uHTS format for early drug discovery
3. Protocols for organoids compound screening in HTS and uHTS format
4. Organoids in target identification and validation

## 6.1 Introduction

High-throughput screening (HTS) is a powerful technique used to rapidly evaluate large numbers of chemical compounds, with the goal of identifying molecules with potential therapeutic effects. Usually, HTS is performed with 2D cell cultures, which, although effective, fail to replicate the complex architecture and cellular diversity of human tissues. This limitation has spurred the development of 3D cell culture systems, such as organoids, to mimic more closely *in vivo* conditions. Organoids — self-organizing, stem cell-derived 3D structures — provide a physiologically relevant model for drug discovery and disease research, offering substantial advantages over conventional 2D cultures in HTS applications.

Historically, drug screening assays rely on HTS assays with 2D cell cultures to gain valuable insight in a timely manner. However, over the last decade, significant efforts have been directed toward integrating organoids into HTS workflows. The synergy between organoid technology and HTS enhances drug discovery pipelines, particularly through high-content screening, which enables multidimensional analysis of organoid responses to pharmacological agents. High-content screening facilitates the quantification of morphological alterations, viability, gene expression profiles, and other biomarkers. Furthermore, organoid-based HTS allows for large-scale compound testing, streamlining the identification of lead candidates. These assays can be tailored to evaluate diverse endpoints, including drug-induced changes in morphology, metabolic activity, and intracellular signaling pathways. Crucially, the integration of organoids with HTS not only accelerates the identification of compounds with therapeutic efficacy but also enables early detection of toxicity, thereby refining candidate selection and reducing reliance on animal models during preclinical development.

## 6.2 High-Throughput Screening Technologies Overview

### 6.2.1 *High-Throughput Screening in Drug Discovery*

HTS is a crucial technology in drug discovery, enabling the testing of thousands to millions compounds for biological activity. By automating the process of testing compound libraries against biological targets, HTS accelerates the identification of promising drug candidates. HTS typically employs robotics, liquid handling systems, and automated data analysis platforms.

HTS has led to several notable successes in drug discovery, some of them discussed here. Imatinib (Gleevec) was identified through HTS as a potent inhibitor of the BCR-ABL fusion protein, which is central in the pathogenesis of chronic myelogenous leukemia. Specifically, imatinib was identified in a screening setting to identify phenylamino-pyrimidines compounds that target PDGF-receptor autophosphorylation [1]. Later, optimization of the class of phenylamino-pyrimidines compounds yielded Imatinib, a highly potent and selective BCR-ABL kinase inhibitor [2]. While not the primary focus of the initial study, imatinib's role in the screening process highlights the utility of HTS platforms. Finally, this discovery led to its development as a targeted therapy, transforming the treatment for chronic myelogenous leukemia. Another example is Maraviroc, a selective CCR5 antagonist, active against human immunodeficiency virus type 1 (HIV-1), which was discovered using a high-throughput screen following the identification of an imidazopyridine CCR5 ligand [3, 4]. Maraviroc is now used in combination with anti-retroviral medications to treat HIV infection. An example in cystic fibrosis, Lumacaftor and Ivacaftor, which target CFTR protein (with F508del mutation), were both discovered using HTS, where compounds were tested to improve folding and function of the defective CFTR protein [5]. Both drugs are now combined in a treatment to improved lung function in patients with cystic fibrosis. Finally, another example is the discovery of Nutlin, a protein-protein interaction inhibitor that disrupts the interaction between p53-MDM2, which leads to the stabilization of p53, a tumor suppressor that regulates cell growth inhibition and apoptosis, important for cancer treatment. The discovery of the compound was done by a cell-based HTS assay system [6].

### 6.2.2 *Automation Requirement for High-Throughput Screening Campaigns*

Successful HTS campaigns rely on a robust and fully integrated automation system to manage the large numbers of compounds tested and the massive amount of data generated. A key component is a high-precision liquid handling system, which ensures accurate and consistent dispensing of small volumes of compounds and reagents into multi-well assay plates, typically 384-well or 1536-well formats. Robotic arms are essential for the automated movement and transfer of plates between various stations, which could include incubators, plate washers, and readers, minimizing human error and increasing throughput. For data acquisition, automated plate readers equipped to detect a variety of biological responses, such as fluorescence, luminescence, absorbance, or time-resolved fluorescence, are required to provide rapid and sensitive measurements. Finally, comprehensive data analysis software is critical to process, manage and interpret the massive amount of data generated, enabling the identification of potential hits based on biological or chemical parameters. All together, these components form a unified automation infrastructure that enables efficient and reproducible large-scale compound screening.

### 6.2.3 *Target-Based and Phenotypical Screening*

HTS can be classified into two main types: target-based screening that focuses on specific known molecular targets involved in a disease, such as the effect of compounds on a specific known protein; and phenotypic screening, which assesses the overall effect of compounds on a biological system without focusing on a specific target, such as studying the effect of compounds on cancer cell growth. In the last approach, after a hit compound is found, a target identification should be performed to uncover its mechanism of action [7]. In some cases, a combination of both approaches may be used to maximize the efficiency of the drug discovery process.

## 6.3 Applications of Organoids in High-Throughput Screening

### 6.3.1 *Drug Discovery*

Organoids are increasingly being utilized for HTS assays, particularly for drug discovery. One of the most significant advantages of organoid-based HTS is the ability to mimic tissue-specific responses to compounds, providing more accurate data compared to 2D cell cultures, and enabling researchers to screen drugs in a more physiologically relevant biological context. It can model a complex disease biology, including interactions between different cell types, and give a more accurate prediction of drug efficacy in human diseases. It maintains tissue architecture, cellular heterogeneity, and gene expression profiles found *in vivo* and therefore is an advanced model for studying biology and for drug discovery. It also has the ability to use patient-derived organoids for tailored drug response, in a personalized medicine approach. Organoid-based HTS can identify toxicity and off-target effects in a more organ-specific context. Organoids can replicate key organ functions such as drug metabolism, offering insights into potential side effects that would be missed using 2D cell culture models. However, there are some challenges, such as variability between organoids batches, growing organoids in large numbers suitable for HTS, and the cost for maintaining and culturing organoid systems.

Despite technical, financial and other challenges for organoid-based HTS, much efforts have been made to advance drug discovery using organoids as summarized in Table 6.1 below.

### 6.3.2 *Technology Advancement Enabling High-Throughput Screening with Organoids*

As organoid-based HTS becomes more prevalent, significant advances in automation, imaging, and data analysis are being made to facilitate large-scale screening.

<u>HTS automation instrumentation</u> is essential for scaling up HTS assays. In our previous study [20], a HTS platform for 3D organoids was developed. This platform streamlined the process of miniaturization of 3D organoid cultures into a 384-well HTS and a 1536-well ultra-HTS (uHTS) plate format and the execution of screening large number of compounds, enabling rapid and reproducible results. Such a technology platform makes it feasible to use 3D organoids for large-scale drug discovery efforts [20]. The detailed procedures will be described in the following sections of this chapter.

Unlike traditional 2D cell culture, 3D organoid culture requires a semi-solid form of extracellular matrix (ECM) to support organoid growth within a 3D architecture. ECM is vital to support epithelial stem cell proliferation, differentiation, and propagation and

**Table 6.1** Summary of the HTS drug discovery campaigns using organoids in different diseases over the last seven years.

| Well Format | Number of Compounds Screened | Organoid Models | Species | Reference |
|---|---|---|---|---|
| 96- | Not reported | Kidney organoids, acute kidney injury | Human | Oishi *et al.*, 2025 [8] |
| 96- | 169 | Triple negative breast cancer | Human | Rao *et al.*, 2024 [9] |
| 1536- | 179 | Melanoma and renal cell carcinoma | Human | Ortiz Jordan *et al.*, 2024 [10] |
| 384- | 6,000 | Pancreatic cancer | Human/ Murine | Duan *et al.*, 2023 [11] |
| 96- | 139 | Colorectal cancer | Human | Luo *et al.*, 2023 [12] |
| 384- | 1,400 | Patient-derived intestinal organoids, cystic fibrosis | Human | de Poel *et al.*, 2023 [13] |
| 384- | 1,400 | Patient-derived intestinal organoids, cystic fibrosis | Human | Spelier *et al.*, 2023 [14] |
| Not reported | 29 | Gallbladder carcinoma | Human | Yuan *et al.*, 2022 [15] |
| 384- | 45 | Breast cancer | Human | Guillen *et al.*, 2022 [16] |
| 96- | 1,816 | Renal cell carcinoma | Human | Cao *et al.*, 2022 [17] |
| 384- | 238 | Liver organoid, drug-induced liver injury | Human | Shinozawa *et al.*, 2021 [18] |
| 96- | 141 | Breast cancer | Human/ Murine | Zhou *et al.*, 2021 [19] |
| 384- and 1536- | 10,240 | Colon cancer (KRASG12D) | Human | Du *et al.*, 2020 [20] |
| 384- | Not reported | Pluripotent stem cells lung organoid, COVID-19 | Human | Han *et al.*, 2020 [21] |
| 96- | 5,000 | Cardiac organoid, cardiovascular disease | Human | Mills *et al.*, 2019 [22] |
| 384- | Not reported | Head and neck squamous cell carcinoma | Human | Driehuis *et al.*, 2019 [23] |
| 384- and 1536- | 3,300 | Pancreatic cancer | Human | Hou *et al.*, 2018 [24] |
| 96- | 55 | Patient-derived organoids, gastrointestinal cancer | Human | Vlachogiannis *et al.*, 2018 [25] |

to maintain their form as an organoid. Matrix components include laminin, collagen IV, entactin, and heparan sulfate proteoglycans that may induce ECM signaling suitable for organoid formation. Currently, the most commonly used ECM for organoid culture is a soluble form of gelatinous protein mixture extracted from mouse Engelbreth-Holm-Swarm tumor tissue, which provides a natural ECM hydrogel that polymerizes at 37°C to form a reconstituted basement membrane. However, handling ECM for automated HTS operations presents challenges as it is supplied as frozen stock, stored at −80°C, maintains soluble form at cold temperatures (4°C), and solidifies easily while processing at room temperature. HTS requires robust assay platforms amendable to automation with minimal day-to-day or batch-to-batch variations. In an HTS setting, a liquid dispenser is generally used to automatically dispense cells or reagents into 384/1536-well plates. Most of the dispensers, e.g., the Multidrop Combi dispenser, use specialized dispensing tubing or cassettes. One end of the tubing is inserted into a conical tube containing cells or reagents and the other end with 8-channel pipetting tips that is attached into instrument in alignment with the Society for Biomolecular Screening standard plate dimensions for precisely dispensing into 96/384/1536-well plates. Due to the high viscosity of the soluble form of BME gel and its polymerization feature upon exposure to warm environment, such as room temperature, it is easy to block the dispensing tubing and tips, especially for low volume dispensing tubing (<10 μL). Dead volume is also required to fill up the tubing before dispensing into microplates. Therefore, an extra volume of at least 2 mL is normally required. The cost of BME gel or Matrigel and organoid culture medium is relatively high. Therefore, in order to enable 3D organoid screening using Matrigel or BME as a supporting matrix, miniaturization to achieve reduced volume and robust readouts is essential, yet challenging. Currently, testing has only been conducted at small scale, e.g. <100 compounds, as proof-of-concept to examine the response of 3D organoids in ECM to drugs [26–30]. Our procedure described in detail in this chapter represents a major advancement in culturing the organoids in a 3D matrix in 384-well and 1536-well plate format that enables HTS and uHTS campaign for early compound/drug screening.

Microscopy and imaging technologies are critical for monitoring organoid morphology in HTS assays. Image-based high-content screening systems are capable of capturing images of organoids in 384-well and 1536-well plates in an automated fashion, allowing for monitoring the growth of organoids, size, morphology, and cellular behavior.

Data analysis: The amount of data produced in organoid-based HTS requires sophisticated computational tools. Software like BREEZE, CellHTS2, and SynergyFinder are available commercially to facilitate HTS data analysis [31]; they can also be developed in-house, or using a Microsoft Excel add-on function.

HTS data analysis involves processing and interpreting the massive datasets generated during HTS to identify compounds with desired biological activity. This process includes data quality checks and identification of false positives. The goal is to identify "hits," which are compounds that show promising activity and can be further investigated in drug discovery. HTS data analysis usually includes: i) Data collection and preprocessing of "raw data" which is often in the form of spreadsheets such as Excel or .csv files. ii) Quality control of HTS. A large-scale HTS campaign usually runs at a single point, therefore the quality of the assay for each screening plate is evaluated using the "controls" in each screening plate. Controls (assay signal and background) without testing compounds are included in each screening plate by one column for each control, e.g., 16 replicates for 384-well plate and 32 replicates for 1536-well plate. HTS quality, such as well-to-well, plate-to-plate and day-to-day variations, is then evaluated by calculating the Z' factor based on the average and the standard derivation of the controls in each plate. A Z' value between 0.5 and 1 suggests the assay/plate is robust and reliable for evaluating the effect of screening compounds for HTS [32]. iii) Primary hit identification: a threshold, or hit cut-off, is set to define which compounds are considered as "hits" in a primary screening campaign.

Example HTS data analysis will be described in the following sections of this chapter.

## 6.4 Protocol for Miniaturizing the Organoids Culture into 384- and 1536-well Plate for High-Throughput Screening/ultra-High-Throughput Screening: Human Colon Organoids as an Example

In this protocol, we utilized genetically engineered organoids to model colorectal cancer with an oncogenic KRAS mutation as a model system for HTS and uHTS platform development [20]. KRAS mutations are amongst the most pervasive genetic alterations in human cancer [33]. Colorectal cancer is one of the most common cancers worldwide [34]. However, the direct therapeutic targeting of constitutively active mutant KRAS has proven challenging despite considerable efforts. Attempts to develop targeted therapies for this genomic subset of patients have been largely unsuccessful, although therapeutic targeting of KRASG12C tumors has now advanced to phase II clinical trials, offering much hope for patients [35]. Thus, establishing a screening platform to target cancers with KRAS mutations is expected to have significant implications.

The procedures described here can be applied to other organoid types. However, the culture medium may vary and should be optimized according to the specific organoid.

### 6.4.1 *Materials/Reagents and Organoids Culture Medium Preparation*

Materials: BME gel (Cultrex Reduced growth factor basement membrane extract, Type 2 (RGF BME-2), Cat. 3533-005-02) was purchased from Trevagen (Franklin Lakes, NJ, USA). Advanced DMEM/F12 medium, N2 supplement, B-27 supplement, HEPES, and GlutaMAX-I, Penicillin and streptomycin, G-418 and hygromycin B were obtained from Invitrogen (Carlsbad, CA, MA, USA). [Leu15]-Gastrin 1 Human, nicotinamide, N-acetylcysteine, human insulin, human transferrin and fetal bovine serum (FBS) were obtained from Sigma-Aldrich (St. Louis, MO, USA). A83-01 was acquired from R & D Systems Inc (Minneapolis, MN, USA). SB202190, Y-27632 and CHIR99021 were purchased from Cayman Chemical (Ann Arbor, Michigan, USA). FGF10 and EGF were purchased from PeproTech (Rocky Hill, New Jersey, USA). TrypLE express and phosphate-buffered saline (PBS) were obtained from Gibco-Thermo Fisher Scientific Inc.

WRN (Wnt3A, RSPO1, Noggin)-conditioned medium: prepared using L-WRN cells that were purchased from ATCC (CRL-3276). The L-WRN cells were derived by transfecting L-Wnt3A cells (ATCC CRL-2647) with an R-spondin 3 and noggin co-expressing vector. Briefly, the cells purchased from ATCC were recovered and cultured with Dulbecco's Modified Eagle's medium (ATCC, Cat. 30-2002) supplemented with 10% FBS, 0.5 mg/mL G-418 and 0.5 mg/mL hygromycin B. Once the cells reached confluence, they were sequentially split and cultured in T-150 flasks (25 mL cell suspension). Upon reaching confluence, the medium was collected by centrifugation (2,000 × g, 5 min) and stored at 4°C. This is the batch 1 of conditioned medium. The remaining cells in the T-150 flasks were continuously cultured by adding 25 mL of medium for 24 hours to repeat the process of collecting additional batches of conditioned medium, which are combined and stored in aliquots at –20°C before use.

Medium for human colon organoid culturing and passaging: the complete organoid culture medium was prepared, which includes the following components: advanced DMEM/F-12 Cell Culture Medium with 50% WRN-conditioned medium, HEPES (1 mM, pH 7.4), 1X glutamax, nicotinamine (10 mM), N-acetylcysteine (1 mM), 1X B27 supplement, 1X N2 supplement, [Leu15]-Gastrin I Human (10 nM), A83-01 (0.5 μM), SB 202190 (10 μM), human transferrin (7.5 μg/mL), human recombinant EGF (50 ng/mL), recombinant human FGF (100 ng/mL) and normocin (100 μg/mL).

Organoid starting/passing medium: prepared by adding Y-27632 (Rho kinase inhibitor; 10 μM) and CHIR 99021 (GSK-3 inhibitor; 2.5 μM) into complete organoid culture medium.

## 6.4.2 *Experimental Procedures*

Here we describe the detailed experimental procedures and tips for setting up a 3D organoid compound HTS, from recovery of organoids from frozen stock, to organoid culture expansion, to 3D organoid culture for compound screening in 384-well HTS and 1536-well uHTS format and HTS data analysis.

### 6.4.2.1 *Recovery of Organoids from Frozen Stock*

Human colon $KRAS^{G12D}$ organoids were generated by engineering normal colon tissue organoids and characterized as previously described [36].

1) The frozen organoids vials were thawed quickly in a 37°C water bath and washed 5 times using PBS (500 g × 5 min).

2) The cell pellets were then re-suspended in ice-cold BME gel and placed in the center of a 24-well plate (50 μL droplet/well).
3) After incubating at 37°C till the BME gel was solidified, organoid passaging medium (0.5 mL) was added to the wells.
4) The organoids were incubated in the cell culture incubator at 37°C with 5% $CO_2$.
5) The medium was replaced and refreshed with complete organoid culture medium every 3 days.

The example images of organoid growth and characterization are shown in Figure 6.1.

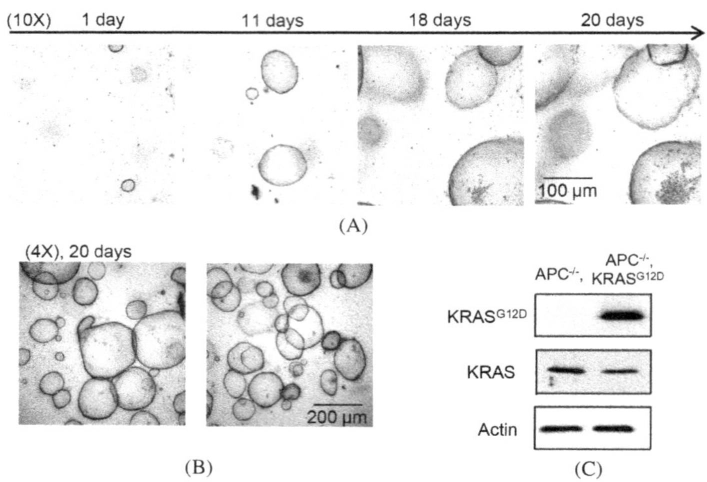


**Figure 6.1** Morphological evaluation and biochemical confirmation of human colon organoids from cryo-preserved frozen samples. (A) Recovered human colon APC-/-; KRASG12D organoids from frozen stocks. Frozen vials of organoids were thawed at 37°C, re-suspended in BME gel and plated into a 24-well plate as a 50 μL droplet per well. The medium was refreshed every 3–4 days. The growth of organoids was monitored with the ImageXpressmicro automated-imaging system (10× objective). (B) Robust growth of human colon APC-/-; KRASG12D organoids (4× objective). Representative images from two different wells of a 24-well plate are shown. All the images shown are merged images of Z-stack using ImageXpress software. (C) The KRASG12D protein expression of human colon APC-/-; KRASG12D organoids was confirmed using anti-KRASG12D antibody in comparison to that of APC-/-; KRASWT organoids. Organoids were collected for Western blot analysis with anti-KRASG12D specific antibody. Reproduced with permission from [20].

### 6.4.2.2 *Organoid Culture Expansion*

1) The organoids/BME gels growing in 24-well plates as described above were collected by pipetting and placed in a 15-mL conical tube.
2) The organoids/BME gels were washed with PBS once (1000 rpm, 5 min).
3) TrypLE express was added and incubated in a 37°C water bath for 15 min to dissociate the cells.
4) Trypsinization was stopped with FBS, and digested cell clusters were washed 3 times with PBS.

Tip: During the PBS washing, the tube containing cells in PBS was mixed well by inverting upside down for more than 5 times to dissociate the cells further mechanically.

5) The cell pellets were re-suspended in ice-cold BME gel at desired volume (normally 1:3 ratio splitting) and re-plated as 50 μL droplet per well in a 24-well plate.
6) The organoids were initially cultured with 0.5 mL/well passaging medium for 3 days after re-plating, then refreshed with 0.5 mL/well completed organoid culture medium every 3 days.

### 6.4.2.3 *3D Organoid Culture for Compound Screening in 384-well High-Throughput Screening and 1536-well Ultra-High-Throughput Screening Format*

The overall workflow is outlined in Figure 6.2 and is described in detail below.

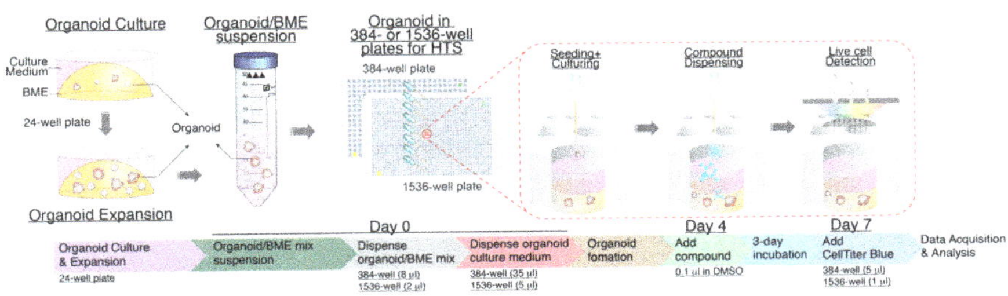


**Figure 6.2** Workflow of 3D organoid culture for compound screening in 384-well HTS and 1536-well uHTS formats. Reproduced with permission from [20].

#### 6.4.2.3.1 3D Organoid Culture for Compound Screening in 384-well High-Throughput Screening Format

***Step 1: Plating organoids into 384-well plate***

1) The organoids growing in a 24-well plate were harvested as described above and re-suspended in ice-cold BME gel to form the cells/BME gel mixture.
2) 8 μL per well of cell/BME gel mixture were dispensed into 384-well plates using multidrop Combi dispenser (Thermo Fisher Scientific).

Tip: to avoid the BME gel solidifying during dispensing, the dispensing cassette was pre-chilled at 4°C and the 50 mL conical tube containing cell/BME gel mixture was placed in ice during dispensing process.

3) The plates were immediately centrifuged at low speed, e.g., 300 × g for 1 min to ensure the uniform distribution of the cells/BME gel in the wells across the entire plate.

Tip: centrifugation also helps to remove any bubbles during dispensing.

4) After incubating the plates in a cell culture incubator for 30 min, 35 μL of warm completed organoid culture medium were dispensed to each well.
5) The plates were sealed with a gas-permeable plate sealer (Breathe-Easy Sealing Film, Diversified Biotech, Cat. #BEM-1) and incubated in the cell incubator.

***Step 2: Compound screening in 384-well HTS format***

1) Organoids plated and cultured in 384-well plates as described above were incubated for 3–5 days at 37°C to allow organoid formation.

Tip: check under microscope for organoid formation. Example images of organoids growing in 384-well plate are shown in Figure 6.3B.

2) Library compounds diluted in DMSO (0.1 μL) were added to each well using the pin-tool integrated with Beckman NX automated liquid handling system (Beckman Coulter, Danaher Corporation).

Tip: To avoid inserting the pin-tool into the cells/BME gel layer at the bottom of the well, the pin-tool dispense height was carefully optimized and set at the height

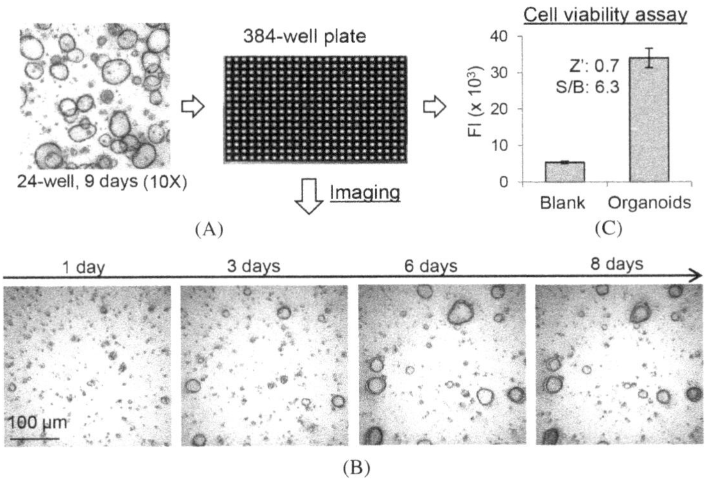


**Figure 6.3** Culturing of human colon organoids in a 384-well plate format. (A) Scheme for miniaturizing organoid culture in a 384-well plate. Organoids growing in BME gel in a 24-well plate were collected and re-suspended in ice-cold BME gel. A organoid cells/BME gel mixture (8 μL/well) was dispensed into a 384-well plate. After incubation for 30 min at 37°C, warm organoid culture medium (35 μL) was dispensed to each well. The plate was incubated for up to 8 days without replacing the medium. (B) The organoids growing in a 384-well plate were monitored using ImageXpress micro and showed progressing growth over the time. (C) The growth of organoids in the 384-well plate was quantified by CellTiter Blue cell viability assay and showed robust FI signals for HTS with Z' of 0.7 and S/B ratio of 6.3. Reproduced with permission from [20].

at which the bottom of the pin-tool was above the cells/BME gel layer but still inside the medium layer for accurate compound transfer.

(Note: The Emory Enriched Bioactive Library, which contains a total of 2,036 compounds, was used as an example for HTS. The collection includes the U.S. Food and Drug Administration (FDA)-approved and bioactive compounds with known activities, targeting more than 20 signaling pathways [37].)

3) The plates were centrifuged at 600 × g for 5 min to ensure uniform distribution of the compound into the wells. The final compound concentration was 4.6 μM and the final DMSO was 0.2%.
4) The plates were sealed with a gas-permeable plate sealer and incubated in the cell culture incubator.

***Step 3: Organoid viability assay in 384-well HTS format***

The viability of the organoids in the 384-well plate was determined by CellTiter Blue reagent (Promega, Madison, WI) at the end of the organoid culturing process.

1) After incubation with compounds for 3 days, the CellTiter Blue reagent (5 μL/well) was dispensed to each well and incubated at 37°C for 4 hours.
2) The fluorescence intensity (FI) was measured using the PHERAstar FSX multi-label plate reader (BMG LABTECH) with excitation at 540/20 nm and emission at 590/20 nm.

The growth of organoids in the 384-well plate was monitored using images and viability assay, with representative examples shown in Figures 6.3 and 6.5.

#### 6.4.2.3.2 3D Organoids Culture for Compound Screening in 1536-well ultra-High-Throughput Screening Format

Note: The procedures are similar to those of the 384-well plate as described above except volume (total volume of ~8 μL per well), which could be challenging for labs without HTS automation instruments.

***Step 1: Plating organoids into 1536-well plate***

1) Organoids growing in 24-well plates were harvested and mixed with ice-cold BME gel as described above.
2) 2 μL/well of cells/BME gel mixture (about 400 cells) were dispensed into a black wall clear bottom 1536-well plate (Corning Cat. 3893#) using Multidrop Combi dispenser.

Tip: The dispensing cassette was pre-chilled at 4°C and the cell/BME gel mixture was placed in ice during dispensing.

3) The plates were immediately centrifuged at low speed, e.g., 300 × g for 1 min to ensure uniform distribution of the cells/BME gel in the wells across the entire plate.

Tip: centrifugation also helps to remove any bubbles during dispensing.

4) After incubating the plate for 30 min to allow the BME gel to solidify, 5 μL warm organoid growth medium were dispensed to each well.
5) The plate was sealed with a gas-permeable sealer and incubated in a cell culture incubator.

***Step 2: Compound screening in 1536-well uHTS format***

1) Organoids plated and cultured in 1536-well plates as described above were incubated for 3–5 days at 37°C to allow organoid formation.

Tip: check under microscope for organoid formation as per example images in Figure 6.5A.

2) Library compounds diluted in DMSO (0.1 μL) were added to each well using the pin-tool integrated with Beckman NX automated liquid handling system (Beckman Coulter, Danaher Corporation).

Tip: To avoid inserting the pin-tool into the cells/BME gel layer at the bottom of the well, the pin-tool dispense height was carefully optimized and set at the height at which the bottom of the pin-tool was above the cells/BME gel layer while but still inside the medium layer for accurate compound transfer.

(Note: here we use screening with a diverse chemical library of 10,240 compounds in 1536-well format as an uHTS example as shown in Figure 6.5.)

3) The plates were centrifuged at 600 × g for 5 min to ensure uniform distribution of the compound into the wells.
4) The plates were sealed with a gas-permeable plate sealer and incubated in a cell culture incubator.

***Step 3: Organoid viability assay in 1536-well HTS format***

The viability of the organoids in 1536-well plate was determined by CellTiter Blue reagent (Promega, Madison, WI) at the end of the organoid culturing process.

1) After incubation with compounds for 3 days, the CellTiter Blue reagent (1 μL/well) was dispensed to each well and incubated at 37°C for 6 hours.

2) The FI was measured using the PHERAstar FSX multi-label plate reader (BMG LABTECH) with excitation at 540/20 nm and emission at 590/20 nm.

The growth of organoids in the 1536-well plate was monitored using images and viability assay as shown in Figure 6.5.

#### 6.4.2.4 *High-Throughput Screening/ultra-High-Throughput Screening Data Analysis*

Screening data were analyzed using the CambridgeSoft Bioassay software, or Microsoft Excel.

1) The performance of the organoid viability assay in the 384-well and 1536-well plates for HTS or uHTS, respectively, was evaluated by Z' factor and S/B ratio which were calculated by the following equations:

$$Z' = 1 - (3 \times SD_{\text{DMSO control}} + 3 \times SD_{\text{blank}}) / (FI_{\text{DMSO control}} - FI_{\text{blank}})$$

$$S/B = FI_{\text{DMSO control}} / FI_{\text{blank}}$$

where $SD_{\text{DMSO}}$ and $SD_{\text{blank}}$ are the standard deviations, and $FI_{\text{DMSO control}}$ and $FI_{\text{blank}}$ are the corresponding average FI signal for the wells with DMSO control or blank with medium only without cells, respectively.

While S/B is useful for describing the assay dynamic range, it does not incorporate the variability of the highest or lowest signals. An assay with a reasonable S/B value can still be of poor quality if the variability of either signal or both are high [38]. The Z' factor is considered the best metric to describe assay quality because it incorporates the mean values of both highest and lowest control signals as well as their variabilities. A Z' factor between 0.5 and 1.0 indicates that the assay is robust for HTS [32].

2) The effect of compounds on the growth of organoids was expressed as % of Control or % of Inhibition based on per plate and calculated as per the following equations:

$$\% \text{ of Control} = (FI_{\text{compound}} - FI_{\text{blank}}) / (FI_{\text{DMSO control}} - FI_{\text{blank}}) \times 100$$

$$\% \text{ of Inhibition} = 100 - \% \text{ of Control}$$

### 6.4.3 *Results*

Example screening data for 384-well HTS is shown in Figure 6.4 and for 1536-well uHTS in Figure 6.5. Organoids have exhibited similar growth in both the 384-well and 1536-well formats. Robust assay performance has been achieved in both HTS and uHTS format with Z' > 0.5 and S/B > 4.

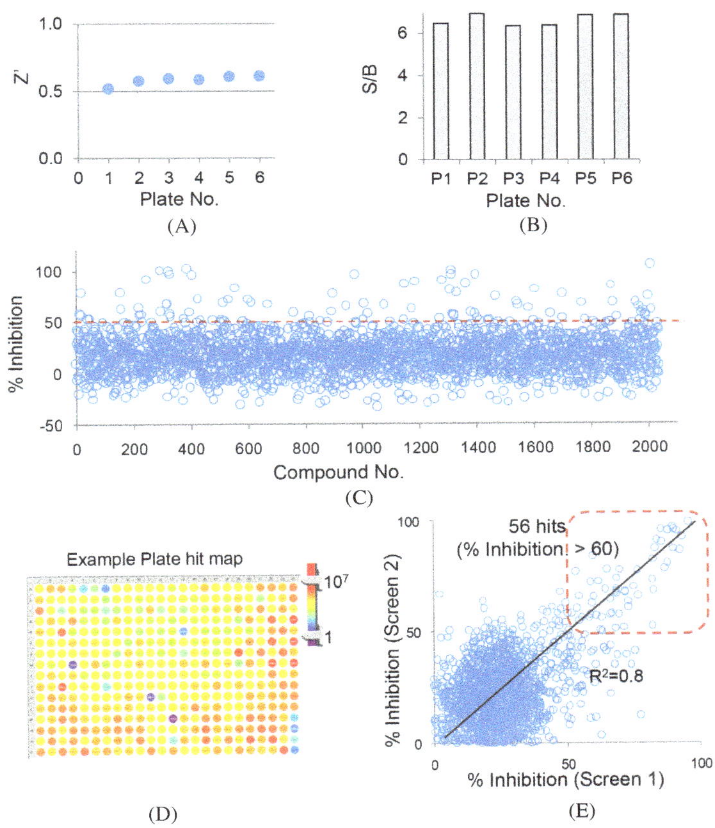


**Figure 6.4** Screening of the 2,036 Emory Enriched Bioactive Library compounds with the human colon organoids in a 384-well plate format. (A) Scatter plot of the HTS with human colon APC-/-; KRASG12D organoids. These organoids cultured in 384-well plates were treated with library compounds (0.1 μL, 4.6 μM final). The plates were incubated for 3 days and subjected to CellTiter Blue cell viability assay. The effect of compound on the growth of KRASG12D organoids were calculated as % of Inhibition based on per plate, analyzed using Cambridge BioAssay software. (B) Performance evaluation with Z' factors and (C) S/B across six 384-well screening plates. (D) An example plate hit map. (E) Correlation between two independent screens. Reproduced with permission from [20].

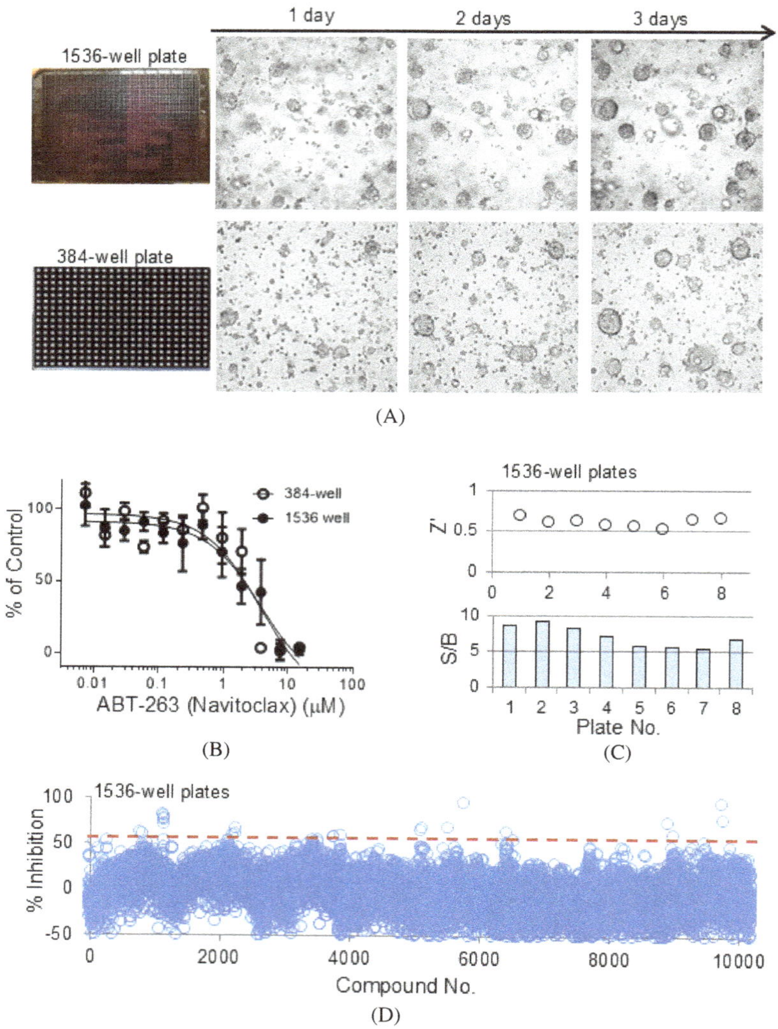


**Figure 6.5** Miniaturized 3D organoid assays in a 1536-well plate format for uHTS. (A) Growth comparison of human colon $APC^{-/-}$; $KRAS^{G12D}$ organoids in 1536- vs 384-well plates was shown. (B) The effect of compounds, ABT-263 as an example, exhibited very similar inhibitory effect on the growth of $APC^{-/-}$; $KRAS^{G12D}$ organoids between 384- and 1536-well plate formats. (C) Performance evaluation for the uHTS viability assay with organoids, showing Z' (> 0.5) and S/B (> 5) scores across the screening plates. (D) Scatter plot of primary screening of 10,240 diversity compound library in a 1536-well uHTS format. Screening data were analyzed using Cambridge BioAssay software. The effect of compounds on the growth of $APC^{-/-}$; $KRAS^{G12D}$ organoids were calculated as % Inhibition per plate. Reproduced with permission from [20].

In summary, our application of the HTS viability assay with KRASG12D-carrying 3D organoids described here was validated in a pilot screen of 2,036 FDA-approved and bioactive compounds (Figure 6.4). To further increase the throughput, after optimization, we have successfully miniaturized our 3D organoid culture into a 1536-well uHTS format (Figure 6.5). The robustness and assay performance of the miniaturized uHTS viability assay for screening were assessed by a 10,240 compound screen. Combining the power of primary organoids with a defined genetic background and advanced HTS technologies, the miniaturized 3D organoid culture platform provides an enabling technology to accelerate basic and translational research using physiologically relevant disease models.

## 6.5 Organoids for Target Identification and Validation

Organoids have a unique position in target identification. Like traditional 2D cell culture, organoids are easily amenable to genetic modulation or to disease-relevant environmental exposures but have the added advantages of cell heterogeneity and 3D cultures such as cell-cell and ECM interactions and soluble factor gradients more similar to *in vivo* models which are not so easily manipulated. Generation of *in vitro* models also requires extensive knowledge of disease biology, which may not be available for disease in early stages of research. Organoids developed from human cells can also fill the gap where *in vitro* models do not adequately recapitulate human biology and/or disease [39, 40]. Moreover, given the ability of source cells to proliferate, these qualities allow disease state and disease progress to be modeled at large scale. Combing high-throughput capabilities with organoid culture provides a powerful system to study and modulate biological processes across many conditions [41–43]. Since organoid model systems can be reproduced across research groups, studies can be replicated and built upon each other with a common background. Possible therapeutic targets can then be discovered by either analyzing expression changes of targets in cases versus control organoids [44] or by modulating potential targets, such as through knockdown or overexpression screens, and detecting changes in phenotype of organoids [45]. Through cultivation of organoids, researchers can model biology in human cells where *in vivo* models fail, monitor response to stimuli and disease progress in real time and across time, expand testing for rare diseases or where clinical samples are limited, and identify key regulators of disease biology at large scale.

CRISPR/Cas9 screens, in which large portions of the genome are knocked down or overexpressed in CRISPR/Cas9 expressing eukaryotic cells with pools of targeted gRNA before monitoring phenotypic changes, have become a critical tool in target and drug discovery [45–48]. Combining CRISPR screens with organoid technology can be a powerful tool for target and drug discovery [49]. Such a system is demonstrated through the work of Berlind *et al.* who have developed a neural organoid model to identify key regulators of neuronal excitotoxicity in tauopathy patient organoids [50]. Taking advantage of key traits of organoids — the study of multiple interacting cell types and application of exogenous disease modulators, Berlind *et al.* created and then treated human-induced pluripotent stem cell (hiPSC)-derived cortical organoids, containing a mix of deep- and superficial-layer neurons, radial glia, and astrocytes [51, 52] with the excitatory neurotransmitter glutamate. Response to treatment was gauged by cell survival through expression of reporter construct Synapsin1::eGFP and oligomeric tau production. This model was taken a step further by enriching for neurons using the established NGN2 overexpression system [53] in an iPSC line stably expressing dCas9-BFP-KRAB [54] before transduction with a genome-wide lentiviral single-guide RNA (sgRNA) library. As these neuron-enriched cultures contained only neuronal cell types, they are considered spheroids but were able to recapitulate the neurotoxicity behaviors seen in the mixed-cell type organoids and contain diverse neuronal cell types. Several enriched gene targets were then identified by next-generation sequencing. In this case, enrichment suggests that knockdown of a given gene improved survival of glutamate-treated neurons. In this manner, several top regulators were identified and then validated with treatment by targeted anti-sense oligomers in organoids. Organoids were also generated by Berlind *et al.* containing tau protein alterations including *MAPT* gene knockout or the neurodegenerative *MAPT* V337M mutation, disease-relevant modulations much easier accomplished in a cell culture model than in an *in vitro* model. To further elucidate the mechanism by which KCTD20 effects excitatory neuron toxicity in a pathological tau context, single-cell RNA-seq was performed on the tau V337M mutant organoids following glutamate treatment in the presence or absence of addition of a KCTD20 anti-sense oligomer to abrogate KCTD20 expression. Several genes and pathways, exocytosis in particular, were identified as downstream targets of KCTD20 and potential areas for future therapeutic targeting. This organoid model offers a unique opportunity to model excitotoxicity in health and disease context and novel approaches to limit subsequent neurodegeneration.

Brain organoids have been especially amenable to solving gaps in experimental techniques. The study of brain processes has been limited by the difficulty of acquiring biological samples and replicating the complexity of the human brain, but pluripotent stem cells under the right culture conditions generate brain organoids that recreate the cellular heterogeneity and complex intercellular networks, signaling, extracellular matrices, and spatial networks [43, 55–58]. In a self-organizing process, neurons form the initial neural network. Further specialization of brain regions or cell types is possible with the addition of other external factors. As such, these organoids also offer the advantage of studying selected cell types in isolation while maintaining targeted heterogeneity and 3D culture context. Lai *et al.* developed an organoid model for traumatic brain injury which addresses gaps in previously used models that include the inability to study brain intrinsic mechanisms over secondary insults, injury susceptibility across different neuronal subtypes, and failure to identify therapeutic approaches by large-scale screens [59]. Human iPSC-derived cortical organoids were developed that contained multiple brain cell types including deep- and upper-layer cortical neurons and astrocytes [51]. High-intensity focused ultrasound (HIFU) was applied to the organoids to mimic a severe primary brain injury, and this injury model recapitulated key traumatic brain injury-related clinical and post-mortem biomarkers [60] and pathological changes, including neuronal death, tau phosphorylation, and TDP-43 proteinopathy. Moreover, neuronal cell death was monitored through expression of a SYN1::EGFP lentiviral reporter which labels excitatory neurons. Single-cell RNA sequencing was performed on sham and HIFU-treated organoids. The transcriptional profiles of injured deep-layer excitatory neurons were enriched in pathways involved in neurodegenerative diseases such as amyotrophic lateral sclerosis. As described in Berlind *et al.*, spheroids enriched for neuronal cell types were developed and transduced with a genome-wide lentiviral sgRNA library. Proteins with mechanosensitive ion channel activity were strongly enriched from the sgRNAs protective of HIFU injury. KCNJ2, an inward-rectifying potassium channel, was a top hit. KCNJ2 expression and activity was reduced in organoids by employing CRISPRi, antisense oligomers, and chemical inhibitors. The inhibition of KCNJ2 mitigated the effects of HIFU-induced injury, providing a neuron-specific therapeutic pathway for treatment of traumatic brain injury.

The expansion of large-scale omics studies in which genetic and expression (transcripts and proteins) of biological samples are comprehensively assessed has greatly broadened the target discovery field across disease types [44, 60, 61]. While rare diseases are by definition infrequent in occurrence, the many number of rare diseases means an overall impact to approximately 10% of the human population [62]. Drug discovery and target identification in rare diseases is challenged by the high cost combined with low market share and difficulty in obtaining subjects for clinical trials [63–65]. Given their reproducibility, scalability, and cost efficiency, organoids can fill the gap in availability of limited clinical samples and clinically relevant models to study rare diseases [66]. Kawaski *et al.* established a biobank of gastroenteropancreatic (GEP) neuroendocrine neoplasm (NEN) organoids [67]. GEP-NEN is a rare cancer type, and indeed only 39 fresh clinical samples were able to be collected by this group over five years. Expansion of these organoids permitted in-depth multi-omics analyses including whole-genome sequencing, RNA sequencing, methylation microarray analysis, and assay for transposase-accessible chromatin using sequencing. Based on the results of these analyses, Kawaski *et al.* were able to recapitulate the GEP-NEN biology from normal colonic organoids, providing another model for the study of GEP-NEN. The multi-omics study of GEP-NEN organoids identified key regulators and potential therapeutic targets of subtypes of this cancer. Use of organoid culture from rare disease backgrounds can establish new targets and extend our capabilities to study these diseases.

Because of the feasibility of genetic and environmental modulation as well as the collection of data across multiple time points, organoid cultures are ideal for studying disease progress. Organoids can be used to study cell behavior over time following a disease stimulus or even model aging [68, 69]. Wang *et al.* were able to develop the Laboratory Engineered Glioblastoma-like Organoid (LEGO) [70]. A core set of tumor suppressors were knocked out with the CRISPR/Cas9 system in normal human-derived iPSCs in spectrum of loss-of-function mutation combinations before differentiating cells by a cerebral organoid protocol that generates heterogeneous neural cell populations and maintains differentiation hierarchies. By using multiple mutation combinations in an isogenic background, tumorigenic heterogeneity could be modeled in this study. DNA methylome, metabolome, lipidome, proteome, and phospho-proteome analysis of these LEGOs across timepoints further expanded the utility of this model by allowing for study of disease progression that is unobtainable through *in vivo* models. This temporal multi-omics analysis of multiple tumor-driving genes connects genetic diversity to observed phenotypic heterogeneity and maps the timeline of molecular changes in glioblastoma multiforme. Each of these molecular changes is an opportunity for therapeutic targeting. In fact, Wang *et al.* identified possible actionable targets with a drug-gene interaction database across different LEGO subgroups. The predictions held when testing compounds across LEGO subgroups/genotypes. This work provides proof of principle that engineered organoids are suitable for target discovery.

## 6.6 Challenges and Future Perspectives

Despite significant progress, several challenges remain in the implementation of organoid-based HTS, presenting important areas for future development:

Standardization

A key challenge in organoid-based HTS is the lack of standardized protocols. Differences in culture conditions, organoid size, and assay readouts can result in variability and hinder reproducibility across studies and laboratories. Establishing universally accepted protocols and quality control measures is critical to ensure consistent and reliable outcomes. Future efforts should focus on developing standardized guidelines for organoid generation, characterization, and assay execution to facilitate cross-study comparisons and regulatory acceptance.

Scalability

Scaling up organoid production to meet the demands of large-scale HTS campaigns remains technically challenging. The process often requires highly skilled personnel and meticulous optimization, limiting throughput and increasing operational complexity. Advances in automation, bioreactor technologies, and microfluidic platforms hold promise for improving scalability and reducing the dependence on manual expertise, paving the way for broader adoption in drug discovery pipelines.

Model Complexity

While organoids successfully recapitulate many structural and functional aspects of native tissues, they still lack certain physiological features, such as full vascularization and interactions with immune cells and other stromal components. Incorporating additional cellular components, engineering vascularized or immune-competent organoid models, and integrating organ-on-chip technologies represent important future directions to enhance the physiological relevance and translational potential of organoid-based assays.

In summary, addressing these challenges through technological innovation, standardization, and model refinement will be essential to fully realize the potential of organoid-based HTS in drug discovery and personalized medicine.

## Key Opinion Points

1. 3D organoids, as physiologically relevant models for screening, are highly preferred over 2D cell cultures to enhance the success and translational potential of HTS-driven drug discovery efforts.
2. Organoid-based screening platforms as a new generation of physiologically relevant models are expected to bridge the gap between traditional 2D cultures and *in vivo* mouse models to facilitate drug discovery and personalized medicine.
3. Even though optimizing conditions to enable scale-up of organoid culture will be valuable, miniaturization of the 3D organoid culturing system to a 1536-well format will not only enable screening a large number of chemicals with a limited number of organoids, but also will drastically reduce the cost of large-scale screening.
4. The use of genetically transformed oncogene mutation organoids derived from primary wild-type organoids has numerous advantages over transformed cell lines. The primary wild-type organoids maintain native differentiation and 3D tissue architecture and allow oncogene mutant-targeting screening to be performed in well-defined human genetic backgrounds devoid of confounding mutations, which commonly occur in long-term passaging of 2D cancer cell lines.
5. For our organoid cultures, we used Cultrex® Reduced growth factor BME as supporting ECM, which is processed to reduce matrix-associated growth factors and provide a defined model system for organoid culture. BME has been used successfully for supporting many tissues or tumor-derived organoid culture as a 3D scaffold [28, 77, 78]. However, we do not expect technical challenges with using other types of ECM, such as Matrigel.

6. Reduced volume in 384-/1536-well format allows cost-saving for expensive BME or other ECM matrix and organoid culture medium.
7. The established protocols for miniaturized 3D organoid culture described in this chapter in 384- and 1536-well formats could be adapted for other types of organoids. However, success of adapting organoids culture into HTS format requires personnel who are familiar and skilled with HTS automation instrumentation.

## Acknowledgments

We thank members of the Fu lab and the Emory Chemical Biology Discovery Center for their helpful discussions and support.

## Funding

This research was supported by NCI's Cancer Target Discovery and Development (CTD[2]) Network (grant number: 1U01CA217875 to Fu, H and 1U01CA217851 to Kuo, C), the RAS Synthetic Lethal Network (RSLN) (grant number: 1U01CA199241-01 to Kuo, C), the Emory-Sage-SGC-Jax TREAT-AD (NIA U54AG065187 supporting E.L.Z.) and Emory Lung Cancer SPORE (NIH P50CA217691), Winship Cancer Institute (NIH 5P30CA138292) and Emory WHSC 10X Single Cell Sequencing Seed Grant (X.M. & Y.D.).

## References

1. Zimmermann J, *et al.* Phenylamino-pyrimidine (PAP) — derivatives: a new class of potent and highly selective PDGF-receptor autophosphorylation inhibitors. Bioorg Med Chem Lett. 1996;6(11):1221–1226.
2. Zimmermann J, Buchdunger E, Mett H, Meyer T, Lydon NB. Potent and selective inhibitors of the Abl-kinase: phenylamino-pyrimidine (PAP) derivatives. Bioorg Med Chem Lett. 1997;7(2):187–192.
3. Dorr P, *et al.* Maraviroc (UK-427,857), a potent, orally bioavailable, and selective small-molecule inhibitor of chemokine receptor CCR5 with broad-spectrum anti-human immunodeficiency virus type 1 activity. Antimicrob Agents Chemother. 2005;49(11): 4721–4732.
4. Wood A, Armour D. The discovery of the CCR5 receptor antagonist, UK-427,857, a new agent for the treatment of HIV infection and AIDS. Prog Med Chem. 2005;43:239–271.

5. Pedemonte N, *et al.* Small-molecule correctors of defective DeltaF508-CFTR cellular processing identified by high-throughput screening. J Clin Invest. 2005;115(9):2564–2571.
6. Li J, Zhang S, Gao L, Chen Y, Xie X. A Cell-Based High-Throughput Assay for the Screening of Small-Molecule Inhibitors of p53–MDM2 Interaction. SLAS Discov. 2011;16(6):450–456.
7. Wang S, Wang Z, Fang L, Lv Y, Du G. Advances of the Target-Based and Phenotypic Screenings and Strategies in Drug Discovery. Int J Drug Discov Pharmacol. 2022;1(1):2.
8. Oishi H, Tabibzadeh N, Morizane R. Advancing preclinical drug evaluation through automated 3D imaging for high-throughput screening with kidney organoids. Biofabrication. 2024;16(3).
9. Rao X, *et al.* Unveiling Epigenetic Vulnerabilities in Triple-Negative Breast Cancer through 3D Organoid Drug Screening. Pharmaceuticals (Basel). 2024;17(4).
10. Ortiz Jordan LM, *et al.* Protocol for high throughput 3D drug screening of patient derived melanoma and renal cell carcinoma. SLAS Discov. 2024;29:100141.
11. Duan X, *et al.* A pancreatic cancer organoid platform identifies an inhibitor specific to mutant KRAS. Cell Stem Cell. 2024;31(1):71–88.e78.
12. Luo Z, *et al.* Establishment of a large-scale patient-derived high-risk colorectal adenoma organoid biobank for high-throughput and high-content drug screening. BMC Med. 2023;21:336.
13. de Poel E, *et al.* FDA-approved drug screening in patient-derived organoids demonstrates potential of drug repurposing for rare cystic fibrosis genotypes. J Cyst Fibros. 2023;22(4):548–559.
14. Spelier S, *et al.* High-throughput functional assay in cystic fibrosis patient-derived organoids allows drug repurposing. ERJ Open Res. 2023;9(2).
15. Yuan B, *et al.* Patient-derived organoids for personalized gallbladder cancer modelling and drug screening. Clin Transl Med. 2022;12(2):e678.
16. Guillen KP, *et al.* A human breast cancer-derived xenograft and organoid platform for drug discovery and precision oncology. Nat Cancer. 2022;3(2):232–250.
17. Cao C, *et al.* Phenotypical screening on metastatic PRCC-TFE3 fusion translocation renal cell carcinoma organoids reveals potential therapeutic agents. Clin Transl Oncol. 2022;24(7):1333–1346.
18. Shinozawa T, *et al.* High-Fidelity Drug-Induced Liver Injury Screen Using Human Pluripotent Stem Cell-Derived Organoids. Gastroenterology. 2021;160(3):831–846.e10.
19. Zhou Z, *et al.* An organoid-based screen for epigenetic inhibitors that stimulate antigen presentation and potentiate T-cell-mediated cytotoxicity. Nat Biomed Eng. 2021;5(12):1320–1335.

20. Du Y, *et al.* Development of a miniaturized 3D organoid culture platform for ultra-high-throughput screening. J Mol Cell Biol. 2020;12(8):630–643.
21. Han Y, *et al.* Identification of SARS-CoV-2 inhibitors using lung and colonic organoids. Nature. 2021;589(7841):270–275.
22. Mills RJ, *et al.* Drug Screening in Human PSC-Cardiac Organoids Identifies Pro-proliferative Compounds Acting via the Mevalonate Pathway. Cell Stem Cell. 2019; 24(6):895–907.e6.
23. Driehuis E, *et al.* Oral Mucosal Organoids as a Potential Platform for Personalized Cancer Therapy. Cancer Discov. 2019;9(7):852–871.
24. Hou S, *et al.* Advanced Development of Primary Pancreatic Organoid Tumor Models for High-Throughput Phenotypic Drug Screening. SLAS Discov. 2018;23(6):574–584.
25. Vlachogiannis G, *et al.* Patient-derived organoids model treatment response of metastatic gastrointestinal cancers. Science. 2018;359(6378):920–926.
26. Gao D, *et al.* Organoid cultures derived from patients with advanced prostate cancer. Cell. 2014;159(1):176–187.
27. van de Wetering M, *et al.* Prospective derivation of a living organoid biobank of colorectal cancer patients. Cell. 2015;161(4):933–945.
28. Sachs N, *et al.* A Living Biobank of Breast Cancer Organoids Captures Disease Heterogeneity. Cell. 2018;172(1–2):373–386.e10.
29. Li L, *et al.* Human primary liver cancer organoids reveal intratumor and interpatient drug response heterogeneity. JCI Insight. 2019;4(2).
30. Schutte M, *et al.* Molecular dissection of colorectal cancer in pre-clinical models identifies biomarkers predicting sensitivity to EGFR inhibitors. Nat Commun. 2017;8:14262.
31. Nunes C, *et al.* HTSplotter: An end-to-end data processing, analysis and visualisation tool for chemical and genetic in vitro perturbation screening. PLoS One. 2024;19(1):e0296322.
32. Zhang JH, Chung TD, Oldenburg KR. A Simple Statistical Parameter for Use in Evaluation and Validation of High Throughput Screening Assays. J Biomol Screen. 1999;4(2):67–73.
33. Wood LD, *et al.* The genomic landscapes of human breast and colorectal cancers. Science. 2007;318(5853):1108–1113.
34. Ferlay J, *et al.* Cancer incidence and mortality worldwide: sources, methods and major patterns in GLOBOCAN 2012. Int J Cancer. 2015;136(5):E359–E386.
35. Canon J, *et al.* The clinical KRAS(G12C) inhibitor AMG 510 drives anti-tumour immunity. Nature. 2019;575(7781):217–223.
36. Ootani A, *et al.* Sustained in vitro intestinal epithelial culture within a Wnt-dependent stem cell niche. Nat Med. 2009;15(6):701–706.

37. Mo X, *et al.* HTiP: High-Throughput Immunomodulator Phenotypic Screening Platform to Reveal IAP Antagonists as Anti-cancer Immune Enhancers. Cell Chem Biol. 2019;26(3):331–339.e3.
38. Markossian S, *et al.*, eds. Assay Guidance Manual. Bethesda (MD): Eli Lilly & Company and the National Center for Advancing Translational Sciences; 2004.
39. Kim J, Koo BK, Knoblich JA. Human organoids: model systems for human biology and medicine. Nat Rev Mol Cell Biol. 2020;21(10):571–584.
40. Lee SY, Koo IS, Hwang HJ, Lee DW. In Vitro three-dimensional (3D) cell culture tools for spheroid and organoid models. SLAS Discov. 2023;28(1):119–137.
41. Ryoo H, Kimmel H, Rondo E, Underhill GH. Advances in high throughput cell culture technologies for therapeutic screening and biological discovery applications. Bioeng Transl Med. 2024;9(3):e10627.
42. Eglen RM, Reisine T. Human iPS Cell-Derived Patient Tissues and 3D Cell Culture Part 1: Target Identification and Lead Optimization. SLAS Technol. 2019;24(1):3–17.
43. Eglen RM, Reisine T. Human iPS Cell-Derived Patient Tissues and 3D Cell Culture Part 2: Spheroids, Organoids, and Disease Modeling. SLAS Technol. 2019;24(1):18–27.
44. Jose A, *et al.* Integration of pan-omics technologies and three-dimensional in vitro tumor models: an approach toward drug discovery and precision medicine. Mol Cancer. 2024;23:50.
45. Hosseini SA, *et al.* CRISPR/Cas9 as precision and high-throughput genetic engineering tools in gastrointestinal cancer research and therapy. Int J Biol Macromol. 2022;223(Pt A):732–754.
46. Shalem O, *et al.* Genome-scale CRISPR-Cas9 knockout screening in human cells. Science. 2014;343(6166):84–87.
47. Wang T, Wei JJ, Sabatini DM, Lander ES. Genetic screens in human cells using the CRISPR-Cas9 system. Science. 2014;343(6166):80–84.
48. Behan FM, *et al.* Prioritization of cancer therapeutic targets using CRISPR-Cas9 screens. Nature. 2019;568(7753):511–516.
49. Mukhare R, *et al.* Integration of Organoids With CRISPR Screens: A Narrative Review. Biol Cell. 2025;117:e70006.
50. Berlind JE, *et al.* KCTD20 suppression mitigates excitotoxicity in tauopathy patient organoids. Neuron. 2025;S0896-6273(25)00415-9. [Epub ahead of print]
51. Paşca AM, *et al.* Functional cortical neurons and astrocytes from human pluripotent stem cells in 3D culture. Nat Methods. 2015;12(7):671–678.
52. Gordon A, *et al.* Long-term maturation of human cortical organoids matches key early postnatal transitions. Nat Neurosci. 2021;24(3):331–342.

53. Lin HC, *et al.* NGN2 induces diverse neuron types from human pluripotency. Stem Cell Reports. 2021;16(9):2118–2127.
54. Tian R, *et al.* CRISPR Interference-Based Platform for Multimodal Genetic Screens in Human iPSC-Derived Neurons. Neuron. 2019;104(2):239–255.e12.
55. Zhao Y, Wang T, Liu J, Wang Z, Lu Y. Emerging brain organoids: 3D models to decipher, identify and revolutionize brain. Bioact Mater. 2025;47:378–402.
56. Kanton S, *et al.* Organoid single-cell genomic atlas uncovers human-specific features of brain development. Nature. 2019;574(7778):418–422.
57. Lancaster MA, *et al.* Cerebral organoids model human brain development and microcephaly. Nature. 2013;501(7467):373–379.
58. Maisumu G, *et al.* Brain organoids: building higher-order complexity and neural circuitry models. Trends Biotechnol. 2025;S0167-7799(25)00120-4. [Epub ahead of print]
59. Lai JD, *et al.* KCNJ2 inhibition mitigates mechanical injury in a human brain organoid model of traumatic brain injury. Cell Stem Cell. 2024;31(4):519–536.e8.
60. Matthews H, Hanison J, Nirmalan N. "Omics"-Informed Drug and Biomarker Discovery: Opportunities, Challenges and Future Perspectives. Proteomes. 2016;4(3):28.
61. Paananen J, Fortino V. An omics perspective on drug target discovery platforms. Brief Bioinform. 2020;21(6):1937–1953.
62. The Lancet Diabetes. Spotlight on rare diseases. Lancet Diabetes Endocrinol. 2019;7(2):75.
63. Yates N, Hinkel J. The economics of moonshots: Value in rare disease drug development. Clin Transl Sci. 2022;15(4):809–812.
64. Yoo HW. Development of orphan drugs for rare diseases. Clin Exp Pediatr. 2024;67(7): 315–327.
65. Mellerio JE. The challenges of clinical trials in rare diseases. Br J Dermatol. 2022;187(4): 453–454.
66. Parvatam S, *et al.* Human-based complex in vitro models: their promise and potential for rare disease therapeutics. Front Cell Dev Biol. 2025;13:1526306.
67. Kawasaki K, *et al.* An Organoid Biobank of Neuroendocrine Neoplasms Enables Genotype-Phenotype Mapping. Cell. 2020;183(5):1420–1435.e21.
68. Torrens-Mas M, *et al.* Organoids: An Emerging Tool to Study Aging Signature across Human Tissues. Modeling Aging with Patient-Derived Organoids. Int J Mol Sci. 2021;22(11):6022.
69. Verstegen MMA, *et al.* Clinical applications of human organoids. Nat Med. 2025;31(3): 409–421.
70. Wang C, *et al.* A multidimensional atlas of human glioblastoma-like organoids reveals highly coordinated molecular networks and effective drugs. NPJ Precis Oncol. 2024;8:19.

71. Weaver VM, *et al.* beta4 integrin-dependent formation of polarized three-dimensional architecture confers resistance to apoptosis in normal and malignant mammary epithelium. Cancer Cell. 2002;2(3):205–216.
72. Kim M, *et al.* Patient-derived lung cancer organoids as in vitro cancer models for therapeutic screening. Nat Commun. 2019;10:3991.
73. Castellon EA. Patient-derived organoids: New co-clinical model to predict treatment response in cancer? Oral Dis. 2019;25(4):928–930.
74. Yang H, Sun L, Liu M, Mao Y. Patient-derived organoids: a promising model for personalized cancer treatment. Gastroenterol Rep (Oxf). 2018;6(4):243–245.
75. Drost J, Clevers H. Organoids in cancer research. Nat Rev Cancer. 2018;18(7):407–418.
76. Li X, *et al.* Oncogenic transformation of diverse gastrointestinal tissues in primary organoid culture. Nat Med. 2014;20(7):769–777.
77. Crespo M, *et al.* Colonic organoids derived from human induced pluripotent stem cells for modeling colorectal cancer and drug testing. Nat Med. 2017;23(7):878–884.
78. Suzuki K, *et al.* Single cell analysis of Crohn's disease patient-derived small intestinal organoids reveals disease activity-dependent modification of stem cell properties. J Gastroenterol. 2018;53(9):1035–1047.

https://doi.org/10.1142/9789819817597_0007

Chapter 7

# Patient-Derived Organoids and Personalized Medicine

Xiaoxiao Wang[1,†], Yufei Wang[1,†], Le Cheng[1], Zhaowu Ma[1,2], Xiaoguang Chen[1,*], Louis Zizhao Wang[3,4]

[1]*School of Basic Medicine, Health Science Center, Yangtze University, Jingzhou 434023, China*

[2]*International Science and Technology Cooperation Base for Molecular Pharmacology of Anticancer Natural Drugs in Hubei, Yangtze University, Jingzhou 434023, China*

[3]*Department of Gastroenterology and Hepatology, Changi General Hospital, Singapore 529889, Singapore*

[4]*SingHealth Duke-NUS Academic Medical Centre, Singapore 168582, Singapore*

**Abstract:** As a malignant disease with extremely high heterogeneity, cancer treatment has long been confronted with core challenges such as "significant inter-individual differences in treatment efficacy, high risk of ineffective treatment, and difficulty in controlling toxic and side effects". Patient-derived cancer organoids (PDOs) — 3D mini-tumors cultured from patients' biopsy samples — have brought revolutionary breakthroughs to personalized oncology research by virtue of their advantage in accurately recapitulating the biological characteristics of tumors. This chapter emphasizes the crucial role of PDOs in predicting the efficacy of chemotherapy, targeted therapy, immunotherapy, radiotherapy, and emerging treatments. By simulating tumor heterogeneity and dynamic changes during treatment, PDOs provide preclinical research support for the optimization of treatment strategies, dosage adjustment, and drug resistance analysis. Research evidence covering a variety of cancer types shows that these organoids can facilitate the formulation of individualized treatment plans, improve treatment outcomes, and reduce toxic reactions. Although there are still challenges in standardization at present, PDOs are expected to transform the

[*]Corresponding author. Email: chen_xg@yangtzeu.edu.cn
[†]These authors contributed equally to this work.

development landscape of precision oncology by bridging laboratory research and clinical application, and promote the advancement of personalized cancer diagnosis and treatment.

**Keywords:** personalized therapy, patient-derived organoids, targeted therapies, immunotherapy, chemotherapy, radiotherapy, neoadjuvant therapy

## Key Points

1. Patient-derived organoids overcome the limitations of conventional models (like cell lines and patient-derived xenografts) by preserving patient-specific genetic backgrounds, tumor heterogeneity, and microenvironment components. This enables a more accurate *in vitro* platform for evaluating individual patient responses to diverse therapies, directly supporting personalized treatment strategy customization.
2. Patient-derived organoids allow for the modeling of dose-response relationships specific to an individual's tumor. This capability facilitates the preclinical determination of optimal therapeutic dosages for various modalities (targeted therapy, chemo, radio, etc.), enabling the development of truly personalized and potentially more effective treatment regimens before clinical application.
3. By faithfully recapitulating the phenotypic, genetic, and transcriptomic features of the original tumor, including its microenvironment, patient-derived organoids serve as powerful tools for investigating the fundamental mechanisms of cancer. This includes elucidating therapeutic targets, signaling pathway dysregulation, immune evasion tactics, and resistance mechanisms, thereby accelerating the development of novel and more effective therapeutic approaches.

## 7.1 Introduction

Personalized medicine has become a fundamental pillar of modern oncology, focusing on tailoring treatment strategies according to the unique characteristics of each patient's disease. However, tumor heterogeneity — both intra- and inter-tumoral — remains a significant challenge in cancer therapy. Conventional models, such as cell lines and animal models, often fail to fully recapitulate the complexity of human tumors, resulting in suboptimal predictions of treatment responses. In recent years, patient-derived organoids (PDOs) have emerged as a promising platform to address this gap. Unlike traditional "one-size-fits-all" approaches, PDO models facilitate the advancement of personalized medicine by comprehensively incorporating patient-specific genetic backgrounds, tumor heterogeneity, and dynamic treatment responses [1]. In clinical practice, effective disease management necessitates accounting for interpatient variability and implementing dynamic adjustments to drug dosages or therapeutic strategies based on individual treatment responses. However, prior to clinical application, compounds must undergo rigorous preclinical evaluation. Traditional preclinical models, such as 2D cell lines and patient-derived xenografts (PDXs), are constrained by significant limitations: 2D cultures lack critical tumor microenvironment components, while PDX models exhibit inherent immune deficiencies. These shortcomings impede drug development progress. As an innovative 3D *in vitro* research model, organoids exhibit rapid growth and stable differentiation capabilities. Compared to 2D cell lines and PDX models, PDOs maintain phenotypic and genetic heterogeneity consistent with their source tissues, enabling the identification of patient-specific genomic, epigenetic, and transcriptomic variations [2]. Furthermore, the strong concordance in drug response profiles between PDOs and their corresponding primary tumors allows for continuous assessment of therapeutic efficacy and prospective prediction of treatment outcomes [3–5]. This approach not only reduces potential drug side effects but also helps avoid unnecessary treatments, thereby improving therapeutic outcomes and patient quality of life [6–8]. PDOs thus present significant opportunities for applications in personalized medicine (Figure 7.1), with their research applications summarized in Table 7.1.

Focusing on PDOs, this chapter addresses their increasingly pivotal role in personalized cancer therapy, particularly within key modalities: targeted therapy, radiotherapy, immunotherapy, chemotherapy, and neoadjuvant therapy. PDOs offer a superior preclinical platform due to their faithful recapitulation of tumor biology, enabling enhanced prediction of drug response, determination of optimal dosing, efficient drug screening, and investigation of resistance pathways. We analyze how PDO utilization refines treatment personalization, leading to improved clinical outcomes and optimized patient care. Finally, we underscore the transformative implications of PDOs for precision medicine and explore their future prospects in oncology.

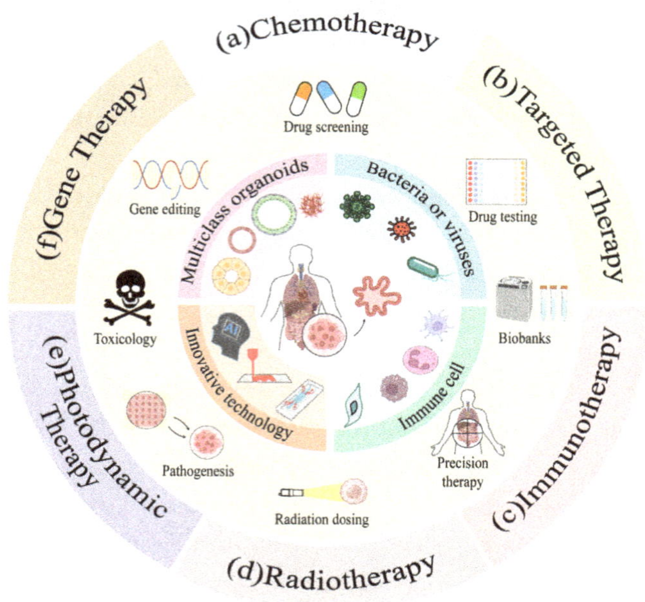


**Figure 7.1** Specific applications of PDOs in tumor personalized therapy. (a) Chemotherapy: PDOs are used for drug screening and testing to predict patient responses to cytotoxic agents like 5-FU and oxaliplatin. (b) Targeted therapy: PDOs identify effective targeted drugs (e.g., KRAS inhibitors) and resistance mechanisms. (c) Immunotherapy: Co-cultures with immune cells evaluate checkpoint inhibitors (e.g., anti-PD-1) and CAR-T/NK therapies. (d) Radiotherapy: PDOs assess tumor radiosensitivity and optimize radiation dosing. (e) Photodynamic therapy: PDOs model light-activated treatments combined with drugs or immunotherapy. (f) Gene therapy: PDOs can undergo gene editing and other manipulations to simulate tumor genetic characteristics and screen therapeutic regimens targeting specific gene mutations.

**Table 7.1** Research applications of PDO in personalized medicine.

| PDO types | Treatment | Key Findings | Reference |
| --- | --- | --- | --- |
| Ovarian clear cell carcinoma | Chemotherapy | The PDO model can encompass the heterogeneity of patient tumors and their clinical response to chemotherapy drugs, and it can also accurately assess the potential of new drugs, such as the HDAC inhibitor belinostat. | [6] |

**Table 7.1** (*Continued*)

| PDO types | Treatment | Key Findings | Reference |
|---|---|---|---|
| Colorectal cancer and gastroesophageal cancer | Chemotherapy | PDOs can encapsulate the patient's clinical treatment response. | [82] |
| Gastric cancer | Chemotherapy | The drug sensitivity testing of PDOs shows dose-response curves consistent with the current standard dosing for gastric cancer cytotoxic therapies. | [83] |
| Ovarian cancer | Chemotherapy | PDOs can be used for drug screening and to capture the responses of different tumor subtypes to platinum-based chemotherapy. | [84] |
| Esophageal and oropharyngeal squamous cell carcinoma | Chemotherapy | The 3D organoids are significantly correlated with the adverse reactions of patients in neoadjuvant chemotherapy or chemoradiotherapy before surgery. | [85] |
| Breast cancer | Chemotherapy | The response of the PDO model to the two chemotherapy drugs, doxorubicin and mitoxantrone, varies greatly among patient samples. | [86] |
| Lung cancer | Chemotherapy | The cellular heterogeneity of PDO is reflected in their different responses to cisplatin or etoposide. | [87] |
| Gastric cancer | Chemotherapy | The cellular heterogeneity of PDO is reflected in their different responses to cisplatin or etoposide. | [12] |
| Esophageal and gastric adenocarcinoma | Chemotherapy | A PDO-derived threshold was defined, which distinguished responders from non-responders to neoadjuvant chemotherapy in esophagogastric adenocarcinoma patients with high sensitivity, specificity, and accuracy in an independent validation cohort. | [13] |
| Pancreatic cancer | Chemotherapy | PDOs exhibit heterogeneous responses to standard-of-care drugs and categorize them into high-, medium-, or low-response groups, accurately predicting treatment responses in treatment-naive patients. | [14] |

(*Continued*)

**Table 7.1** (*Continued*)

| PDO types | Treatment | Key Findings | Reference |
|---|---|---|---|
| Peritoneal metastatic colorectal cancer | Chemotherapy | Organoids are relevant models for studying chemotherapy sensitivity in peritoneal metastasis of colorectal cancer and can be used for large-scale drug screening strategies or personalized medicine. | [88] |
| Gynecological cancers (such as ovarian cancer and endometrial cancer) | Chemotherapy | The PDO model can accurately reflect the patient's sensitivity to platinum-based chemotherapy and other relevant drugs, and even predict drug resistance. | [89] |
| Urothelial carcinoma | Chemotherapy | Organoids can help assess the response of urothelial carcinoma to various anticancer drugs (such as gemcitabine and paclitaxel) and can serve as a drug screening platform. | [90] |
| Renal cell carcinoma | Chemotherapy | Most PDOs are resistant to conventional chemotherapy drugs (such as cisplatin, 5-FU, and gemcitabine). Additionally, several compounds targeting the AKT signaling pathway or the MEK/ERK signaling pathway have shown therapeutic potential. | [91] |
| Colorectal cancer with liver metastasis | Chemotherapy | *In vitro* chemotherapy sensitivity data demonstrate the value of PDO models in predicting patients' chemotherapy responses (FOLFOX or FOLFIRI) and clinical prognosis. | [92] |
| Pancreatic cancer | Chemotherapy | PDOs from different patients exhibit varying responses to chemotherapy drugs (such as FOLFIRINOX and Gem/Pac), and by eliminating ineffective drugs to personalize treatment plans, it may reduce side effects and increase the chances of patients completing the full course of neoadjuvant therapy. | [11] |
| Gastric cancer | Chemotherapy | PDO drug sensitivity testing can predict the clinical response of gastric cancer patients to drugs such as capecitabine and oxaliplatin. | [93] |

Table 7.1 (*Continued*)

| PDO types | Treatment | Key Findings | Reference |
|---|---|---|---|
| Peritoneal metastasis of colorectal cancer | Chemotherapy | PDOs may be a reliable *in vitro* model for evaluating intraperitoneal heated chemotherapy regimens at the individual patient level. | [94] |
| Colorectal cancer | Chemotherapy | PDOs could be used to prevent cancer patients from undergoing ineffective irinotecan-based chemotherapy. | [95] |
| Breast cancer | Chemotherapy | The microtubule-targeting drug-sensitive response signatures of PDOs predict improved distant relapse-free survival for invasive breast cancers treated with adjuvant chemotherapy. | [96] |
| Pancreatic cancer | Chemotherapy | The pathological response of patients to neoadjuvant chemotherapy is associated with the PDO chemotherapy response, particularly to oxaliplatin. | [97] |
| Biliary tract cancer | Chemotherapy | PDOs exhibit different responses to chemotherapy drugs such as gemcitabine, cisplatin, 5-fluorouracil, and oxaliplatin, and these findings were validated in the majority of patients with actual clinical responses. | [98] |
| Endometrial cancer | Targeted therapy | Selective estrogen receptor modulators (such as tamoxifen and raloxifene) have significant individual variations in their effects on the human endometrium. The PDO model can serve as a tool for personalized medicine by identifying patients at an increased risk of developing endometrial lesions. | [99] |
| Lung cancer | Targeted therapy | PDOs recapitulate the tissue structure of primary lung tumors and respond to drugs based on their genomic alterations: BRCA2 mutation organoids for olaparib, EGFR mutation organoids for erlotinib, and EGFR mutation/MET amplification organoids for crizotinib. | [19] |

(*Continued*)

**Table 7.1** (*Continued*)

| PDO types | Treatment | Key Findings | Reference |
|---|---|---|---|
| Hypophysoma | Targeted therapy | PDOs derived from tumors producing corticotropin, prolactin, gonadotropins, and growth hormone exhibit morphological diversity within organoid lines across individual patients and subtypes. Moreover, the PDO model demonstrates patient-specific drug responses within each tumor subtype. | [20] |
| Glioblastoma | Targeted therapy | PDO models derived from different patients exhibit selective responses to drugs. | [100] |
| Small cell carcinoma of the prostate | Targeted therapy | The PDO model has demonstrated the correlation between ALK activation mutations and the pathogenesis of small cell carcinoma of the prostate, and it suggests the therapeutic potential of targeting ALK molecular alterations in prostate small cell carcinoma patients. | [23] |
| Lung cancer | Targeted therapy, chemotherapy | PDO-based drug sensitivity testing accurately predicted the clinical response of this group of advanced lung cancer patients to chemotherapy and targeted therapy. | [24] |
| Breast cancer | Targeted therapy | Combining patient-derived PDOs with mini-PDXs enables rapid and precise screening of drug sensitivity. | [25] |
| Colorectal cancer | Targeted therapy | Combining patient-derived cancer organoids with transcriptomics and chromatin analysis can identify personalized drug targets to overcome oxaliplatin resistance. | [101] |
| Colorectal cancer | Targeted therapy | The PDO model elucidated the interaction between EGF signaling and ERK activation in tumors. | [26] |
| B-cell lymphoma | Targeted therapy | The PDO model revealed the complex crosstalk between diffuse large B-cell lymphoma and the lymphoma microenvironment, and developed combination inhibition therapies targeting multiple aberrant signaling pathways. | [27] |

**Table 7.1** (*Continued*)

| PDO types | Treatment | Key Findings | Reference |
|---|---|---|---|
| Lung adenocarcinoma | Targeted therapy | PDOs can predict the clinical response of individual patients to targeted therapy and identify effective anticancer treatments targeting new molecular targets. | [102] |
| Prostate cancer | Targeted therapy | B7-H3 has been identified as a potential therapeutic target for advanced prostate cancer. | [21] |
| Glioblastoma | Targeted therapy | PDOs can be used for personalized drug screening, allowing for the rapid identification of potential effective treatment options tailored to specific patients. | [103] |
| Colorectal cancer | Targeted therapy | PDOs can effectively assess the efficacy of different drugs and drug combinations in a preclinical setting, particularly in personalized targeted therapies for RAS mutations. | [104] |
| Glioblastoma | Targeted therapy | PDOs can reflect the gene expression characteristics of patient-derived tumor cells, making drug sensitivity testing more personalized. | [105] |
| Ovarian cancer | Targeted therapy, Chemotherapy | PDOs summarize the patient's clinical response to platinum-based chemotherapy and demonstrate the drug response heterogeneity to targeted therapies, including PARPi. | [106] |
| Colorectal cancer | Targeted therapy, Chemotherapy | A scoring method ("chemotherapy map") has been established to identify *in vitro* responders based on PDOs, with the "chemotherapy map" predicting treatment response with a sensitivity and specificity of 75%. | [107] |
| Pancreatic cancer | Targeted therapy | The PDO model identifies genotype-based personalized drug targets (integrin-linked kinase) and can test the efficacy of candidate targeted drugs in organoids. | [108] |

(*Continued*)

**Table 7.1** (*Continued*)

| PDO types | Treatment | Key Findings | Reference |
|---|---|---|---|
| Lymph node / Melanoma | Immunotherapy | PDO responses to immune checkpoint blockade are highly correlated with the clinical responses of patients. | [30] |
| Chordoma | Immunotherapy | PDOs can predict individual patient responses to PD-1/PD-L1 checkpoint inhibitors. | [31] |
| Lung cancer | Immunotherapy | A combined phenotypic and transcriptomic FascRNA-seq platform has been established to analyze the dynamic response of the local tumor immune microenvironment under immune checkpoint blockade therapy. | [32] |
| Cholangiocarcinoma | Immunotherapy | A PDO and immune cell co-culture method has been developed to predict which ICIs are most effective for individual patients. | [109] |
| Esophageal squamous cell carcinoma | Immunotherapy | It was revealed that the loss of TP53, CDKN2A, and NOTCH1 induces immune evasion in esophageal tumors and the initiation of esophageal squamous cell carcinoma, suggesting that CCL2 blockade could be a viable option for targeting PCN-type. | [110] |
| Colorectal cancer | Immunotherapy | PDOs can help predict the response of tumors with different genetic backgrounds to immunotherapy, such as the combination of PD-1 and CTLA-4 inhibitors. | [34] |
| Colorectal cancer | Immunotherapy | Through co-culture of PDO and allogeneic CD8 T cells, it was found that the heterogeneity and plasticity of CEA expression seem to confer low sensitivity of PDO to cibisatamab (a T cell bispecific antibody). | [36] |
| Common epithelial cancer | Immunotherapy | PDOs can detect tumor-specific defects that block T cell recognition and may serve as a tool for selecting T cells for adoptive cell therapy. | [111] |

Table 7.1 (*Continued*)

| PDO types | Treatment | Key Findings | Reference |
|---|---|---|---|
| Cervical cancer | Immunotherapy | The PDOs-tumor-infiltrating lymphocyte co-culture system demonstrates a clear response corresponding to established immune therapy efficacy markers, such as the ratio of CTLs. | [37] |
| Glioblastoma | Immunotherapy | PDOs maintain many key characteristics of glioblastoma and can be rapidly deployed to study patient-specific therapeutic strategies. | [112] |
| Prostate cancer | Immunotherapy | PDOs can accurately simulate the complex microenvironment of prostate cancer to assess patient-specific immune therapy responses. By combining adaptive T cells and CAR immunotherapy, they contribute to the development of personalized treatment strategies for patients. | [113] |
| Colorectal cancer | Immunotherapy | The PDO-based *in vitro* platform allows for the personalized assessment of the efficacy and tumor specificity of chimeric antigen receptors. | [40] |
| Clear cell renal cell carcinoma | Immunotherapy | Immune cell responses can be assessed on the PDO model, and the efficacy of immune therapy drugs (such as toripalimab) can be screened. | [114] |
| Pancreatic ductal adenocarcinoma | Immunotherapy | Adenoviral cytotoxicity in PDOs can predict anti-tumor efficacy in subcutaneous xenograft models and provide information on the response of primary tumors and metastatic sites. | [41] |
| Colorectal cancer | Radiotherapy | The response of colorectal cancer patients to neoadjuvant chemoradiotherapy is closely related to the intrinsic tissue radiosensitivity of their PDO. | [45] |

(*Continued*)

**Table 7.1** (*Continued*)

| PDO types | Treatment | Key Findings | Reference |
|---|---|---|---|
| Cervical cancer | Radiotherapy | Adenocarcinoma and large cell neuroendocrine carcinoma organoids exhibit resistance to radiotherapy, while squamous cell carcinoma and villous adenocarcinoma organoids show significant response to radiotherapy. | [115] |
| Colorectal cancer | Radiotherapy | The response of patients to chemoradiotherapy highly matches the response of PDOs, with an accuracy of 84%, sensitivity of 78%, and specificity of 92%. | [52] |
| Nasopharyngeal carcinoma | Radiotherapy | Hypoxic nasopharyngeal carcinoma PDOs exhibit high radiation resistance, requiring higher doses of radiation to compensate for the hypoxia. | [48] |
| Pancreatic cancer | Radiotherapy | PDOs are suitable for assessing *in vitro* radiation response, showing a dose-response correlation. | [47] |
| Lung cancer, colorectal cancer and pancreatic cancer | Chemoradiotherapy | Using PDO growth rate and optical metabolic imaging to determine treatment thresholds can predict individual patient responses to chemoradiotherapy. | [116] |
| Colorectal cancer | Chemoradiotherapy | PDOs demonstrate clinically relevant responses to chemotherapy and radiotherapy, reflecting the treatment efficacy observed in patients. | [54] |
| Glioblastoma | Radiotherapy | PDOs may provide a key method for understanding the dynamic mechanisms of resistance in glioblastoma. | [117] |
| Squamous cell carcinoma of the head and neck | Chemoradiotherapy | The PDO model shows different responses to current drugs used in the treatment of squamous cell carcinoma of the head and neck, such as cisplatin, carboplatin, and cetuximab, as well as some targeted therapies that are not yet widely used in clinical practice. | [118] |

Table 7.1 (*Continued*)

| PDO types | Treatment | Key Findings | Reference |
|---|---|---|---|
| Human intestinal organoids | Radiotherapy | Human intestinal organoids can be used for personalized assessment of the gastrointestinal response to radiation through transcriptome analysis. | [50] |
| Small/large intestine organoids (normal tissue) | Radiotherapy | It reveals the inherent radiosensitivity of small intestinal stem cells and colon stem cells. | [46] |
| Carcinoma of esophagus | Chemoradiotherapy | PDOs can predict the response to standard chemotherapy, $\gamma$-irradiation, and newer non-standard treatment methods. | [119] |
| Head and neck squamous cell carcinoma | Photodynamic therapy | Head and neck cancer organoids faithfully recapitulate the EGFR expression levels of their corresponding tissues and, importantly, demonstrate a significant correlation between EGFR expression levels and response to EGFR-targeted photodynamic therapy. | [62] |
| Breast cancer | Photodynamic therapy | PDOs can evaluate the therapeutic effect of immunophotodynamic therapy. | [63] |
| Glioblastoma | Photodynamic therapy | Through systematic optimization using PDO models, the optimal treatment parameters for 5-aminolevulinic acid-mediated photodynamic therapy were established while effectively preventing phototoxic damage to normal brain tissue. | [65] |
| Cholangiocarcinoma | Photodynamic therapy | Cholangiocarcinoma organoids exhibit distinct photodynamic activity that effectively differentiates between organoids derived from strictured-but-normal bile ducts and those from cholangiocarcinoma patients. | [67] |
| Bladder cancer | Photodynamic therapy combined with radiotherapy | The therapeutic intervention exhibited differential cellular effects across various bladder cancer organoid models, with malignant organoids (particularly G3/G4 grades) demonstrating significantly higher response rates. | [64] |

(*Continued*)

**Table 7.1** (*Continued*)

| PDO types | Treatment | Key Findings | Reference |
|---|---|---|---|
| Pancreatic cancer | Photodynamic therapy combined with chemotherapy | Photodynamic therapy demonstrates a unique mechanism of action by generating non-overlapping cytotoxic effects with chemotherapy, which not only significantly enhances immediate cytotoxicity against metastatic pancreatic cancer organoids but also improves long-term therapeutic outcomes. | [69] |
| Breast cancer | Gene therapy | The DNA copy number variations and sequence alterations in organoids faithfully mirror those in the original tumor tissues, enabling *in vitro* drug screening that correlates well with *in vivo* xenograft responses and patient outcomes. | [7] |
| Primary sclerosing cholangitis | Gene therapy | The organoid model faithfully retains disease-specific pro-inflammatory gene signatures, thereby providing a direct research platform for evaluating patient responses to potential gene therapy regimens. | [71] |
| Colon | Gene therapy | Through targeted deletion of the mismatch repair gene MLH1 in colon organoids, it was demonstrated that mutation accumulation is driven by replication errors. The mutational spectra generated in these organoids closely resemble those observed in colorectal cancers with DNA mismatch repair deficiency. | [72] |
| Cystic fibrosis | Gene therapy | Using the CRISPR/Cas9 genome editing system, the CFTR gene locus was corrected via homologous recombination in intestinal stem cells derived from cystic fibrosis patients. Functional assays of the corrected organoids demonstrated their potential for predicting individual patients' responsiveness to gene therapy. | [73] |

*Note*: **5-FU:** 5-Fluorouracil. **FOLFOX:** 5-FU + Oxaliplatin. **FOLFIRI:** Folinic acid + 5-FU + Irinotecan. **FOLFIRINOX:** 5-FU + Leucovorin + Irinotecan + Oxaliplatin. **ICBs:** Immune checkpoint blockers. **PCN:** Precancerous niche. **CTLs:** Cytotoxic T lymphocytes. **CAR:** Chimeric antigen receptor.

## 7.2 Patient-derived Organoids Guide Personalized Chemotherapy

Chemotherapy remains a cornerstone of cancer treatment, utilizing cytotoxic agents — such as DNA-damaging compounds and antimetabolites — to inhibit tumor cell proliferation or induce apoptosis. However, due to tumor heterogeneity and inter-individual variability in pharmacokinetics, patient responses to chemotherapy often differ markedly, resulting in suboptimal efficacy or significant adverse effects. PDOs offer a promising platform to assess the direct effects of chemotherapeutic agents on cancer cells, enabling the capture of personalized tumor responses and informing treatment decision-making. For example, PDOs derived from pancreatic ductal adenocarcinoma (PDAC) have demonstrated chemosensitivity profiles that align closely with clinical responses in individual patients [9]. In a similar study, researchers generated PDAC organoid models and tested their responses to four commonly used chemotherapeutic agents. The organoids exhibited varying degrees of drug sensitivity — showing greater sensitivity to gemcitabine and cisplatin — and combination therapies were more effective than single-agent treatments [10]. Such variability in drug response is likely attributable to both inter- and intra-tumoral heterogeneity, which PDOs are well-suited to model. Thorel *et al.* [6] developed seven models from a single ovarian clear cell carcinoma case, including 2D cell lines, PDOs, and PDXs. Both PDX and PDO models recapitulated tumor heterogeneity and mirrored clinical responses to chemotherapy agents such as carboplatin, doxorubicin, and gemcitabine. Notably, PDOs offered superior predictive capacity for evaluating novel therapeutic agents, including the HDAC inhibitor belinostat, underscoring their value as preclinical models.

Hennig *et al.* [11] further demonstrated the utility of PDOs in guiding personalized treatment regimens by identifying and excluding ineffective drugs, thereby potentially reducing toxicity and improving adherence to neoadjuvant therapy. Similarly, Seidlitz *et al.* [12] reported heterogeneous responses among gastric cancer organoids to conventional chemotherapies — including 5-fluorouracil, oxaliplatin, irinotecan, epirubicin, and docetaxel. Drug sensitivity was concentration-dependent and varied by organoid line; for instance, DD109 responded to 5-FU only at high concentrations, whereas DD191 and DD282 were sensitive at lower doses. These findings suggest that establishing efficacy thresholds for individual organoid lines could optimize therapeutic strategies. More recently, Schmäche *et al.* [13] established a PDO-derived threshold to stratify pathological responses to neoadjuvant chemotherapy in patients with esophagogastric adenocarcinoma. This threshold successfully distinguished responders from non-responders with high sensitivity (90%), specificity (100%), and accuracy (92%) in an independent validation cohort. In another study, PDOs derived from 54 treatment-naïve pancreatic cancer patients were subjected to single-agent drug viability assays, and a combination therapy prediction score was developed. The organoids exhibited heterogeneous responses to standard-of-care agents, and the scoring system accurately predicted clinical outcomes with 91.1% accuracy [14].

Tumor recurrence following chemotherapy remains a significant clinical obstacle, largely due to an incomplete understanding of resistance mechanisms driven by the complex interplay between tumor heterogeneity and the tumor microenvironment. Organoid technology offers a powerful platform for investigating patient-specific mechanisms of drug resistance, allowing for detailed characterization of tumor cell resistance patterns and supporting the development of tailored therapeutic strategies. Chen *et al.* [15] established PDO models integrated with single-cell RNA sequencing, identifying genes (e.g., STMN1, VEGFA, and NDRG1) and transcription factors (E2F1, BRCA1, MYBL2, CDX2, and CDX1) associated with oxaliplatin resistance. These findings provide a molecular framework for the development of personalized targeted therapies. Similarly, Laoukili *et al.* [16] compared drug responses between organoids derived from colorectal cancer peritoneal metastases and their matched primary tumors. Metastatic organoids exhibited greater resistance to oxaliplatin, with glutamate-cysteine ligase identified as a potential mediator, underscoring the presence of metastasis-specific resistance mechanisms. Additional studies have demonstrated the pivotal role of the tumor microenvironment in modulating chemosensitivity. Stigliani *et al.* [17] explored how microenvironmental conditions affect drug responses within specific genetic contexts. Their findings revealed that acidic extracellular conditions significantly enhanced organoid viability — particularly in TP53 wild-type models — and reduced the efficacy of gemcitabine/erlotinib treatment. These adaptive responses may underlie primary chemoresistance in localized tumor regions characterized by hypoxic or acidic niches.

## 7.3 Patient-derived Organoids Guide Targeted Therapy

Targeted therapy represents a major advancement in cancer treatment by selectively inhibiting key molecular drivers of tumorigenesis — such as kinases, epigenetic regulators, and cyclins — to suppress malignant cell proliferation. Unlike conventional chemotherapy, which broadly affects all rapidly dividing cells, targeted agents act specifically on tumor-associated molecular alterations (e.g., HER2 amplification, ALK fusions), thereby minimizing off-target toxicity and preserving normal tissue function. The integration of companion diagnostic technologies further enhances therapeutic precision by enabling pre-treatment patient stratification — a critical advantage for individuals with advanced-stage cancer and a narrow therapeutic window. However, the emergence of acquired resistance, driven by tumor heterogeneity and clonal evolution, continues to limit the long-term efficacy of targeted therapies, highlighting the need for more adaptive and durable treatment strategies. In this context, PDO models have emerged as invaluable tools in the pursuit of personalized cancer therapy. Ideally, precision oncology should encompass comprehensive tumor genomic profiling, identification of genotype-specific therapeutic targets, and the selection of corresponding targeted agents [18]. PDOs are uniquely capable of capturing both inter- and intratumoral heterogeneity, offering unprecedented opportunities to validate genomically guided therapies, facilitate high-throughput drug screening, and uncover novel therapeutic targets. For example, molecular targeted therapies in lung cancer are often developed based on distinct genetic alterations. Kim *et al.* [19] established a biobank of 80 lung cancer organoid strains encompassing five histological subtypes. This organoid biobank faithfully recapitulated the histopathological and genetic features of the original tumors and enabled the prediction of patient-specific drug responses through tailored *in vitro* assays. In Cushing's disease, a rare endocrine disorder caused by pituitary neuroendocrine tumors, progress has been limited by the absence of preclinical models that accurately replicate the tumor microenvironment. Addressing this gap, Chakrabarti *et al.* [20] generated human pituitary tumor organoids from patient-derived tissues. These organoids preserved the morphological diversity and lineage-specific characteristics of the original tumors across various subtypes. High-throughput drug screening using these organoids revealed subtype-specific drug responses, establishing them as a novel and physiologically relevant platform for modeling Cushing's disease and identifying potential targeted therapies. In the context of prostate cancer, Guo *et al.* [21] employed PDO models to uncover frequent overexpression of the B3-H7 gene in advanced cases, nominating it as a candidate therapeutic target. Collectively, these studies underscore the pivotal role of PDOs in bridging the gap between genomic insights and the development of clinically actionable targeted therapies.

A pivotal application of personalized targeted therapy lies in the use of PDOs for drug sensitivity assays, offering a unique opportunity to evaluate individual patient responses to various therapeutic agents and thereby enabling tailored treatment strategies. For instance, cystic fibrosis — a genetic disorder caused by mutations in the CFTR gene — results in severe dysfunction across the pulmonary, digestive, and urogenital systems [3]. Berkers *et al.* [22] demonstrated a strong correlation between forskolin-induced swelling responses in rectal organoids derived from cystic fibrosis patients and their clinical responses to CFTR modulator therapies. This study established that organoid-based *in vitro* assays can prospectively identify effective treatments for individuals with diverse CFTR mutations.

In a landmark case report, Carneiro *et al.* [23] described a patient with refractory small cell prostate carcinoma harboring an activating ALK F1174C mutation who achieved remarkable clinical benefit from ALK inhibitor therapy. Prostate organoid models were generated to assess responses to the ALK inhibitors crizotinib and alectinib, with alectinib demonstrating superior efficacy in suppressing ALK F1174C-positive cell proliferation. Furthermore, a real-world study involving 212 lung cancer organoids from 107 patients revealed that organoid-based drug sensitivity testing accurately predicted clinical responses to both chemotherapy and targeted therapies in advanced lung cancer patients, underscoring its potential as a precision medicine tool [24]. In breast cancer, Cui *et al.* [25] developed a comprehensive organoid biobank representing diverse molecular subtypes and, for the first time, integrated PDOs with mini-PDXs to explore their combined utility as platforms for drug screening. This approach identified alpelisib plus fulvestrant as a promising therapeutic combination, which was validated by monitoring dynamic changes in PI3K/AKT/mTOR signaling and estrogen receptor expression.

A mechanistic understanding of targetable pathways remains central to therapeutic selection. Ponsioen *et al.* [26] developed real-time, quantitative drug response assays in KRAS- and BRAF-mutant colorectal cancer organoids, demonstrating that oncogenic signaling was significantly suppressed following EGFR inhibition. These findings underscore the clinical relevance of incorporating EGFR inhibitors into combination regimens for colorectal cancer. Similarly, in B-cell malignancies, Shah *et al.* [27] established lymphoma organoid models that faithfully recapitulated the complex crosstalk between diffuse large B-cell lymphoma and its tumor microenvironment. This model facilitated the development of innovative combination therapies targeting multiple aberrant pathways, effectively overcoming microenvironment-mediated resistance to MALT1 inhibitors.

## 7.4 Patient-derived Organoids Guide Immunotherapy

Over the past decade, immunotherapy has emerged as a pivotal approach in cancer treatment, demonstrating transformative potential, particularly through immune checkpoint inhibitors (ICIs), immune cell therapies, and oncolytic viral therapies. PDO models not only faithfully recapitulate human disease but also serve as valuable tools for evaluating the efficacy of these therapies, enabling patient stratification to identify those most likely to respond. Furthermore, by developing immunocompetent patient-derived tumor organoids and employing immune cell co-culture techniques, researchers can effectively replicate the intricate tumor immune microenvironment (Figure 7.2). This approach allows direct observation of immune cell-tumor cell interactions, facilitating the assessment of immunotherapy efficacy and supporting the development of more personalized treatment strategies [28].

ICIs have demonstrated significant clinical benefits across a range of tumor types. However, substantial interpatient heterogeneity means many patients do not respond to ICIs, highlighting the urgent need for predictive methods to identify suitable candidates for personalized immunotherapy, thereby minimizing unnecessary toxicity and reducing economic burden. Emerging evidence indicates that PDO models can effectively recapitulate patient-specific responses to ICIs.

Notably, Votanopoulos *et al.* [30] developed an immunocompetent PDO model incorporating lymph nodes and melanoma tissues, revealing an 85% concordance between organoid responses to ICIs and corresponding clinical outcomes. This model offers promising avenues for personalized treatment strategies. Similarly, Scognamiglio *et al.* [31] established chordoma-derived organoids to assess PD-1/PD-L1 checkpoint inhibitor sensitivity. They observed a dose-dependent reduction in tumor size within 24 hours of nivolumab treatment in PD-L1-positive organoids, including those with heterogeneous PD-L1 expression, suggesting that even patients with limited PD-L1 expression may benefit from anti-PD-1 therapy. Therefore, PDOs represent a promising functional model that may predict response to PD-1/PD-L1 inhibitors in chordoma patients, potentially overcoming the limitations of standard PD-L1 immunohistochemistry. These findings underscore the potential of organoid-based drug testing to guide individualized immunotherapy.

Recent technological advances have further enhanced the utility of organoid models in immunotherapy research. A novel functional association single-cell RNA sequencing platform was applied to primary lung cancer organoids preserving tumor immune microenvironment heterogeneity. This approach enabled correlation analyses between single-organoid transcriptomic profiles and PD-1 responses, providing new insights into tumor immune microenvironment dynamics during immune checkpoint blockade therapy [32].

Combination immunotherapy strategies have shown particular clinical promise. Dual inhibition of PD-1 and CTLA-4 has been shown to improve response rates in metastatic melanoma [33], and similar approaches are being explored in digestive system cancers. Chalabi *et al.* [34] used a co-culture of early-stage colorectal cancer PDOs with peripheral blood mononuclear cells to evaluate neoadjuvant immunotherapy. The combination of PD-1 and CTLA-4 inhibitors yielded a robust pathological response in mismatch repair-deficient tumors, whereas only partial responses were observed in mismatch repair-proficient cases. These findings underscore the importance of patient stratification in immunotherapy, as a one-size-fits-all strategy remains inadequate.

The clinical translation of organoid-based immunotherapy testing is actively under investigation. An ongoing clinical trial (NCT05404321) evaluates PDOs for predicting responses to ICI-chemotherapy combinations in triple-negative breast cancer. This study employs 3D tumor-like organoids co-cultured with autologous immune cells, with results systematically compared to clinical outcomes [35]. Such approaches have the potential to significantly advance precision immunotherapy by enabling *ex vivo* assessment of treatment response prior to clinical intervention.

Recent years have also seen remarkable progress in immune cell-based therapies, which offer unique advantages in cancer treatment. Carcinoembryonic antigen (CEA), highly expressed on colorectal cancer cells, represents an ideal therapeutic target [36].

Gonzalez-Exposito *et al.* [36] developed a co-culture system of colorectal cancer PDOs and CD8+ T cells stratified by CEA expression levels. Their results revealed that high CEA expression correlated with sensitivity to the bispecific antibody cibisatamab (targeting CEA and CD3), whereas low CEA expression associated with resistance. Functional analyses implicated enhanced Wnt/β-catenin signaling in CEA-low tumor cells as a potential immune evasion mechanism. These phenotypic and immune response assessments deepen our understanding of immune escape and offer insights for overcoming therapeutic resistance, laying the foundation for more effective personalized treatments. In cervical cancer, Huang *et al.* [37] developed an organoid co-culture model to evaluate individual responses to adoptive T cell therapy. By expanding tumor-infiltrating lymphocytes and co-culturing them with PDOs, they successfully simulated tumor–lymphocyte interactions, demonstrating distinct responses aligned with established immunotherapy biomarkers, highlighting the model's predictive potential for adoptive T cell therapy outcomes.

Chimeric antigen receptor (CAR)-T cell therapy has achieved remarkable success in leukemia, receiving FDA approval [38]. Wang *et al.* [39] optimized CAR-T cells targeting glypican-3 in hepatocellular carcinoma. Co-culture with hepatocellular carcinoma organoids showed significant tumor growth inhibition. To evaluate the specificity of CAR natural killer (NK) cells, Schnalzger *et al.* [40] tested CAR-NK-92 cytotoxicity against colorectal cancer and normal organoids. CAR-NK-92 cells effectively eliminated tumor cells — even within challenging tumor microenvironments characterized by low tumor-associated antigen expression — while sparing normal organoids, thus minimizing off-target toxicity. Collectively, these studies highlight the transformative potential of PDO models in optimizing immune cell-based therapies. By faithfully recapitulating tumor–immune interactions, organoid platforms enable mechanistic investigations and accelerate clinical translation toward safer, more effective personalized immunotherapies.

Oncolytic virus therapy, an emerging immunotherapeutic strategy, is currently under clinical evaluation. Notably, organoid models have been employed to assess the antitumor immune responses elicited by these therapies, demonstrating promising results [41]. Giulia *et al.* [41] provided compelling evidence that oncolytic adenoviruses can efficiently replicate, proliferate, and induce cancer cell death in tumor organoids, while sparing normal organoids from cytotoxicity. Importantly, PDAC-derived PDOs exhibited heterogeneous sensitivity to these viral agents. Furthermore, the organoid platform validated the enhanced therapeutic efficacy of combining oncolytic adenoviruses with standard chemotherapeutic agents.

Remarkably, oncolytic viruses also show potential to overcome therapy resistance. Miao *et al.* [42] demonstrated that the combination of oncolytic adenoviruses with bromodomain inhibitors (iBet-762 and OTX-015) creates an immunologically favorable tumor microenvironment and restores drug sensitivity in resistant cancer cells. This combinatorial approach achieved superior clinical outcomes compared to standard-of-care treatments. Beyond their direct oncolytic effects, these viruses serve as versatile drug delivery vehicles to potentiate immunotherapy. A recent study engineered an oncolytic adenovirus encoding a PD-L1-targeting Fc fusion peptide, which not only augmented the antitumor activity of ICIs but also significantly mitigated immune-related adverse events [43].

Collectively, PDOs have emerged as invaluable tools for predicting immunotherapy responses, elucidating mechanisms of immune evasion, and facilitating the development of novel immunotherapeutic strategies. Their capacity to faithfully recapitulate patient-specific tumor–immune interactions positions them as essential platforms in advancing precision immuno-oncology.

## 7.5 Patient-derived Organoids Guide Radiotherapy

Radiotherapy remains a cornerstone of cancer treatment, utilizing high-energy radiation (e.g., X-rays and particle beams) to induce DNA damage in tumor cells, thereby eliminating malignancies or inhibiting their growth. When combined with targeted therapies, immunotherapy, or chemotherapy as an adjuvant approach, radiotherapy has demonstrated remarkable clinical efficacy [44]. Given the inherent inter-individual variability in radiosensitivity, personalized radiotherapy regimen design is crucial. PDOs have emerged as valuable tools in this context, faithfully recapitulating patient-specific tumors and normal tissue responses to radiation. Hsu *et al.* [45] systematically evaluated the radiosensitivity of organoids derived from both normal intestinal tissue and colorectal tumors. Their findings revealed that adenoma PDOs originating from intestinal stem cell populations retained the radioresistant phenotype of normal colorectal organoids. During malignant transformation, the capacity for homologous recombination-mediated DNA repair is often diminished, resulting in significantly increased radiosensitivity in tumor-derived PDOs. This discovery opens the door to PDO-based testing for radiation dose optimization, enabling personalized radiotherapy planning while minimizing normal tissue toxicity. In a pioneering study, researchers developed a robust organoid-based model to simulate dose-dependent radiation effects on intestinal tissues. Utilizing clonogenic survival assays in combination with mathematical modeling, they generated comprehensive radiation dose–response curves, allowing accurate quantification of intrinsic radiosensitivity and tissue-specific radiation tolerance [46]. Building on this framework, Goor *et al.* [47] irradiated pancreatic cancer PDOs with doses ranging from 0 to 40 Gy. Viability assays conducted at 7 and 10 days post-irradiation demonstrated >50% survival at 12 Gy and revealed strong dose–response correlations up to 14 Gy, reinforcing the utility of PDOs as reliable *in vitro* models for assessing radiation response. Notably, Lucky *et al.* [48] explored the impact of hypoxia on radioresistance using recurrent nasopharyngeal carcinoma organoids. Their findings revealed that hypoxic nasopharyngeal carcinoma PDOs exhibited pronounced resistance to radiation, necessitating higher radiotherapy doses to achieve therapeutic efficacy. These results highlight the potential of PDOs to inform dose adjustments that account for microenvironment-mediated resistance, particularly in recurrent or treatment-refractory tumors.

Beyond conventional photon-based radiotherapy, proton therapy is gaining increasing clinical importance due to its favorable dose-distribution properties. Kristin *et al.* [49] demonstrated that both proton and photon irradiation elicited similarly heterogeneous response patterns in PDOs, allowing for patient stratification based on differential radiosensitivity. In a comprehensive comparison of radiation modalities, Ali *et al.* [50] examined the effects of photon, proton, and carbon ion irradiation (at 4 Gy) on intestinal organoids. Each radiation type induced distinct transcriptional signatures, enabling clear discrimination between healthy organoids and those derived from Fanconi anemia patients based on radiosensitivity. This represents a critical advancement toward defining safe and effective radiation dose thresholds for vulnerable patient populations.

Radiotherapy is renowned for its potent local control, clinical efficacy, and cost-effectiveness, yet its therapeutic outcomes exhibit significant inter-patient variability.

Consequently, radiotherapy is frequently combined with chemotherapy to enhance treatment responses. BRAF mutation is a relatively rare mutation, and patients with this mutation often exhibit resistance to conventional chemotherapy. Mu and his research team [51] demonstrated this point using a colorectal cancer organoid model. Notably, the organoids showed a strong response to concurrent chemoradiotherapy. Furthermore, a phase III clinical trial revealed that rectal cancer organoid responses strongly correlated with patient outcomes following chemoradiation, achieving 84% accuracy, 78% sensitivity, and 92% specificity [52], solidifying PDOs as robust predictive tools. Sanjit *et al.* [53] further showed that the expression of OCT4 and SOX2 is significantly upregulated in pancreatic cancer organoids following radiation therapy at doses of 4 and 8 Gy, mediating pancreatic cancer growth and treatment resistance. However, when radiotherapy is combined with 5-FU treatment, the resistance is reversed, and the organoids undergo cell death. Targeting SOX2/OCT4 alongside chemoradiation may thus significantly improve pancreatic cancer management. PDOs also facilitate identification of patients likely to benefit from neoadjuvant chemoradiotherapy, optimizing therapeutic strategies while minimizing overtreatment. Karuna *et al.* [54] developed an *ex vivo* radiation platform featuring neoadjuvant chemoradiotherapy-resistant organoids from recurrent/poor-responder patients, enabling pretreatment response prediction to spare resistant individuals from unnecessary toxicity. Current organoid models often overlook the tumor microenvironment's critical role in radiotherapy responses. Radiation-induced stromal and immune alterations within the tumor microenvironment contribute to radioresistance and recurrence, suggesting potential synergy between radiotherapy and immunotherapy [55, 56]. For instance, cancer-associated fibroblast (CAF)- secreted interleukin-1 (IL-1) promotes radioresistance in colorectal cancer organoids by inducing DNA damage and CAF senescence. Vitamin D receptor antagonists and minocycline can block IL-1 and reverse CAF polarization, thereby enhancing radiosensitivity [55]. These findings establish a framework for improving radiotherapy in stroma-rich tumors. Additionally, radiotherapy markedly increases intra-tumoral M2 macrophage polarization — a key tumor microenvironment alteration faithfully recapitulated in organoid models. Combining radiotherapy with immunomodulators thus holds therapeutic promise. Notably, radiosensitizers are increasingly used alongside radiotherapy to enhance efficacy at lower, safer doses. Misun *et al.* [57] evaluated short-chain fatty acids as radiosensitizers in colorectal cancer organoids, revealing butyrate's dual capacity to potentiate radiation effects while protecting normal organoids. Thymoquinone, a bioactive compound in Nigella sativa oil, radiosensitizes various cancers [58]. Samar *et al.* [58] demonstrated that 3 μM thymoquinone combined with 2 Gy radiotherapy significantly impaired colorectal cancer organoid clonogenicity without normal tissue toxicity.

## 7.6 Patient-Derived Organoids Guide Emerging Therapies

### 7.6.1 *Photodynamic Therapy*

Photodynamic therapy (PDT) has emerged as a minimally invasive approach garnering significant attention in cancer therapeutics. This biphasic treatment modality operates through a photochemical mechanism involving three key components: light of specific wavelengths, oxygen, and photosensitizers, which collectively generate reactive oxygen species to induce targeted cell death or vascular damage [59]. PDOs, with their remarkable ability to recapitulate native tissue architecture and optical properties, enable precise evaluation of light absorption dynamics. The application of 3D organoid systems has opened new avenues for investigating PDT in oncology, particularly through high-throughput image-based analyses that yield robust statistical data on photosensitizer efficacy and PDT outcomes [60, 61]. PDT demonstrates versatility as both a standalone treatment and an adjuvant to conventional therapies, with documented applications in superficial and select deep-seated tumors.

Organoid models of superficial tumors, including head and neck, breast, and bladder cancers, have pioneered combination studies with PDT. Driehuis *et al.* demonstrated that head and neck squamous cell carcinoma-derived organoids faithfully recapitulated native EGFR expression levels, crucially revealing a significant correlation between EGFR expression and response to EGFR-targeted PDT [62]. Beyond direct tumoricidal effects, PDT-induced release of tumor-associated antigens can activate systemic immune responses against metastatic disease. Ye *et al.* [63] developed IT-4F nanoparticles featuring an acceptor-donor-acceptor (A-D-A) structure for immunogenic PDT in breast cancer, with organoid-based validation showing marked growth inhibition post-treatment. For bladder cancer preservation strategies employing both PDT and ionizing radiation [64], combination therapy elicited heterogeneous cellular responses across tumor grades — particularly showing enhanced efficacy in high-grade (G3/G4) organoids through distinct cytotoxic, cell death, and immunogenic mechanisms. These findings underscore organoids' potential in evaluating PDT-based combination therapies. Technological advances now extend PDT applications to deep-seated tumors. Pedrosa *et al.* [65] established a glioblastoma PDO-normal brain coculture system to optimize 5-aminolevulinic acid-mediated PDT parameters, achieving tumor-specific cytotoxicity while preventing normal tissue phototoxicity. In cholangiocarcinoma, where PDT is incorporated in the National Comprehensive Cancer Network guidelines for biliary decompression [66], Fujiwara *et al.* [67] demonstrated significantly higher photodynamic activity in cholangiocarcinoma versus non-neoplastic bile duct organoids, suggesting organoid-based profiling could stratify PDT-eligible patients. Sorafenib-PDT combinations synergistically enhanced reactive oxygen species accumulation in cholangiocarcinoma organoids, permitting dose reduction while maintaining efficacy [68]. For stroma-rich pancreatic cancer, Broekgaarden *et al.* [69] systematically evaluated PDT-oxaliplatin (L-OHP) combinations in metastatic models, revealing non-overlapping toxicity mechanisms that enhanced both immediate cytotoxicity and long-term outcomes. Organoid platforms also enable high-throughput photosensitizer screening for optimal tumor-specific accumulation and activation kinetics [60], facilitating precision PDT development.

### 7.6.2 *Gene Therapy*

Gene therapy represents a transformative therapeutic strategy that involves the introduction, deletion, or modification of genetic material to treat or prevent disease. This approach aims to correct or replace mutated genes, restore normal cellular or tissue function, or induce therapeutic effects via the expression of functional genes. Compared to conventional cell lines and animal models, PDOs offer superior fidelity in modeling individual genetic mutations, drug responses, and disease phenotypes — making them an ideal platform for advancing personalized gene therapy. For example, Sachs *et al.* [7] established a biobank of over 100 breast cancer organoid lines and demonstrated that DNA copy number variations and sequence alterations in the organoids closely matched those of the corresponding primary tumors. Drug sensitivity testing using these models enabled the identification of optimal treatment strategies, underscoring the value of organoids in personalized gene therapy research. In another notable study, van de Wetering *et al.* [70] generated 20 matched tumor–normal organoid pairs from colorectal cancer patients and developed an automated high-throughput drug screening platform to test 83 compounds. Genomic and transcriptomic analyses revealed the heterogeneity of organoid responses and established correlations between oncogenic mutations and drug sensitivities.

Organoid systems have also been employed in gene editing studies to interrogate the functional consequences of specific mutations. For instance, researchers established cholangiocyte organoids from patients with primary sclerosing cholangitis, which retained disease-specific pro-inflammatory gene signatures. This personalized model offers a direct platform to assess patient-specific responses to candidate gene therapies [71]. Further demonstrating the utility of organoids in mechanistic studies, Jarno *et al.* [72] used CRISPR-Cas9 to delete the mismatch repair gene MLH1 in colon organoids. Whole-genome sequencing revealed that mutation accumulation was driven by replication errors, and the resulting mutational spectra closely resembled those found in mismatch repair-deficient colorectal cancers. These findings open new avenues for understanding tumor evolution and therapeutic vulnerabilities. Importantly, organoid-based gene therapy is not limited to oncology. In cystic fibrosis, researchers applied Cas9-mediated homologous recombination to introduce wild-type CFTR alleles into intestinal organoids derived from two patients carrying the common ΔF508 mutation. The genetically corrected organoids exhibited rapid luminal expansion in response to forskolin-induced swelling, whereas un-transfected controls showed no such response [73]. This study illustrates the potential of organoids for functional validation of gene correction in monogenic diseases.

## 7.7 Challenges and Future Perspectives

PDO models have emerged as a powerful and innovative platform for advancing personalized oncology. These biopsy-derived 3D cultures exhibit strong clinical utility, particularly through serial drug sensitivity testing, which enables accurate prediction of therapeutic responses [3]. The value of PDOs is reflected in three major clinical benefits: (1) reduction of ineffective treatments, (2) decreased incidence of adverse drug reactions, and (3) improved quality of life for patients [1]. By characterizing the biological profiles of individual tumors, PDOs facilitate personalized treatment selection, allowing clinicians to identify the most effective agents and dosages for tailored regimens. Importantly, PDO models also allow for *in vitro* testing of various drug combinations, enabling the design of individualized combination strategies. This capability offers a time- and cost-efficient alternative to traditional multi-phase clinical trials. Compared to conventional "one-size-fits-all" treatment paradigms, PDOs represent a paradigm shift in precision oncology, enabling more accurate, efficient, and patient-specific therapeutic decision-making [1, 44].

Despite their promising potential, several key challenges must be addressed before widespread clinical implementation can be achieved. First, the successful establishment of clinically usable PDOs often hinges on obtaining a sufficient quantity of viable tumor cells. The process of organoid generation from patient biopsies remains time-consuming — typically requiring 2–4 weeks for expansion and drug testing — and is associated with relatively low success rates [74, 75]. This time constraint limits the feasibility of integrating PDO-based testing into urgent treatment timelines, particularly for aggressive or rapidly progressing cancers. Second, standardization and validation of organoid culture protocols are critical for ensuring reproducibility and reliability in clinical applications [74]. However, due to significant inter- and intra-tumoral heterogeneity, developing a universal culture protocol remains challenging. Future efforts should focus on creating subtype-specific and tissue-specific protocols tailored to distinct molecular and histopathological features, thereby improving both the efficiency and fidelity of tumor organoid cultures [75]. Third, the translation of PDO-derived biomarkers and predictive models into routine clinical practice remains a formidable obstacle. Existing drug screening platforms and computational prediction models often overlook inter-individual pharmacokinetic variability — including differences in drug absorption, distribution, metabolism, and excretion — which are critical determinants of treatment efficacy and safety [76]. Addressing this limitation will require integration of pharmacokinetic profiling and testing on normal tissue-derived organoids to identify patient-specific therapeutic windows and minimize toxicity [76, 77]. Finally, ethical considerations surrounding organoid biobanking must be carefully managed. These include issues related to informed consent, privacy, long-term storage, and ownership of patient-derived tissues and data [78]. Clear regulatory guidelines and transparent governance frameworks will be essential to ensure ethical compliance in both research and clinical applications.

In conclusion, while technical, biological, and ethical challenges remain, ongoing advancements in organoid culture, standardization, and integration with multi-omics and pharmacological profiling hold promise for overcoming these limitations. As such, PDOs are poised to become a cornerstone of precision oncology — enabling more accurate, efficient, and personalized cancer treatment strategies, and offering a valuable platform for translational research and therapeutic development.

## Key Opinion Points

1. Standardization and preservation of tumor heterogeneity: As PDOs gain increasing traction in both clinical and research settings, the development of standardized and reproducible organoid derivation protocols is essential. These techniques must faithfully preserve the intrinsic genetic and phenotypic heterogeneity of primary tumors to ensure clinical relevance and predictive accuracy [79].
2. Preclinical applications and translational potential: PDOs hold substantial promise in preclinical research and drug discovery. Their close biological resemblance to patient tumors enhances the interpretability of preclinical findings, particularly in the context of drug sensitivity and resistance mechanisms. This may significantly improve the translational success of novel therapeutics [80].
3. Limitations of traditional models and the need for patient-specific systems: Conventional biomedical models, such as animal models and 2D cell cultures, remain widely used in disease mechanism studies and drug development. However, these systems often fall short due to interspecies differences and the absence of a physiologically relevant tumor microenvironment. Overcoming these limitations is essential for precision medicine and requires addressing two core challenges: (1) elucidating the influence of human genetic diversity on disease progression and therapeutic responses, and (2) establishing advanced *in vitro* systems that maintain long-term patient-specific tumor characteristics. These needs underscore the growing importance of organoid-based models as a next-generation platform bridging cellular and organ-level biology [3].
4. Modeling acquired resistance and longitudinal response: Beyond identifying the most effective therapies for individual patients, PDOs offer the unique capability to model acquired drug resistance. By retaining the genetic diversity of the primary tumor, PDOs can give rise to resistant subclones under selective drug pressure — mirroring resistance patterns that emerge during treatment *in vivo*. Further research is required to validate the predictive fidelity of

these models and to integrate resistance monitoring into real-time therapeutic decision-making [81].

## References

1. Soto-Gamez A, Gunawan JP, Barazzuol L, Pringle S, Coppes RP. Organoid-based personalized medicine: from tumor outcome prediction to autologous transplantation. Stem Cells. 2024;42(6):499–508.
2. Takahashi T. Organoids for drug discovery and personalized medicine. Annu Rev Pharmacol Toxicol. 2019;59:447–462.
3. Tang XY, Wu S, Wang D, Chu C, Hong Y, Tao M, *et al.* Human organoids in basic research and clinical applications. Signal Transduct Target Ther. 2022;7(1):168.
4. Kim SY, van de Wetering M, Clevers H, Sanders K. The future of tumor organoids in precision therapy. Trends Cancer. 2025.
5. Zhu Z, Shen J, Ho PC, Hu Y, Ma Z, Wang L. Transforming cancer treatment: integrating patient-derived organoids and CRISPR screening for precision medicine. Front Pharmacol. 2025;16:1563198.
6. Thorel L, Morice PM, Paysant H, Florent R, Babin G, Thomine C, *et al.* Comparative analysis of response to treatments and molecular features of tumor-derived organoids versus cell lines and PDX derived from the same ovarian clear cell carcinoma. J Exp Clin Cancer Res. 2023;42(1):260.
7. Sachs N, de Ligt J, Kopper O, Gogola E, Bounova G, Weeber F, *et al.* A living biobank of breast cancer organoids captures disease heterogeneity. Cell. 2018;172(1–2):373–386.e10.
8. Xu H, Jiao D, Liu A, Wu K. Tumor organoids: applications in cancer modeling and potentials in precision medicine. J Hematol Oncol. 2022;15(1):58.
9. Grossman JE, Muthuswamy L, Huang L, Akshinthala D, Perea S, Gonzalez RS, *et al.* Organoid sensitivity correlates with therapeutic response in patients with pancreatic cancer. Clin Cancer Res. 2022;28(4):708–718.
10. Gong M, Meng H, Tan D, Li P, Qin J, An Q, *et al.* Establishment of organoid models for pancreatic ductal adenocarcinoma and screening of individualized therapy strategy. Anim Models Exp Med. 2023;6(5):409–418.
11. Hennig A, Baenke F, Klimova A, Drukewitz S, Jahnke B, Brückmann S, *et al.* Detecting drug resistance in pancreatic cancer organoids guides optimized chemotherapy treatment. J Pathol. 2022;257(5):607–619.
12. Seidlitz T, Merker SR, Rothe A, Zakrzewski F, von Neubeck C, Grützmann K, *et al.* Human gastric cancer modelling using organoids. Gut. 2019;68(2):207–217.

13. Schmäche T, Fohgrub J, Klimova A, Laaber K, Drukewitz S, Merboth F, *et al.* Stratifying esophago-gastric cancer treatment using a patient-derived organoid-based threshold. Mol Cancer. 2024;23(1):10.
14. Beutel AK, Schütte L, Scheible J, Roger E, Müller M, Perkhofer L, *et al.* A prospective feasibility trial to challenge patient-derived pancreatic cancer organoids in predicting treatment response. Cancers. 2021;13(11).
15. Chen G, Gong T, Wang Z, Wang Z, Lin X, Chen S, *et al.* Colorectal cancer organoid models uncover oxaliplatin-resistant mechanisms at single cell resolution. Cell Oncol. 2022;45(6):1155–1167.
16. Laoukili J, Constantinides A, Wassenaar ECE, Elias SG, Raats DAE, van Schelven SJ, *et al.* Peritoneal metastases from colorectal cancer belong to consensus molecular subtype 4 and are sensitised to oxaliplatin by inhibiting reducing capacity. Br J Cancer. 2022;126(12):1824–1833.
17. Stigliani A, Ialchina R, Yao J, Czaplinska D, Dai Y, Andersen HB, *et al.* Adaptation to an acid microenvironment promotes pancreatic cancer organoid growth and drug resistance. Cell Rep. 2024;43(7):114409.
18. Shiihara M, Furukawa T. Application of patient-derived cancer organoids to personalized medicine. J Pers Med. 2022;12(5).
19. Kim M, Mun H, Sung CO, Cho EJ, Jeon HJ, Chun SM, *et al.* Patient-derived lung cancer organoids as in vitro cancer models for therapeutic screening. Nat Commun. 2019;10(1):3991.
20. Chakrabarti J, Pandey R, Churko JM, Eschbacher J, Mallick S, Chen Y, *et al.* Development of human pituitary neuroendocrine tumor organoids to facilitate effective targeted treatments of Cushing's disease. Cells. 2022;11(21).
21. Guo C, Figueiredo I, Gurel B, Neeb A, Seed G, Crespo M, *et al.* B7-H3 as a therapeutic target in advanced prostate cancer. Eur Urol. 2023;83(3):224–238.
22. Berkers G, van Mourik P, Vonk AM, Kruisselbrink E, Dekkers JF, de Winter-de Groot KM, *et al.* Rectal organoids enable personalized treatment of cystic fibrosis. Cell Rep. 2019;26(7):1701–1708.e3.
23. Carneiro BA, Pamarthy S, Shah AN, Sagar V, Unno K, Han H, *et al.* Anaplastic lymphoma kinase mutation (ALK F1174C) in small cell carcinoma of the prostate and molecular response to alectinib. Clin Cancer Res. 2018;24(12):2732–2739.
24. Wang HM, Zhang CY, Peng KC, Chen ZX, Su JW, Li YF, *et al.* Using patient-derived organoids to predict locally advanced or metastatic lung cancer tumor response: a real-world study. Cell Rep Med. 2023;4(2):100911.

25. Cui Y, Ran R, Da Y, Zhang H, Jiang M, Qi X, *et al.* The combination of breast cancer PDO and mini-PDX platform for drug screening and individualized treatment. J Cell Mol Med. 2024;28(9):e18374.
26. Ponsioen B, Post JB, Buissant des Amorie JR, Laskaris D, van Ineveld RL, Kersten S, *et al.* Quantifying single-cell ERK dynamics in colorectal cancer organoids reveals EGFR as an amplifier of oncogenic MAPK pathway signalling. Nat Cell Biol. 2021; 23(4):377–390.
27. Shah SB, Carlson CR, Lai K, Zhong Z, Marsico G, Lee KM, *et al.* Combinatorial treatment rescues tumour-microenvironment-mediated attenuation of MALT1 inhibitors in B-cell lymphomas. Nat Mater. 2023;22(4):511–523.
28. Grönholm M, Feodoroff M, Antignani G, Martins B, Hamdan F, Cerullo V. Patient-derived organoids for precision cancer immunotherapy. Cancer Res. 2021;81(12):3149–3155.
29. Mei J, Liu X, Tian HX, Chen Y, Cao Y, Zeng J, *et al.* Tumour organoids and assembloids: patient-derived cancer avatars for immunotherapy. Clin Transl Med. 2024;14(4):e1656.
30. Votanopoulos KI, Forsythe S, Sivakumar H, Mazzocchi A, Aleman J, Miller L, *et al.* Model of patient-specific immune-enhanced organoids for immunotherapy screening: feasibility study. Ann Surg Oncol. 2020;27(6):1956–1967.
31. Scognamiglio G, De Chiara A, Parafioriti A, Armiraglio E, Fazioli F, Gallo M, *et al.* Patient-derived organoids as a potential model to predict response to PD-1/PD-L1 checkpoint inhibitors. Br J Cancer. 2019;121(11):979–982.
32. Liu C, Li K, Sui X, Zhao T, Zhang T, Chen Z, *et al.* Patient-derived tumor organoids combined with function-associated scRNA-Seq for dissecting the local immune response of lung cancer. Adv Sci. 2024;11(31):e2400185.
33. Larkin J, Hodi FS, Wolchok JD. Combined nivolumab and ipilimumab or monotherapy in untreated melanoma. N Engl J Med. 2015;373(13):1270–1271.
34. Chalabi M, Fanchi LF, Dijkstra KK, Van den Berg JG, Aalbers AG, Sikorska K, *et al.* Neoadjuvant immunotherapy leads to pathological responses in MMR-proficient and MMR-deficient early-stage colon cancers. Nat Med. 2020;26(4):566–576.
35. Divoux J, Florent R, Jacobs M, Lequesne J, Grellard JM, San C, *et al.* The TRIPLEX study: use of patient-derived tumor organoids as an innovative tool for precision medicine in triple-negative breast cancer. BMC Cancer. 2023;23(1):883.
36. Gonzalez-Exposito R, Semiannikova M, Griffiths B, Khan K, Barber LJ, Woolston A, *et al.* CEA expression heterogeneity and plasticity confer resistance to the CEA-targeting bispecific immunotherapy antibody cibisatamab (CEA-TCB) in patient-derived colorectal cancer organoids. J Immunother Cancer. 2019;7(1):101.

37. Huang H, Pan Y, Huang J, Zhang C, Liao Y, Du Q, *et al.* Patient-derived organoids as personalized avatars and a potential immunotherapy model in cervical cancer. iScience. 2023;26(11):108198.
38. June CH, Sadelain M. Chimeric antigen receptor therapy. N Engl J Med. 2018; 379(1):64–73.
39. Wang Y, Gao Y, Niu C, Wang B, Zhao S, Roex G, *et al.* Chimeric antigen receptor clustering via cysteines enhances T-cell efficacy against tumor. Cancer Immunol Immunother. 2022;71(11):2801–2814.
40. Schnalzger TE, de Groot MH, Zhang C, Mosa MH, Michels BE, Röder J, *et al.* 3D model for CAR-mediated cytotoxicity using patient-derived colorectal cancer organoids. EMBO J. 2019;38(12).
41. Raimondi G, Mato-Berciano A, Pascual-Sabater S, Rovira-Rigau M, Cuatrecasas M, Fondevila C, *et al.* Patient-derived pancreatic tumour organoids identify therapeutic responses to oncolytic adenoviruses. EBioMedicine. 2020;56:102786.
42. Miao T, Symonds A, Hickman OJ, Wu D, Wang P, Lemoine N, *et al.* Inhibition of bromodomain proteins enhances oncolytic HAdVC5 replication and efficacy in pancreatic ductal adenocarcinoma (PDAC) models. Int J Mol Sci. 2024;25(2).
43. Hamdan F, Ylösmäki E, Chiaro J, Giannoula Y, Long M, Fusciello M, *et al.* Novel oncolytic adenovirus expressing enhanced cross-hybrid IgGA Fc PD-L1 inhibitor activates multiple immune effector populations leading to enhanced tumor killing in vitro, in vivo and with patient-derived tumor organoids. J Immunother Cancer. 2021;9(8).
44. Wang Y, Li Y, Sheng Z, Deng W, Yuan H, Wang S, *et al.* Advances of patient-derived organoids in personalized radiotherapy. Front Oncol. 2022;12:888416.
45. Hsu KS, Adileh M, Martin ML, Makarov V, Chen J, Wu C, *et al.* Colorectal cancer develops inherent radiosensitivity that can be predicted using patient-derived organoids. Cancer Res. 2022;82(12):2298–2312.
46. Martin ML, Adileh M, Hsu KS, Hua G, Lee SG, Li C, *et al.* Organoids reveal that inherent radiosensitivity of small and large intestinal stem cells determines organ sensitivity. Cancer Res. 2020;80(5):1219–1227.
47. van Goor I, Raymakers L, Andel DSH, Brosens LAA, Kranenburg O, Leusen JHW, *et al.* Radiation response assessment of organoids derived from patients with pancreatic cancer. Clin Transl Radiat Oncol. 2024;48:100829.
48. Lucky SS, Law M, Lui MH, Mong J, Shi J, Yu S, *et al.* Patient-derived nasopharyngeal cancer organoids for disease modeling and radiation dose optimization. Front Oncol. 2021;11:622244.

49. Pape K, Lößner AJ, William D, Czempiel T, Beyreuther E, Klimova A, *et al.* Sensitization of patient-derived colorectal cancer organoids to photon and proton radiation by targeting DNA damage response mechanisms. Cancers. 2022;14(20).
50. Nowrouzi A, Sertorio MG, Akbarpour M, Knoll M, Krunic D, Kuhar M, *et al.* Personalized assessment of normal tissue radiosensitivity via transcriptome response to photon, proton and carbon irradiation in patient-derived human intestinal organoids. Cancers. 2020;12(2).
51. Mu P, Mo S, He X, Zhang H, Lv T, Xu R, *et al.* Unveiling radiobiological traits and therapeutic responses of BRAF(V600E)-mutant colorectal cancer via patient-derived organoids. J Exp Clin Cancer Res. 2025;44(1):92.
52. Yao Y, Xu X, Yang L, Zhu J, Wan J, Shen L, *et al.* Patient-derived organoids predict chemoradiation responses of locally advanced rectal cancer. Cell Stem Cell. 2020;26(1):17–26.e6.
53. Roy S, Dukic T, Keepers Z, Bhandary B, Lamichhane N, Molitoris J, *et al.* SOX2 and OCT4 mediate radiation and drug resistance in pancreatic tumor organoids. Cell Death Discov. 2024;10(1):106.
54. Ganesh K, Wu C, O'Rourke KP, Szeglin BC, Zheng Y, Sauvé CG, *et al.* A rectal cancer organoid platform to study individual responses to chemoradiation. Nat Med. 2019;25(10):1607–1614.
55. Nicolas AM, Pesic M, Engel E, Ziegler PK, Diefenhardt M, Kennel KB, *et al.* Inflammatory fibroblasts mediate resistance to neoadjuvant therapy in rectal cancer. Cancer Cell. 2022;40(2):168–184.e13.
56. Kim JK, Wu C, Del Latto M, Gao Y, Choi SH, Kierstead M, *et al.* An immunocompetent rectal cancer model to study radiation therapy. Cell Rep Methods. 2022;2(12):100353.
57. Park M, Kwon J, Shin HJ, Moon SM, Kim SB, Shin US, *et al.* Butyrate enhances the efficacy of radiotherapy via FOXO3A in colorectal cancer patient-derived organoids. Int J Oncol. 2020;57(6):1307–1318.
58. Al Bitar S, Ballout F, Monzer A, Kanso M, Saheb N, Mukherji D, *et al.* Thymoquinone radiosensitizes human colorectal cancer cells in 2D and 3D culture models. Cancers. 2022;14(6).
59. Correia JH, Rodrigues JA, Pimenta S, Dong T, Yang Z. Photodynamic therapy review: principles, photosensitizers, applications, and future directions. Pharmaceutics. 2021;13(9).
60. Ma HL, Urbaczek AC, Zeferino Ribeiro de Souza F, Bernal C, Rodrigues Perussi J, Carrilho E. Replicating endothelial shear stress in organ-on-a-chip for predictive hypericin photodynamic efficiency. Int J Pharm. 2023;634:122629.

61. Deiana M, Andrés Castán JM, Josse P, Kahsay A, Sánchez DP, Morice K, *et al.* A new G-quadruplex-specific photosensitizer inducing genome instability in cancer cells by triggering oxidative DNA damage and impeding replication fork progression. Nucleic Acids Res. 2023;51(12):6264–6285.
62. Driehuis E, Spelier S, Beltrán Hernández I, de Bree R, SM W, Clevers H, *et al.* Patient-derived head and neck cancer organoids recapitulate EGFR expression levels of respective tissues and are responsive to EGFR-targeted photodynamic therapy. J Clin Med. 2019;8(11).
63. Ye Y, Zhao S, Pang E, Tang Y, Zhu P, Gao W, *et al.* Indacenodithienothiophene-based A-D-A-type phototheranostics for immuno-phototherapy. J Nanobiotechnol. 2025; 23(1):309.
64. Reinhold A, Glasow A, Nürnberger S, Weimann A, Telemann L, Stolzenburg JU, *et al.* Ionizing radiation and photodynamic therapy lead to multimodal tumor cell death, synergistic cytotoxicity and immune cell invasion in human bladder cancer organoids. Photodiagn Photodyn Ther. 2025;51:104459.
65. Pedrosa L, Bedia C, Diao D, Mosteiro A, Ferrés A, Stanzani E, *et al.* Preclinical studies with glioblastoma brain organoid co-cultures show efficient 5-ALA photodynamic therapy. Cells. 2023;12(8).
66. Benson AB, D'Angelica MI, Abrams T, Abbott DE, Ahmed A, Anaya DA, *et al.* NCCN Guidelines® Insights: biliary tract cancers, version 2.2023. J Natl Compr Canc Netw. 2023;21(7):694–704.
67. Fujiwara H, Takahara N, Tateishi K, Tanaka M, Kanai S, Kato H, *et al.* 5-aminolevulinic acid-mediated photodynamic activity in patient-derived cholangiocarcinoma organoids. Surg Oncol. 2020;35:484–490.
68. Huang YP, Wang YX, Zhou H, Liu ZT, Zhang ZJ, Xiong L, *et al.* Surufatinib combined with photodynamic therapy induces ferroptosis to inhibit cholangiocarcinoma in vitro and in tumor models. Front Pharmacol. 2024;15:1288255.
69. Broekgaarden M, Rizvi I, Bulin AL, Petrovic L, Goldschmidt R, Massodi I, *et al.* Neoadjuvant photodynamic therapy augments immediate and prolonged oxaliplatin efficacy in metastatic pancreatic cancer organoids. Oncotarget. 2018;9(16):13009–13022.
70. van de Wetering M, Francies HE, Francis JM, Bounova G, Iorio F, Pronk A, *et al.* Prospective derivation of a living organoid biobank of colorectal cancer patients. Cell. 2015;161(4):933–945.
71. Yao Q, Chen W, Yu Y, Gao F, Zhou J, Wu J, *et al.* Human placental mesenchymal stem cells relieve primary sclerosing cholangitis via upregulation of TGR5 in Mdr2(-/-) mice and human intrahepatic cholangiocyte organoid models. Research (Wash D C). 2023;6:0207.

72. Drost J, van Boxtel R, Blokzijl F, Mizutani T, Sasaki N, Sasselli V, *et al.* Use of CRISPR-modified human stem cell organoids to study the origin of mutational signatures in cancer. Science. 2017;358(6360):234–238.
73. Schwank G, Koo BK, Sasselli V, Dekkers JF, Heo I, Demircan T, *et al.* Functional repair of CFTR by CRISPR/Cas9 in intestinal stem cell organoids of cystic fibrosis patients. Cell Stem Cell. 2013;13(6):653–658.
74. Rossi R, De Angelis ML, Xhelili E, Sette G, Eramo A, De Maria R, *et al.* Lung cancer organoids: the rough path to personalized medicine. Cancers. 2022;14(15).
75. Werner RS, Kirschner MB, Opitz I. Primary lung cancer organoids for personalized medicine-are they ready for clinical use? Cancers. 2021;13(19).
76. Feng F, Shen B, Mou X, Li Y, Li H. Large-scale pharmacogenomic studies and drug response prediction for personalized cancer medicine. J Genet Genom. 2021;48(7):540–541.
77. Xiang D, He A, Zhou R, Wang Y, Xiao X, Gong T, *et al.* Building consensus on the application of organoid-based drug sensitivity testing in cancer precision medicine and drug development. Theranostics. 2024;14(8):3300–3316.
78. Li Y, Tang P, Cai S, Peng J, Hua G. Organoid based personalized medicine: from bench to bedside. Cell Regen (Lond). 2020;9(1):21.
79. LeSavage BL, Suhar RA, Broguiere N, Lutolf MP, Heilshorn SC. Next-generation cancer organoids. Nat Mater. 2022;21(2):143–159.
80. Veninga V, Voest EE. Tumor organoids: opportunities and challenges to guide precision medicine. Cancer Cell. 2021;39(9):1190–1201.
81. Bartfeld S, Clevers H. Stem cell-derived organoids and their application for medical research and patient treatment. J Mol Med (Berl). 2017;95(7):729–738.
82. Vlachogiannis G, Hedayat S, Vatsiou A, Jamin Y, Fernández-Mateos J, Khan K, *et al.* Patient-derived organoids model treatment response of metastatic gastrointestinal cancers. Science. 2018;359(6378):920–926.
83. Gao M, Lin M, Rao M, Thompson H, Hirai K, Choi M, *et al.* Development of patient-derived gastric cancer organoids from endoscopic biopsies and surgical tissues. Ann Surg Oncol. 2018;25(9):2767–2775.
84. Kopper O, de Witte CJ, Lõhmussaar K, Valle-Inclan JE, Hami N, Kester L, *et al.* An organoid platform for ovarian cancer captures intra- and interpatient heterogeneity. Nat Med. 2019;25(5):838–849.
85. Kijima T, Nakagawa H, Shimonosono M, Chandramouleeswaran PM, Hara T, Sahu V, *et al.* Three-dimensional organoids reveal therapy resistance of esophageal and oropharyngeal squamous cell carcinoma cells. Cell Mol Gastroenterol Hepatol. 2019; 7(1):73–91.

86. Nayak B, Balachander GM, Manjunath S, Rangarajan A, Chatterjee K. Tissue mimetic 3D scaffold for breast tumor-derived organoid culture toward personalized chemotherapy. Colloids Surf B Biointerfaces. 2019;180:334–343.
87. Choi SY, Cho YH, Kim DS, Ji W, Choi CM, Lee JC, *et al.* Establishment and long-term expansion of small cell lung cancer patient-derived tumor organoids. Int J Mol Sci. 2021;22(3).
88. Roy P, Canet-Jourdan C, Annereau M, Zajac O, Gelli M, Broutin S, *et al.* Organoids as preclinical models to improve intraperitoneal chemotherapy effectiveness for colorectal cancer patients with peritoneal metastases: preclinical models to improve HIPEC. Int J Pharm. 2017;531(1):143–152.
89. Bi J, Newtson AM, Zhang Y, Devor EJ, Samuelson MI, Thiel KW, *et al.* Successful patient-derived organoid culture of gynecologic cancers for disease modeling and drug sensitivity testing. Cancers (Basel). 2021;13(12).
90. Li Z, Xu H, Gong Y, Chen W, Zhan Y, Yu L, *et al.* Patient-derived upper tract urothelial carcinoma organoids as a platform for drug screening. Adv Sci. 2022;9(4):e2103999.
91. Li Z, Xu H, Yu L, Wang J, Meng Q, Mei H, *et al.* Patient-derived renal cell carcinoma organoids for personalized cancer therapy. Clin Transl Med. 2022;12(7):e970.
92. Mo S, Tang P, Luo W, Zhang L, Li Y, Hu X, *et al.* Patient-derived organoids from colorectal cancer with paired liver metastasis reveal tumor heterogeneity and predict response to chemotherapy. Adv Sci. 2022;9(31):e2204097.
93. Zu M, Hao X, Ning J, Zhou X, Gong Y, Lang Y, *et al.* Patient-derived organoid culture of gastric cancer for disease modeling and drug sensitivity testing. Biomed Pharmacother. 2023;163:114751.
94. Varinelli L, Battistessa D, Guaglio M, Zanutto S, Illescas O, Lorenc EJ, *et al.* Colorectal carcinoma peritoneal metastases-derived organoids: results and perspective of a model for tailoring hyperthermic intraperitoneal chemotherapy from bench-to-bedside. J Exp Clin Cancer Res. 2024;43(1):132.
95. Ooft SN, Weeber F, Dijkstra KK, McLean CM, Kaing S, van Werkhoven E, *et al.* Patient-derived organoids can predict response to chemotherapy in metastatic colorectal cancer patients. Sci Transl Med. 2019;11(513):eaay2574.
96. Chen P, Zhang X, Ding R, Yang L, Lyu X, Zeng J, *et al.* Patient-derived organoids can guide personalized-therapies for patients with advanced breast cancer. Adv Sci. 2021;8(22):e2101176.
97. Demyan L, Habowski AN, Plenker D, King DA, Standring OJ, Tsang C, *et al.* Pancreatic cancer patient-derived organoids can predict response to neoadjuvant chemotherapy. Ann Surg. 2022;276(3):450–462.

98. Ren X, Huang M, Weng W, Xie Y, Wu Y, Zhu S, *et al.* Personalized drug screening in patient-derived organoids of biliary tract cancer and its clinical application. Cell Rep Med. 2023;4(11):101277.
99. Bläuer M, Heinonen PK, Rovio P, Ylikomi T. Effects of tamoxifen and raloxifene on normal human endometrial cells in an organotypic in vitro model. Eur J Pharmacol. 2008;592(1–3):13–18.
100. Lenin S, Ponthier E, Scheer KG, Yeo ECF, Tea MN, Ebert LM, *et al.* A drug screening pipeline using 2D and 3D patient-derived in vitro models for pre-clinical analysis of therapy response in glioblastoma. Int J Mol Sci. 2021;22(9).
101. Tung KL, Chen KY, Negrete M, Chen T, Safi A, Aljamal AA, *et al.* Integrated chromatin and transcriptomic profiling of patient-derived colon cancer organoids identifies personalized drug targets to overcome oxaliplatin resistance. Genes Dis. 2021;8(2):203–214.
102. Kim SY, Kim SM, Lim S, Lee JY, Choi SJ, Yang SD, *et al.* Modeling clinical responses to targeted therapies by patient-derived organoids of advanced lung adenocarcinoma. Clin Cancer Res. 2021;27(15):4397–4409.
103. Ratliff M, Kim H, Qi H, Kim M, Ku B, Azorin DD, *et al.* Patient-derived tumor organoids for guidance of personalized drug therapies in recurrent glioblastoma. Int J Mol Sci. 2022;23(12).
104. Verissimo CS, Overmeer RM, Ponsioen B, Drost J, Mertens S, Verlaan-Klink I, *et al.* Targeting mutant RAS in patient-derived colorectal cancer organoids by combinatorial drug screening. Elife. 2016;5.
105. Reed MR, Lyle AG, De Loose A, Maddukuri L, Learned K, Beale HC, *et al.* A functional precision medicine pipeline combines comparative transcriptomics and tumor organoid modeling to identify bespoke treatment strategies for glioblastoma. Cells. 2021;10(12).
106. Tao M, Sun F, Wang J, Wang Y, Zhu H, Chen M, *et al.* Developing patient-derived organoids to predict PARP inhibitor response and explore resistance overcoming strategies in ovarian cancer. Pharmacol Res. 2022;179:106232.
107. Cartry J, Bedja S, Boilève A, Mathieu JRR, Gontran E, Annereau M, *et al.* Implementing patient derived organoids in functional precision medicine for patients with advanced colorectal cancer. J Exp Clin Cancer Res. 2023;42(1):281.
108. Shiihara M, Ishikawa T, Saiki Y, Omori Y, Hirose K, Fukushige S, *et al.* Development of a system combining comprehensive genotyping and organoid cultures for identifying and testing genotype-oriented personalised medicine for pancreatobiliary cancers. Eur J Cancer. 2021;148:239–250.
109. Zhou G, Lieshout R, van Tienderen GS, de Ruiter V, van Royen ME, Boor PPC, *et al.* Modelling immune cytotoxicity for cholangiocarcinoma with tumour-derived organoids and effector T cells. Br J Cancer. 2022;127(4):649–660.

110. Ko KP, Huang Y, Zhang S, Zou G, Kim B, Zhang J, *et al.* Key genetic determinants driving esophageal squamous cell carcinoma initiation and immune evasion. Gastroenterology. 2023;165(3):613–628.e20.
111. Parikh AY, Masi R, Gasmi B, Hanada KI, Parkhurst M, Gartner J, *et al.* Using patient-derived tumor organoids from common epithelial cancers to analyze personalized T-cell responses to neoantigens. Cancer Immunol Immunother. 2023;72(10):3149–3162.
112. Jacob F, Salinas RD, Zhang DY, Nguyen PTT, Schnoll JG, Wong SZH, *et al.* A patient-derived glioblastoma organoid model and biobank recapitulates inter- and intra-tumoral heterogeneity. Cell. 2020;180(1):188–204.e22.
113. Bartucci M, Ferrari AC, Kim IY, Ploss A, Yarmush M, Sabaawy HE. Personalized medicine approaches in prostate cancer employing patient-derived 3D organoids and humanized mice. Front Cell Dev Biol. 2016;4:64.
114. Xue Y, Wang B, Tao Y, Xia J, Yuan K, Zheng J, *et al.* Patient-derived organoids potentiate precision medicine in advanced clear cell renal cell carcinoma. Precis Clin Med. 2022;5(4):pbac028.
115. Seol HS, Oh JH, Choi E, Kim S, Kim H, Nam EJ. Preclinical investigation of patient-derived cervical cancer organoids for precision medicine. J Gynecol Oncol. 2023;34(3):e35.
116. Pasch CA, Favreau PF, Yueh AE, Babiarz CP, Gillette AA, Sharick JT, *et al.* Patient-derived cancer organoid cultures to predict sensitivity to chemotherapy and radiation. Clin Cancer Res. 2019;25(17):5376–5387.
117. Sundar SJ, Shakya S, Barnett A, Wallace LC, Jeon H, Sloan A, *et al.* Three-dimensional organoid culture unveils resistance to clinical therapies in adult and pediatric glioblastoma. Transl Oncol. 2022;15(1):101251.
118. Driehuis E, Kolders S, Spelier S, Lõhmussaar K, Willems SM, Devriese LA, *et al.* Oral mucosal organoids as a potential platform for personalized cancer therapy. Cancer Discov. 2019;9(7):852–871.
119. Karakasheva TA, Gabre JT, Sachdeva UM, Cruz-Acuña R, Lin EW, DeMarshall M, *et al.* Patient-derived organoids as a platform for modeling a patient's response to chemoradiotherapy in esophageal cancer. Sci Rep. 2021;11(1):21304.

https://doi.org/10.1142/9789819817597_0008

Chapter 8

# Optimizing Organoid-Based Drug Sensitivity Testing: Essential Insights and Best Practices

Yi Zhou[1,2,*], Ling Jiao[2], Wentao Yang[3], Xiaozhen Liu[4]

[1]*Hangzhou AimingMed Technologies Co., Ltd, Hangzhou 310000, China*

[2]*Laboratory of Human Disease and Immunotherapies, West China Hospital, Sichuan University, Chengdu, China*

[3]*Department of Emergency Medicine, West China Hospital, West China School of Medicine of Sichuan University, China*

[4]*Zhejiang Provincial People's Hospital, Hangzhou 310014, China*

**Abstract:** Organoid-based drug sensitivity testing has emerged as a transformative approach in precision oncology, enabling personalized therapeutic decision-making through functional profiling of patient-derived tumor models. This chapter provides a comprehensive overview of the technical workflows, validation metrics, and clinical applications of organoid-based drug sensitivity testing. It details key steps including sample acquisition, organoid cultivation, high-throughput drug screening, and data analysis, while addressing challenges related to standardization and inter-laboratory reproducibility.

Case studies across diverse cancer types—including colorectal, gastric, lung, pancreatic, and breast—highlight the strong concordance between *in vitro* organoid responses and real-world clinical outcomes. The chapter concludes with expert perspectives and future directions to enhance clinical implementation, emphasizing the need for harmonized protocols, integration with genomics, and scalable workflows. Together, these insights underscore the promise of organoid technology as a cornerstone of functional precision medicine.

**Keywords:** patient-derived organoids, drug sensitivity testing, precision medicine, personalized treatment

*Corresponding author. Email: timzhouyi@gmail.com

## Key Points

1. Organoid-based drug sensitivity testing offers a powerful tool for precision oncology by enabling individualized therapeutic selection.
2. Organoids can be established from a variety of clinical specimens; sample collection and processing procedures should be optimized and aligned with clinicians.
3. Culture protocols must be adapted for each tumor type to ensure successful and representative organoid development.
4. Drug sensitivity testing methodology includes drug treatment protocols, data collection techniques, and analytical approaches to assess therapeutic responses.
5. Technical and biological factors can introduce variability in drug sensitivity testing; rigorous control measures are essential to minimize inconsistencies.
6. Robust quality control and standardized methodologies are critical to ensure reproducibility and clinical relevance of organoid-based drug sensitivity testing.

## 8.1 Introduction

In the previous chapter, we reviewed the evolution of precision medicine. At its core, precision medicine aims to tailor therapeutic strategies to the unique genetic, phenotypic, and environmental characteristics of each patient. Organoids exemplify this paradigm by faithfully recapitulating the biological features of individual diseases within a controlled laboratory setting [1]. These 3D models preserve the architectural, molecular, and functional properties of the source tissue, enabling researchers and clinicians to simulate and study patient-specific treatment responses.

In oncology, patient-derived organoids (PDOs) have proven particularly valuable for modeling tumor heterogeneity and predicting therapeutic efficacy. PDOs allow for the assessment of tumor-specific sensitivity to chemotherapeutic agents and targeted therapies, thus enabling the design of individualized treatment regimens prior to clinical application. Importantly, organoids overcome many limitations associated with traditional 2D cell cultures by more accurately mimicking the *in vivo* tumor microenvironment [2]. For example, colorectal cancer organoids have demonstrated strong concordance between *in vitro* drug response profiles and actual patient outcomes, underscoring their predictive potential [3]. The workflow of organoid-based drug sensitivity testing is shown in Figure 8.1.

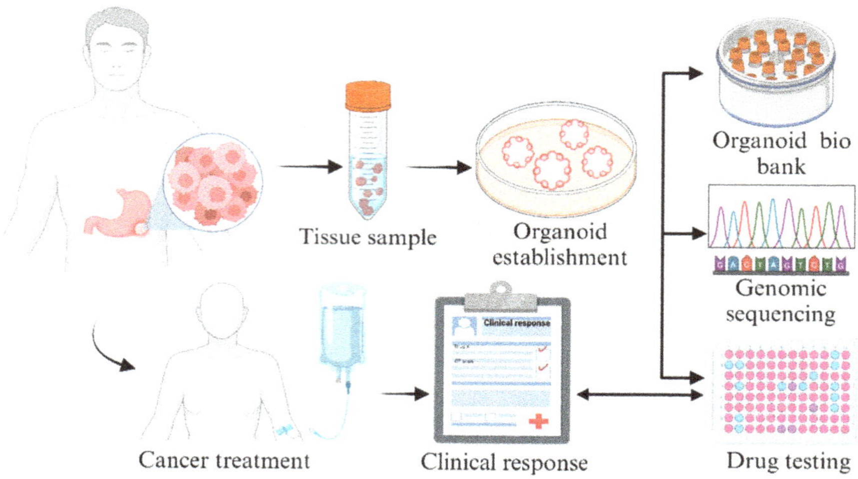


**Figure 8.1** Schematic representation of personalized cancer treatment using organoid-based drug sensitivity testing. Reproduced with permission from [4].

Despite these promising developments, careful consideration is required at every stage of organoid-based drug sensitivity testing — from sample collection and organoid culture to drug screening and data analysis. Variability in tissue source, culture media, and laboratory handling can result in inconsistent organoid growth and unreliable drug response data [5]. Moreover, implementing high-throughput drug screening demands advanced technical infrastructure, trained personnel, and standardized operating procedures. Another key challenge is the complexity of data interpretation; accurately analyzing dose–response relationships, accounting for biological heterogeneity, and evaluating drug synergy often necessitate the use of computational tools such as machine learning and bioinformatics pipelines [6].

## 8.2 Sample Collection and Processing

### 8.2.1 *Tissue Sources*

The development of organoid models begins with the acquisition of high-quality tissue specimens, which serve as the foundation for generating patient-specific organoids. These tissues are generally obtained from three primary sources: primary tumors, metastatic lesions, and biopsy samples. Surgically resected primary tumors are a common and abundant source for organoid derivation. These samples typically contain diverse cell populations, enhancing the biological fidelity of the resulting organoid models. Immediate processing is critical to preserve cell viability and structural integrity [7].

Tissues collected from metastatic sites offer valuable insights into advanced disease progression and therapy resistance. Organoids established from these lesions can recapitulate the genetic and phenotypic characteristics of secondary tumors, making them suitable platforms for investigating drug resistance mechanisms [8].

Minimally invasive biopsies provide an alternative tissue source when surgical resection is not feasible. This approach is particularly relevant in cancers such as pancreatic ductal adenocarcinoma, where surgical options are limited. Despite their smaller size, advances in tissue dissociation techniques have enabled successful organoid generation from biopsy-derived material [9].

The requirement for different samples are summarized in Table 8.1 [10].

**Table 8.1** Common specimen types and requirements for tumor organoid culture.

| Specimen Type | Collection Method | Collection Amount | Remarks |
|---|---|---|---|
| Fresh tumor tissue | Surgery | At least ≥0.5 g in total, recommended to retrieve at least 3 tissue blocks each approximately 1 $cm^3$ in size. | The collection shall target areas rich in cancer cells, avoiding areas mixed with fat, mucus threads, necrotic tissue, fibrous tissue, blood clots, etc. |
| | Endoscopic biopsy | Retrieve more than 3 pieces of tissue, with a total weight of ≥0.5 g. | |
| | Needle biopsy | At least 3 cm in total tissue length (each piece more than 1 cm, at least 3 pieces). | |
| Malignant effusion (pleural or abdominal fluid, etc.) | Aspiration or drainage | 1) For large volumes, obtain fresh drainage fluid of 200–300 mL collected as quickly as possible;<br>2) For small volumes, withdraw as many drainage fluid samples as possible; >50 mL is recommended. | 1) Keep the drainage bag warm and away from light.<br>2) Sample collection is not advisable if imaging results suggest that the amount of fluid in the patient is less than 100 mL. |

### 8.2.2 *Preprocessing Methods*

The preparation of tissue samples is a critical step that directly impacts the success of organoid culture. It typically involves a combination of mechanical and enzymatic dissociation to release viable cells from the extracellular matrix.

Mechanical dissociation involves fragmenting the tissue into smaller pieces to increase surface area for enzymatic action. Instruments such as scalpels, scissors, or tissue grinders are used. Over-processing should be avoided, as it can compromise cell viability and damage tissue architecture [11].

Enzymatic digestion employs proteolytic enzymes like collagenase, dispase, or trypsin to break down the extracellular matrix and release single cells. Parameters such as enzyme concentration, incubation time, and temperature must be carefully optimized to maximize yield without compromising cell integrity [12].

For dense or fibrotic tissues, combining mechanical and enzymatic methods yields higher efficiency. Post-digestion, the sample is typically filtered through mesh strainers to remove debris and generate a uniform single-cell suspension [2]. For difficult-to-digest tissue, sequential digestion with different enzymes are recommended.

### 8.2.3 *Quality Assurance During Sample Processing*

To ensure reproducibility and biological relevance, several quality control measures should be implemented during tissue handling. While it is recommended to perform quality assurance testing prior to initiating organoid culture, clinical samples are often limited in availability, and in many cases cannot be recollected. Therefore, regardless of quality assurance outcomes, it is advisable to proceed with organoid culture to maximize the possibility of generating a viable model and offer the best potential benefit to the patient [13].

#### 8.2.3.1 *Contamination Prevention*

Maintaining sterility throughout the sample collection and processing workflow is essential to prevent bacterial, fungal, or mycoplasma contamination, which can compromise organoid viability and confound downstream analyses. Aseptic techniques include working within a laminar flow hood, using sterile instruments and reagents, and implementing routine cleaning and decontamination protocols. The addition of antibiotic and antifungal agents to tissue processing buffers and culture media provides further protection, particularly during initial culture establishment. Regular microbial screening should also be performed to detect any latent contamination early and maintain the integrity of the organoid culture system [12].

#### 8.2.3.2 *Viability Assessment*

Cell viability is a critical determinant of organoid culture success. It is typically assessed using methods such as trypan blue exclusion, which distinguishes live cells from dead cells based on membrane integrity, or fluorescence-based live/dead assays like calcein-AM/propidium iodide staining. These assays allow for quantification of live cells under a microscope or via cell counter. Accurate viability assessment helps prioritize high-quality cell populations for downstream culture. Only viable, healthy cells are used for organoid seeding to enhance the likelihood of robust organoid formation, minimize contamination by necrotic material, and maintain reproducibility. In the context of limited clinical samples, optimizing the use of viable cells is essential to maximize culture efficiency and data reliability [1].

#### 8.2.3.3 *Genetic and Phenotypic Characterization*

Prior to culture, genomic sequencing or immunohistochemical staining may be performed to verify tumor content and ensure sample relevance to the study objectives [8]. This is especially useful when tissue biobank is available and organoid culture can be established from cryopreserved samples.

## 8.3 Optimization of Organoid Culture Conditions

### 8.3.1 *Cultivation Conditions*

The cultivation of organoids is a meticulous process that requires carefully regulated conditions to ensure successful growth and maintenance. Key factors include the use of extracellular matrices, customized culture media, and controlled environmental parameters.

1. **Extracellular Matrix (ECM):** The ECM provides a 3D scaffold that closely mimics the native tissue microenvironment. Matrigel, a widely used basement

membrane matrix derived from Engelbreth-Holm-Swarm mouse sarcoma cells, supplies critical structural proteins such as laminin and collagen IV, along with growth factors that support proliferation and differentiation [11]. Synthetic hydrogels are also being explored to enhance reproducibility and reduce batch variability [14].

2. **Culture Media:** Organoid culture media must be tailored to the tissue of origin and typically include:
   - **Wnt agonists (e.g., R-spondin):** To maintain stemness.
   - **Epidermal Growth Factor:** To promote proliferation.
   - **Noggin:** To inhibit BMP signaling and support self-renewal.
   - **N2 and B27 supplements:** To provide neuronal and epithelial support [15].

   Ongoing research continues to optimize media formulations for specific tissue types. It is advised to purchase culture medium validated for organoid growth. Key parameters to access the culture medium include success rate of establish organoid culture, rate of proliferation, and support for subculture.
3. **Environmental Factors:** Standard culture conditions include incubation at 37°C in a humidified atmosphere with 5% $CO_2$. For tumor organoids, hypoxic environments may be simulated to better replicate poorly vascularized tumors and increase physiological relevance [12]. But most of the time, organoids are cultured in regular cell culture conditions.

## 8.3.2 *Access of Organoid Culture*

Rigorous assessment is essential to maintain the integrity and reproducibility of organoid cultures.

1. **Morphological Assessment:** Regular monitoring under the microscope helps detect changes in size, shape, and overall morphology. Unusual features may signal contamination or suboptimal growth conditions [2].
2. **Genomic Validation:** Techniques such as whole-genome sequencing or RNA sequencing are employed to verify that organoids retain the genetic characteristics of the original tissue. This is especially important for tumor-derived organoids used in drug testing [8].
3. **Functional Testing:** Functional validation ensures that organoids replicate key physiological functions of the parent tissue. For example, intestinal organoids

should demonstrate absorption and secretion activity, while brain organoids are evaluated for synaptic signaling [1].

### 8.3.3 *Challenges in Cultivation*

Despite substantial progress, several obstacles remain in standardizing and scaling organoid culture:

1. **Batch-to-Batch Variability:** Natural ECM products like Matrigel can vary in composition, affecting reproducibility. ECM from different bands or different batches behave differently. It is advisable to store a validated batch to ensure consistency. Research into defined synthetic matrices is ongoing to address this concern [14].
2. **Tissue-Specific Protocols:** Each tissue type may require a unique set of growth factors and culture conditions. For example, lung organoids differ substantially from hepatic or intestinal organoids in their requirements. Detailed standard operating procedures need to be developed for each tissue type.
3. **Long-Term Maintenance:** Extended culture periods can lead to genetic drift or phenotypic instability. Regular validation and controlled passaging are necessary to maintain the biological relevance of long-term cultures [7]. For organoid-based drug sensitivity test, it is recommended to perform the test within three passages to minimize inconsistency between organoid and the sample of origin.

## 8.4 Drug Testing Methodology

### 8.4.1 *Drug Screening*

Drug screening is a cornerstone of organoid-based drug sensitivity testing (DST), enabling the identification of effective treatments tailored to individual patients. This process involves drug selection, experimental setup, and evaluation of therapeutic efficacy.

1. **Drug Selection:** Screening protocols may include U.S. Food and Drug Administration (FDA)-approved therapies, investigational compounds, or personalized drug combinations based on a patient's tumor profile. Standard chemotherapeutic agents are often included as controls, while novel compounds are explored for targeted or combination strategies. Personalized regimens are

typically aligned with molecular characteristics such as KRAS or TP53 mutations. It is advised to communicate with clinicians to select the panel of drugs for testing [16, 17].

2. **Experimental Setup:** High-throughput screening platforms are widely adopted for their capacity to test multiple agents simultaneously. Robotic liquid handling systems and automated imaging tools enable precise dosing and minimize user variability, increasing reproducibility [18]. Manual handling is also accepted if automated equipment is not available.
3. **Drug Efficacy Evaluation:** Drug response is commonly assessed through viability assays, which measures ATP as an indicator of metabolic activity. Additional tools like live-cell imaging and confocal microscopy offer spatial and temporal insights into drug-induced changes, including apoptosis and proliferation [2].

### 8.4.2 *Testing Platforms*

Microplate reader is typically used for data collection for cell viability assay. Recent advancement suggests high-content imaging systems to be an alternative platform. These platforms integrate advanced microscopy with artificial intelligence-assisted image analysis to extract detailed phenotypic information. In addition to offering deep insights into drug-induced morphological and functional changes, high-content imaging provides a non-invasive method for continuous monitoring of organoid growth and viability over time following drug exposure. Compared to conventional end-point assays measured by microplate readers, this approach enhances temporal resolution and enables dynamic profiling of drug responses [19].

### 8.4.3 *Data Analysis*

Data analysis in organoid DST transforms raw assay outputs into meaningful conclusions about drug efficacy, and finally reports to clinicians for advice on therapy selection.

1. **Dose–Response Curves:** Quantitative analysis of drug responses typically involves generating dose–response curves, from which parameters like IC50 (half-maximal inhibitory concentration), $E_{max}$ (maximum effect), and Hill coefficients are derived. These metrics offer insight into both the potency

and efficacy of each compound tested. Curve-fitting algorithms are used to model the sigmoidal relationship between drug concentration and biological response. These curves are essential for comparing relative sensitivities [20, 21].

2. **Predictive Modeling:** To manage the complexity of organoid DST data, machine learning techniques such as unsupervised clustering, support vector machines, and deep neural networks are increasingly utilized. These models integrate organoid-specific phenotypic, genotypic, and treatment response data to classify tumor subtypes and forecast responses to therapies. In clinical settings, predictive models can aid in stratifying patients and prioritizing drug candidates with the highest likelihood of success [22].
3. **Biological Interpretation:** A comprehensive understanding of drug effects requires integration of DST data with high-throughput molecular datasets, including genomics, transcriptomics, proteomics, and metabolomics. These multi-omics approaches help elucidate the underlying mechanisms of drug sensitivity or resistance. For instance, linking a gene mutation to a poor drug response can inform combination strategies or the need for alternative therapies. Such integrative analyses are crucial for identifying biomarkers and improving the translational relevance of organoid-based platforms [23].

### 8.4.4 *Challenges and Future Directions*

Challenges in organoid-based DST include variability in organoid generation, scalability, and complex data interpretation. Addressing these issues requires the development of standardized protocols, incorporation of artificial intelligence-driven analytics, and refinement of bioengineering tools. Continued collaboration between bioengineers, data scientists, and clinicians will be essential to fully realize the clinical potential of this platform.

## 8.5 Quality Control and Standardization

Robust quality control and standardization are essential to ensure reproducibility and translational value in organoid-based DST. As this platform moves toward clinical adoption, harmonizing experimental variables and analytical approaches becomes increasingly critical.

### 8.5.1 *Sample Management*

Effective sample management begins at the point of collection and extends through culture, testing, and long-term storage. Key considerations include:

1. **Documentation and Metadata:** Each sample should be accompanied by comprehensive metadata including patient ID, diagnosis, treatment history, collection method, and anatomical origin. Accurate recordkeeping supports traceability and data interpretation. Whenever possible, incorporating molecular profiling data, such as sequencing results, is recommended. These data provide additional insights into disease mechanisms and may enhance downstream analyses, such as biomarker identification and therapeutic target discovery.
2. **Labeling and Tracking:** Standardized labeling using barcodes or QR codes, combined with robust digital inventory systems, is essential for minimizing human error and ensuring traceability. A centralized sample tracking system allows real-time updates of sample status, location, and handling history, which facilitates quality assurance and regulatory compliance, especially in clinical research settings.
3. **Sample Integrity:** Prompt processing of freshly collected tissues is vital to maintain high cellular viability and preserve molecular fidelity. Delays can result in cell death, enzymatic degradation, or shifts in gene expression profiles. When immediate processing is not feasible, the use of validated cryopreservation protocols ensures that organoid cultures can still be established later with minimal compromise to quality and reproducibility.

### 8.5.2 *Experimental Standardization*

Reducing inter-experimental and inter-laboratory variability requires rigorous standardization of procedures.

1. **Protocol Harmonization:** The adoption of harmonized protocols for key procedures — such as tissue dissociation, organoid seeding, culture maintenance, drug treatment, and endpoint measurements — is essential for ensuring comparability across studies. Shared standard operating procedures reduce inter-operator variability, enhance reproducibility, and facilitate collaboration between research

centers. Use of validated, peer-reviewed protocols also allows findings to be replicated more easily and increases the robustness of multi-center studies.

2. **Reference Standards:** Establishing defined positive and negative controls and using standardized reagents are critical for benchmarking performance. Consistent application of these standards enables cross-experimental comparison and helps identify batch-specific anomalies.
3. **Technical Replicates:** Incorporating technical replicates across all experimental conditions is fundamental for quantifying biological variability and improving the reliability of drug response data. Performing independent repeat assays on multiple organoid wells ensures that results are not artifacts of localized culture variability. Statistical methods, such as coefficient of variation and reproducibility metrics, can then be applied to assess consistency and validate conclusions with higher confidence.

### 8.5.3 *Data Reporting and Validation*

Transparent and consistent data reporting is essential to ensure reproducibility, support collaborative research, and facilitate data reuse in organoid-based DST.

1. **Reporting Parameters:** All experimental details should be comprehensively documented, including organoid passage number, seeding density, type and concentration of drugs used, duration of drug exposure, assay types, and readout techniques. Metadata such as culture duration, media formulation, and ECM source should also be reported. Clear and detailed documentation improves the interpretability of results and enables accurate replication by other researchers.
2. **Statistical Validation:** Robust statistical methodologies must be applied to analyze and interpret DST results. This includes replicate averaging, assessment of inter- and intra-assay variability, and calculation of confidence intervals. Use of appropriate statistical tests — such as ANOVA, t-tests, or non-parametric equivalents — ensures that conclusions are supported by rigorous analysis. Statistical thresholds for determining significance should be predefined and consistently applied.
3. **Data Sharing:** Whenever possible, experimental data, protocols, and metadata should be deposited into public or consortium-based repositories. Sharing

datasets in accessible formats encourages external validation, fosters transparency, and accelerates method optimization across the field. Initiatives like the Human Cancer Models Initiative and organoid portals support the creation of standardized, open-access organoid data frameworks.

### 8.5.4 *Challenges in Cross-Laboratory Consistency*

Despite ongoing efforts to harmonize organoid workflows, significant challenges persist across different laboratories.

1. **Protocol Variation:** Differences in media composition, ECM products, enzyme sources, and handling procedures can introduce considerable variability in organoid morphology, growth rates, and drug responses. For instance, batch-to-batch inconsistency in Matrigel has been widely recognized as a major source of reproducibility challenges in organoid research [14].
2. **Data Analysis Pipelines:** Variations in the tools and statistical methods used for data processing — such as normalization strategies, curve fitting algorithms, and criteria for hit selection — can lead to inconsistencies in result interpretation. These disparities hinder the development and validation of universal drug response models and complicate multi-center data comparison [24].

## 8.6 Case Studies and Applications

Organoid-based DST has moved beyond proof-of-concept validation and is now utilized in translational research and co-clinical trials. With the ability to recapitulate individual tumor biology *in vitro*, organoids offer a powerful platform to test therapeutic agents under conditions that mimic patient-specific contexts. These systems are particularly suited for precision medicine.

Over the past decade, a growing body of literature has highlighted the effectiveness of organoid-based DST in various cancer types, showing impressive correlations between *in vitro* responses and clinical outcomes. These case studies provide concrete examples of how PDOs can be applied in both academic and clinical settings, paving the way for routine integration into oncology workflows. The examples that follow demonstrate the versatility of the platform across a broad spectrum of tumors, highlighting its predictive accuracy, therapeutic relevance, and practical feasibility.

## 8.6.1 *Colorectal Cancer*

Vlachogiannis *et al.* conducted a landmark study involving 21 patients with metastatic colorectal cancer, from whom 110 organoids were successfully derived [16]. These PDOs were exposed to 55 different therapeutic regimens, reflecting the actual treatment plans administered to the patients. The study aimed to assess the predictive accuracy of organoid-based DST by comparing *in vitro* responses with clinical outcomes.

The results were highly encouraging: the organoid models achieved an overall concordance of 88% with clinical responses. More specifically, the sensitivity of the organoid assay was reported at 100%, indicating that all true responders in clinical settings were correctly identified by the PDOs. The specificity was 93%, meaning that non-responders were also accurately predicted in most cases. The positive predictive value (PPV) stood at 88%, while the negative predictive value (NPV) reached 100%. These findings demonstrate not only the robustness but also the clinical utility of organoid models in identifying effective therapies and avoiding ineffective ones.

In addition to guiding treatment decisions, the study revealed mechanisms of resistance that were not detectable through genomic profiling alone. For instance, some organoids exhibited resistance due to phenotypic plasticity and stem-like cell populations, suggesting a role for microenvironmental factors in drug response. These insights further underscore the advantage of functional testing using PDOs over purely molecular approaches in personalized cancer therapy.

## 8.6.2 *Gastric Cancer*

In a recent study, researchers generated PDOs from both primary gastric tumors and corresponding lymphatic metastatic lesions [25]. This paired approach allowed direct comparison of drug sensitivity between tumor stages and enhanced understanding of clonal evolution and therapeutic resistance.

The study involved organoid generation from 21 gastric cancer patients, yielding a total of 35 organoid lines (including 14 pairs of primary and lymph node-derived samples). These PDOs were characterized through histopathological assessment and genomic sequencing, confirming high concordance with the originating tissues in both structure and mutational profile.

Drug testing was conducted using 15 chemotherapeutic and targeted agents commonly used in gastric cancer management. PDOs were screened for sensitivity to agents such as 5-fluorouracil, oxaliplatin, irinotecan, and trastuzumab. Sensitivity was defined by a reduction in cell viability exceeding 50% *in vitro*. The results showed a clinical concordance rate of approximately 85.7%, with sensitivity and specificity values of 87.5% and 84.6%, respectively. Notably, lymph node-derived PDOs frequently exhibited reduced sensitivity compared to their primary tumor counterparts, highlighting potential differences in drug resistance between tumor stages.

This dual-source strategy demonstrated that PDOs can be effectively used to predict individualized responses and explore tumor heterogeneity. The findings reinforce the potential of PDOs as a precision medicine tool in gastric cancer, enabling informed therapeutic choices and deeper insight into metastatic behavior.

### 8.6.3 *Lung Cancer*

A comprehensive real-world study evaluated the predictive utility of PDOs for therapy selection in advanced non-small cell lung cancer [26]. The study involved 107 patients with locally advanced or metastatic lung cancer and successfully generated 214 lung cancer organoids, primarily derived from malignant pleural effusions.

Each organoid was subjected to DST using a panel of chemotherapeutics and targeted agents tailored to the patients' clinical regimens. Clinical outcomes were measured in parallel, including radiological response and progression-free survival. Among a subset of matched clinical and organoid data (84 patient-organism comparisons), the DST exhibited strong predictive performance. For example, in EGFR-mutant cases treated with osimertinib, the area under the receiver operating characteristic curve reached 0.94, reflecting high accuracy in forecasting treatment efficacy. Across the broader dataset, the concordance between organoid DST results and actual clinical responses exceeded 85%.

In addition to first-line therapy prediction, the organoids were instrumental in guiding second-line options. For instance, in patients with acquired resistance due to RET or MET alterations, DST identified effective combinatorial strategies (e.g., osimertinib plus savolitinib), which were subsequently validated in clinical settings.

This study highlights the scalability and accuracy of organoid platforms in lung cancer, supporting their use in real-time treatment guidance and resistance management.

### 8.6.4 *Glioblastoma*

A precision oncology study utilizing patient-derived glioblastoma organoids (PD-GBOs) for individualized drug response profiling in recurrent glioblastoma [27]. The study established a PD-GBO platform to evaluate therapeutic efficacy *in vitro*, followed by *in vivo* validation using patient-derived xenograft (PDX) models.

Tumor samples were collected from four patients with recurrent glioblastoma. Each sample was used to generate PD-GBOs, which retained key histopathological and molecular characteristics of the original tumors. A panel of 41 FDA-approved drugs — including kinase inhibitors, chemotherapeutic agents, and targeted compounds — was tested for each organoid line. Drug response was assessed via cell viability assays, and data were integrated with transcriptomic profiles to identify actionable targets.

The turnaround time from tumor resection to *in vitro* treatment prediction was 13–15 days. Effective treatment candidates were identified for three out of four patients, demonstrating a 75% success rate in actionable hit generation. These candidates were subsequently validated *in vivo* using PDX models, where they exhibited tumor growth suppression consistent with organoid-based predictions.

This study illustrates the feasibility and clinical relevance of integrating PD-GBOs into a rapid decision-making framework. It further highlights how drug screening in organoids, when combined with genomic profiling and PDX validation, can provide a robust strategy for navigating therapeutic resistance in aggressive and heterogeneous tumors like glioblastoma.

### 8.6.5 *Breast Cancer*

A recent study titled "Establishment of patient-derived organoids for guiding personalized therapies in breast cancer patients" provides a robust demonstration of organoid utility in breast cancer precision medicine [26]. In this prospective clinical investigation, 87 breast cancer patients were enrolled, from whom 69 organoids were successfully cultured, resulting in a culture success rate of approximately 79.3%.

Each PDO line underwent DST against a panel of 12 standard and targeted therapies, including docetaxel, doxorubicin, tamoxifen, palbociclib, and olaparib. The PDOs retained histological and molecular features of their parental tumors, and subtype-specific drug responses were observed. Notably, BRCA1/2-mutant organoids displayed marked sensitivity to PARP inhibitors.

The predictive performance of the PDO assay was assessed by comparing *in vitro* drug responses with clinical outcomes across a subset of patients. The study reported a sensitivity of 83.3%, specificity of 88.0%, PPV of 85.7%, and NPV of 86.2%, achieving an overall concordance rate of 86.9%.

These findings underscore the effectiveness of PDOs in modeling inter-patient heterogeneity and enabling personalized therapeutic decisions. The study demonstrates how breast cancer organoids can be integrated into real-world clinical workflows to improve treatment outcomes, particularly for genetically defined subgroups like BRCA-mutated patients.

### 8.6.6 *Ovarian Cancer*

Researchers developed a syngeneic organoid model system from genetically engineered mouse models that faithfully recapitulate high-grade serous ovarian carcinoma. While the study did not use human PDOs, it employed a platform with high translational relevance to BRCA1-deficient ovarian cancer [28].

The research involved the generation of 25 syngeneic organoid lines engineered with combinations of Trp53, BRCA1, and RB1 mutations. These organoids were subjected to drug screening with a panel of 11 agents, including PARP inhibitors (e.g., olaparib), platinum-based chemotherapy (e.g., cisplatin), and PI3K inhibitors. Using Bliss independence and Loewe additivity models, the study identified synergistic drug combinations tailored to specific genetic alterations.

Although the study was preclinical and did not report human sensitivity, specificity, or predictive values, it demonstrated a strong correlation between organoid responses and *in vivo* therapeutic efficacy in murine transplantation models. Organoids with BRCA1 loss were particularly sensitive to olaparib and showed enhanced tumor control when treated with combination regimens.

This research underscores the potential of genetically defined organoid platforms for the development of personalized combination therapies, particularly in genetically stratified subsets like BRCA-deficient ovarian cancer. It provides a strong foundation for future studies involving PDOs in clinical settings.

### 8.6.7 *Liver Cancer*

In a foundational study researchers successfully established long-term organoid cultures from primary liver cancers, including hepatocellular carcinoma (HCC), cholangiocarcinoma (CCA), and combined HCC/CCA subtypes. The study aimed to model liver cancer heterogeneity and evaluate the utility of organoids in therapeutic screening [29].

A total of 11 patient-derived tumor samples were used to generate subtype-specific organoids. These cultures preserved the histological and molecular features of their original tumors and were characterized via transcriptomic and proteomic profiling. Importantly, the researchers performed drug screening across these models using a panel of 29 agents, including sorafenib (standard of care for HCC), MEK inhibitors, and epigenetic modulators.

Although the study did not report explicit sensitivity, specificity, PPV, or NPV values, the drug response profiles were found to be subtype-specific and consistent with known vulnerabilities. For example, CCA organoids exhibited higher sensitivity to FGFR inhibitors, whereas HCC organoids demonstrated partial response to sorafenib and MEK inhibition. These findings highlight the translational potential of liver cancer PDOs in identifying subtype-guided therapeutic opportunities.

This work laid the groundwork for using liver cancer organoids in both basic research and clinical applications, offering a reproducible platform to study liver tumor biology, test drug efficacy, and develop personalized treatment strategies.

### 8.6.8 *Pancreatic Cancer*

A pivotal study highlighted the translational potential of pancreatic cancer PDOs in predicting clinical drug response [30]. The study established 66 PDO lines from 113 patient samples, yielding a success rate of 58%, and evaluated the organoids' drug sensitivity using a panel of standard-of-care agents including gemcitabine, paclitaxel, 5-fluorouracil, and irinotecan.

Drug sensitivity in PDOs was determined via dose–response assays and correlated with actual patient outcomes using RECIST criteria and progression-free survival data. Among the subset of patients with matched clinical outcomes (n = 35), PDO responses demonstrated a sensitivity of 100%, specificity of 93%, PPV of 94%, and NPV of 100%, with an overall concordance rate of 97%.

This study established PDO-based DST as a feasible and highly accurate approach for guiding pancreatic cancer treatment, particularly in the selection of first-line therapies. It also underscored the ability of organoids to reflect tumor heterogeneity and capture mechanisms of resistance not readily identified through genomic profiling alone.

### 8.6.9 *Summary of Case Study Insights*

The breadth of clinical and translational studies reviewed in this chapter highlights the remarkable utility of organoid-based DST in precision oncology. Across a wide spectrum of tumor types — including colorectal, gastric, lung, pancreatic, breast, liver, and ovarian cancers — organoid models have consistently demonstrated high predictive accuracy in identifying patient-specific therapeutic responses.

The predictive metrics reported across different studies were particularly compelling. Sensitivity, specificity, and concordance rates often exceeded 85%, with several studies reaching or surpassing 90% accuracy in forecasting patient responses. For example, colorectal and pancreatic cancer organoids showed almost perfect alignment with clinical outcomes, while breast and lung cancer PDOs achieved similarly robust predictive values. These metrics affirm the reliability of PDOs as functional proxies for real-world tumor behavior.

However, cancer-specific nuances were observed. In gastric cancer, paired organoids from primary and metastatic lesions revealed differing sensitivities, highlighting intra-patient heterogeneity and clonal evolution. In glioblastoma and ovarian cancer, organoids provided key insights into resistance mechanisms and enabled the design of targeted combination therapies. Meanwhile, liver and pancreatic organoid models illustrated the potential for subtype-specific drug stratification.

Overall, these studies confirm that organoid-based DST is not only feasible across multiple cancer types but also highly informative for guiding individualized treatment strategies. As technologies evolve and standardization improves, PDO platforms are poised to play a central role in functional precision medicine, bridging molecular insights with actionable clinical decisions.

## 8.7 Conclusion

Organoid-based DST has emerged as a valuable platform in the era of precision oncology. By capturing the histological and molecular complexity of individual tumors, organoids offer functional insight that complements genomic profiling and enables more accurate treatment prediction. The breadth of case studies presented in this chapter confirms the versatility of PDO-based testing across multiple tumor types, from common cancers like colorectal and breast to challenging entities like pancreatic and glioblastoma.

Despite these advances, several challenges limit the full integration of organoid technology into routine clinical workflows. First, differences in culture conditions, extracellular matrices, and assay protocols contribute to variability in results, underscoring the need for protocol harmonization. Second, turnaround time and scalability remain concerns, especially for aggressive malignancies where rapid decisions are critical. Third, limited tissue availability and difficulty in culturing some tumor types restrict the generalizability of PDOs. Finally, interpreting the complex data generated from high-content screening and multi-omics integration still requires advanced bioinformatics tools and validation.

Looking forward, future efforts should focus on improving culture efficiency, automating workflows, and embedding standardized quality control measures.

Collaboration across research centers and clinical institutions is also vital for generating large-scale datasets and establishing benchmarks for clinical validation. As these efforts advance, organoid-based DST is poised to become a cornerstone in personalized cancer treatment, bridging preclinical testing and patient-specific therapeutic decision-making.

## Key Opinion Points

- **Standardization Is Essential:** Experts agree that harmonizing culture protocols, drug screening procedures, and analytical frameworks is a top priority to improve reproducibility and clinical translation.
- **Clinical Integration Requires Scalability:** To become a routine part of precision oncology, organoid platforms must achieve faster turnaround times, higher success rates across cancer types, and compatibility with hospital-based workflows.
- **Functional Testing Complements Genomics:** Organoid DST provides dynamic, phenotypic data that captures tumor heterogeneity and drug resistance mechanisms not evident through molecular profiling alone. Experts suggest its integration with sequencing-based methods to enable more comprehensive patient stratification.

## References

1. Lancaster MA, Knoblich JA. Organogenesis in a dish: modeling development and disease using organoid technologies. Science. 2014;345(6194):1247125.
2. Fatehullah A, Tan SH, Barker N. Organoids as an in vitro model of human development and disease. Nat Cell Biol. 2016;18(3):246–254.
3. Qu S, *et al.* Patient-derived organoids in human cancer: a platform for fundamental research and precision medicine. Mol Biomed. 2024;5(1):6.
4. Silva TN, Worthley DL, Woods SL. Precision medicine for gastric cancer: current state of organoid drug testing. Organoids. 2024;3(4):266–280.
5. Hofree M, *et al.* Challenges in identifying cancer genes by analysis of exome sequencing data. Nat Commun. 2016;7:12096.
6. Przybylla R, *et al.* Novel in vitro models for cell differentiation and drug transport studies of the human intestine. Cells. 2023;12(19).
7. van de Wetering M, *et al.* Prospective derivation of a living organoid biobank of colorectal cancer patients. Cell. 2015;161(4):933–945.

8. Sachs N, *et al.* A living biobank of breast cancer organoids captures disease heterogeneity. Cell. 2018;172(1–2):373–386.e10.
9. Tiriac H, *et al.* Organoid profiling identifies common responders to chemotherapy in pancreatic cancer. Cancer Discov. 2018;8(9):1112–1129.
10. Wu Z, *et al.* Expert consensus on patient derived tumor organoid culture and drug sensitivity testing. J Organoid Biosci. 2024;2(2):1–14.
11. Huch M, *et al.* The hope and the hype of organoid research. Development. 2017;144(6): 938–941.
12. Clevers H. Modeling development and disease with organoids. Cell. 2016;165(7): 1586–1597.
13. Sontheimer-Phelps A, *et al.* Human colon-on-a-chip enables continuous in vitro analysis of colon mucus layer accumulation and physiology. Cell Mol Gastroenterol Hepatol. 2020;9(3):507–526.
14. Gjorevski N, *et al.* Designer matrices for intestinal stem cell and organoid culture. Nature. 2016;539(7630):560–564.
15. Sato T, *et al.* Single Lgr5 stem cells build crypt-villus structures in vitro without a mesenchymal niche. Nature. 2009;459(7244):262–265.
16. Vlachogiannis G, *et al.* Patient-derived organoids model treatment response of metastatic gastrointestinal cancers. Science. 2018;359(6378):920–926.
17. Kopper O, *et al.* An organoid platform for ovarian cancer captures intra- and interpatient heterogeneity. Nat Med. 2019;25(5):838–849.
18. Jiang S, *et al.* An automated organoid platform with inter-organoid homogeneity and inter-patient heterogeneity. Cell Rep Med. 2020;1(9):100161.
19. Charles S, *et al.* Non-invasive quality control of organoid cultures using mesofluidic CSTR bioreactors and high-content imaging. Adv Mater Technol. 2025;10(3).
20. Bi J, *et al.* Successful patient-derived organoid culture of gynecologic cancers for disease modeling and drug sensitivity testing. Cancers (Basel). 2021;13(12).
21. Lee SY, *et al.* Correction: Cancer organoid-based diagnosis reactivity prediction (CODRP) index-based anticancer drug sensitivity test in ALK-rearrangement positive non-small cell lung cancer (NSCLC). J Exp Clin Cancer Res. 2023;42(1):332.
22. Fujimura Y, *et al.* Machine learning-based estimation of spatial gene expression pattern during ESC-derived retinal organoid development. Sci Rep. 2023;13(1):22781.
23. Smith CA, *et al.* Single-cell transcriptomics of human organoid-derived enteroendocrine cell populations from the small intestine. J Physiol. 2024.
24. Rezapour M, Narayanan A, Gurcan MN. Machine learning analysis of RNA-Seq data identifies key gene signatures and pathways in Mpox virus-induced gastrointestinal complications using colon organoid models. Int J Mol Sci. 2024;25(20).

25. Yang R, *et al.* Drug-induced senescence by aurora kinase inhibitors attenuates innate immune response of macrophages on gastric cancer organoids. Cancer Lett. 2024;598: 217106.
26. Wang HM, *et al.* Using patient-derived organoids to predict locally advanced or metastatic lung cancer tumor response: a real-world study. Cell Rep Med. 2023;4(2):100911.
27. Ratliff M, *et al.* Patient-derived tumor organoids for guidance of personalized drug therapies in recurrent glioblastoma. Int J Mol Sci. 2022;23(12).
28. Zhang S, *et al.* Genetically defined, syngeneic organoid platform for developing combination therapies for ovarian cancer. Cancer Discov. 2021;11(2):362–383.
29. Broutier L, *et al.* Human primary liver cancer-derived organoid cultures for disease modeling and drug screening. Nat Med. 2017;23(12):1424–1435.
30. Grossman JE, *et al.* Organoid sensitivity correlates with therapeutic response in patients with pancreatic cancer. Clin Cancer Res. 2022;28(4):708–718.

https://doi.org/10.1142/9789819817597_0009

Chapter 9

# Single-Cell Analysis and Omics Techniques

Long Chen[1,2], Wei Jin[1], Xinrui Zhang[1], Jun Zhang[1,2], Liming Chen[2,3,*]

[1]*Department of Biochemistry, School of Life Sciences, Nanjing Normal University, Nanjing, China*

[2]*Jiangsu Institute of Cancer Research, Jiangsu Cancer Hospital, the Affiliated Cancer Hospital of Nanjing Medical University, Nanjing, China*

[3]*Jiangsu Key Laboratory of Innovative Cancer Diagnosis & Therapeutics, Cancer Institute of Jiangsu Province, Nanjing 210009, China*

**Abstract:** The term "omics" refers to a collection of fields that study the molecular composition of organisms. These fields include genomics, transcriptomics, and proteomics. Research has expanded over time from single-omics to multi-omics, incorporating single-cell resolution to gain a more detailed understanding of cellular heterogeneity. In 2013, single-cell sequencing was named "Technology of the Year" and has played a pivotal role in this shift by enabling detailed molecular analyses at the single-cell level. This technology has allowed researchers to explore previously uncharted biological questions to improve our understanding of gene expression, DNA methylation, and protein expression in individual cells. This information is important for the development of organoids with 3D cellular structures. This chapter focuses on how integrating single-cell technologies with multi-omics approaches provides a comprehensive insight into cellular behavior, regulatory mechanisms, and disease processes. It also highlights progress in the field of organoids, where transitioning from one-dimensional methods to more integrated, multi-faceted perspectives captures the complexity of 3D cellular structures at unprecedented levels. This marks the beginning of a new era in the life sciences. Combining single-cell multi-omics and organoid technology has the potential to reveal new therapeutic strategies and improve the precision of medical treatments.

**Keywords:** multi-omics, organoids, single-cell sequencing

[*]Corresponding author. Email: chenliming1981@u.nus.edu

## Key Points

1. With the development of single-cell sequencing technology, from first- to third-generation sequencing platform, high-resolution analysis of the genome and epigenome has been achieved. Integration with organoid models has illuminated the dynamic evolution of cellular heterogeneity, gene regulatory mechanisms, and disease mechanisms, including cancer.
2. Single-cell transcriptome sequencing (scRNA-seq) analyzes cell diversity, developmental trajectory and tumor microenvironment through tools such as Seurat and RNA velocity analysis. These tools promote a deep understanding of gene expression dynamics in precision medicine.
3. Single-cell proteomics has lagged behind due to technical limitations (such as low sensitivity and complex post-translational modification) and relies on fluorescent labeling, antibody detection and mass spectrometry. However, it is still necessary to overcome the bottleneck of protein abundance fluctuation and multi-omics integration.
4. Multi-omics integration technologies, such as G&T-seq and CITE-seq, combine genome, transcriptome, epigenome and proteome data with computational tools and CRISPR screening to comprehensively analyze cellular regulatory networks and disease mechanisms.
5. As 3D disease models, organoids solve the problem of sample scarcity and improve the efficiency of drug screening. However, challenges regarding standardization, repeatability, and cost still hinder the expansion of organoid applications from basic research to precision medicine.

## 9.1 Introduction

With the deepening of biological research, scientists' understanding of life is increasingly shifting from a single, traditional experimental model to a more complex and multi-dimensional level. The rise of this new process, single-cell omics technology, has given us a finer perspective for observing cellular heterogeneity, allowing us to study it at an unprecedented resolution. Cellular heterogeneity refers to the differences in gene expression, metabolic activity and other molecular characteristics of different cells within a population, which is of great significance for the occurrence, development and treatment of diseases.

The emergence of single-cell omics technology allows us to not only explore the differences between the genome and transcriptome at the level of a single cell, but also reveal the dynamic changes of different components (such as RNA, DNA, protein, etc.) in the cell (Figure 9.1). The application of this technology has brought revolutionary advances in many fields such as basic biology, oncology, and neuroscience. Especially in cancer research, single-cell omics technology provides unprecedented tools for the elucidation of the diversity of tumor microenvironment and tumor heterogeneity.

Furthermore, the ongoing advancement of multi-omics technologies has established single-cell multi-omics as an emerging frontier. By simultaneously analyzing the genome, transcriptome, epigenetics and other information of a single cell, researchers can obtain more comprehensive cellular information and reveal the interaction and

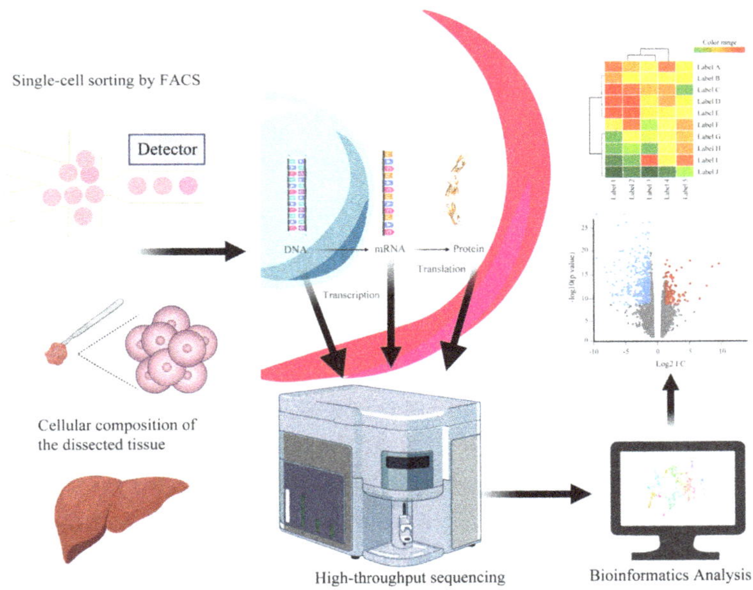


**Figure 9.1** Schematic diagram of single-cell multi-omics process from sample collection, preparation, sequencing to analysis [1]. First. cellular suspension is obtained from the dissected tissue and single cells are sorted by fluorescence-activated cell sorting. Then, high-throughput sequencing is performed on single cells to acquire the data of the transcriptome and proteome. Finally, bioinformatics analysis is utilized to process sequencing and visualize data.

regulatory mechanism between different levels. For instance, integrating single-cell genomics with epigenetic studies can improve our understanding of the intricacies involved in gene expression regulation and shaping phenotypes.

Complementing this, organoid technology offers a transformative platform for life science research. Organoids are 3D cell populations obtained by *in vitro* culture, which can mimic the structure and function of tissues and organs *in vivo*. The maturation of organoid technology enables scientists to faithfully recapitulate developmental processes, pathological states, and drug responses, thereby facilitating drug discovery, disease modeling (including cancer), and regenerative medicine.

## 9.2 The Development of Single-cell Sequencing Technology in Genomics and Epigenomics

The term "genome" refers to the entirety of genetic material within a given organism, comprising DNA (or RNA in certain viruses). The genome contains all the genetic information required by an organism and controls its development, growth, metabolism and physiological functions [2]. The development of omics research is predicated on sequencing technology, wherein DNA sequencing technology, also known as gene sequencing, serves as the foundational bedrock for advancing molecular biology, genetic engineering, and our understanding of life's genetic basis [3, 4].

In 1977, the pioneering scientists Walter Gilbert and Frederick Sanger developed the first sequencing method that allowed them to sequence the bacteriophage φX174, a breakthrough that marked the dawn of genomics, despite the fact that the genome consisted of only 5,375 base pairs. Since then, sequencing technology has undergone a tremendous transformation, from first- to third-generation sequencing methods. The original first-generation sequencing technology was only available for small fragments (700 to 1,000 bases) and is still in use today [5]. However, with the growing demands of modern science, particularly in the fields of genomics and personalized medicine, it is clear that this technology is no longer sufficient. In the mid-2000s, the release of the first truly high-throughput sequencing platform reduced the cost of sequencing the human genome by a factor of 50,000 compared to the Human Genome Project, giving rise to next-generation sequencing technology [6]. This innovative technology signifies a substantial advancement, enabling the simultaneous sequencing of an impressive number of DNA fragments, ranging from thousands to millions, in a single run. These advances have significantly increased sequencing yields while reducing costs and making genomic research more accessible [7]. However, despite the high throughput of next-generation sequencing, the short reads that are often generated can make complex genome assembly difficult. In order to confront this challenge, researchers have introduced methods of single-molecule sequencing, which enable the direct sequencing of longer DNA fragments, frequently exceeding tens of thousands of bases. This improvement in accuracy has led to a reduction in errors introduced by short-read techniques, thereby facilitating more precise genome assembly [8].

All multicellular organisms originate from a single cell. In humans, for example, an adult is made up of about 40 trillion cells, and these cells originate from a fertilized egg, which is formed by combining genetic material from both parents [11]. Through a series of cell divisions and differentiation, the zygote forms a variety of different cell types, which in turn form tissues and eventually develop into a complete individual. It is therefore generally assumed that all cells in an organism have much the same genetic make-up [12]. However, each cell contains not only germline polymorphisms inherited from parents, but also entirely new mutations acquired during germ cell formation, as well as somatic mutations that accumulate during successive cell divisions [13]. These genetic variations are not random; they document the DNA damage and repair processes that occur in the germline and somatic cells. Therefore, studying these genomic mutations not only helps to develop personalized treatment strategies, but also provides valuable insights into evolutionary biology and population genetics through time series analysis [14] (Figure 9.2).

Substantial evidence indicates that the progressive accumulation of genomic abnormalities occurs widely in seemingly healthy cells during aging. This accumulation is believed to be a fundamental cause of numerous human diseases. The widespread application of genomics has had a profound impact on precision medicine. By identifying the genetic variants that contribute most to individual differences, researchers can better understand the genetic basis of disease and develop targeted therapies [15–17].

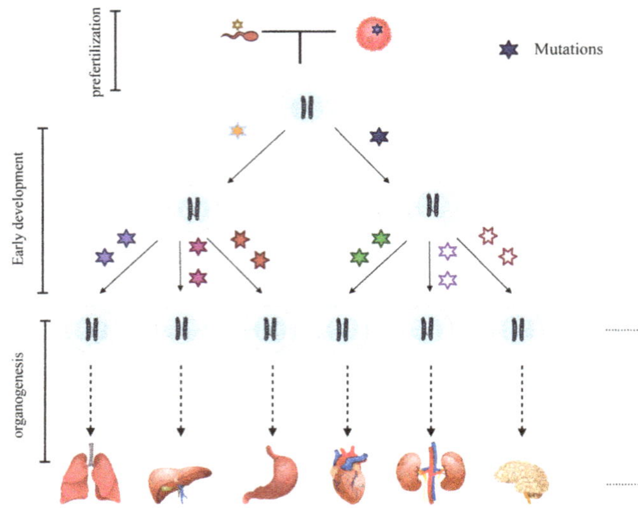


**Figure 9.2** Schematic diagram of somatic mutations occuring during the development of multicellular organisms from fertilization [9]. Different mutations occur at each stage of development, from the union of the sperm and egg to form a fertilized egg, through the early stages, and on to the formation of an organ. Studying these mutations in individual development has important implications for developing personalized therapeutic strategies, as well as for studying evolution and population genetics from a time-series perspective. The star shapes represent mutations.

In recent years, extensive whole-genome sequencing efforts have focused on tumor tissue, systematically classifying somatic mutations in human cancers [18]. In contrast, normal tissues tend to have few, weaker mutations that may occur in only a few cells, making it difficult to identify these weak mutational signals [19]. The advent of single-cell resolution technology has precipitated a paradigm shift in the field of somatic mutation research, enabling the exploration of previously inaccessible intricacies within normal tissues [20, 21]. Historically, disease research has often been limited by sample availability. This field has been revolutionized by the development of organoid technology [22]. Organoid technology enables long-term clonal expansion of stem cells. These 3D structures — which recapitulate *in vivo* tissue physiology — are powerful tools for studying disease pathogenesis, including infectious, genetic, and malignant disorders. Organoids uniquely permit the analysis of somatic mutations in single cells while circumventing whole-genome amplification artifacts [23, 24]. Beyond genomics, single-cell epigenomic profiling are equally critical for delineating gene regulatory dynamics

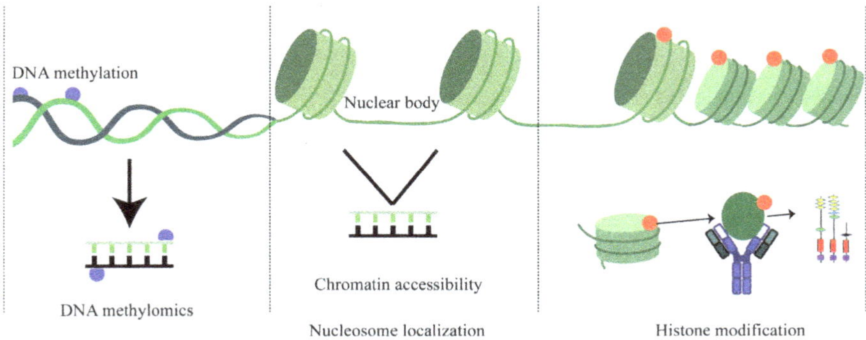


**Figure 9.3** Schematic diagram of major epigenetic events. A series of epigenetic changes were observed in cells, including aberrant genomic methylation, histone modifications and chromatin accessibility. The study of these epigenetic phenomena using single-cell techniques will provide a powerful tool for exploring dynamic changes in gene expression.

underlying cellular phenotypes [25-27]. These methods can explore a wealth of epigenetic information at the single-cell level, ranging from DNA methylation, nucleosome positioning, chromosomal accessibility to histone modifications (Figure 9.3).

Presently, the most widely used method is ATAC-seq, which was developed in 2013 by the laboratories of William J. Greenleaf and Howard Y. Chang at Stanford University. This method is employed to study the physical structure of the genome by identifying open chromatin regions [28]. This technique uses a highly active transposase enzyme that binds to an open chromatin region and inserts a sequencing adapter as it cleaves the region. The sequencing library obtained by this method contains sequences rich in the open chromatin region, and the dynamic remodeling of chromatin structure is one of the main mechanisms influencing which genes are transcribed and when. When chromatin is open, DNA-binding proteins can approach regulatory sequences and enable transcription. Single-cell ATAC-seq (scATAC-seq) captures single cells using the Fluidigm C1 microfluidic platform, fragments open chromatin using the Tn5 transposase, and labels and amplifies libraries using cell-recognition barcode primers, further improving the efficiency of identifying open chromatin regions. This approach can provide information on chromatin accessibility and reveal regions of gene transcription in single cells [29]. But it doesn't stop there. Hundreds of thousands of regulatory elements work synergistically in different contexts to orchestrate gene expression patterns, and scATAC-seq provides information about these different elements, including their cell type specificity, binding site motifs, and whether low-expressed genes such as transcription factors are likely to be turned on [30, 31].

Bisulfite sequencing (BS-seq) remains the gold standard for base-resolution DNA methylation profiling, with bisulfite-specific PCR widely used for targeted analysis [32]. The method relies on bisulfite conversion, where unmethylated cytosines undergo deamination to uracil, while 5-methylcytosine resists conversion. Subsequent sequencing identifies methylation patterns by detecting C-to-T transitions in amplified DNA. The primary benefit of the base switch-based approach is that it facilitates the study of the demethylation of specific CpG sites. Its popularity among researchers stems from its high transformation efficiency (>99%), good reproducibility, and easy access to commercial kits. The prevailing approach in conventional single-cell methylation assays is predicated on the process of bisulfite conversion [33].

Among bisulfite-based methylation profiling methods, Reduced Representation Bisulfite Sequencing (RRBS) offers a cost-effective solution for CpG-rich region analysis, while Whole-Genome Bisulfite Sequencing (WGBS) provides comprehensive coverage at higher expense. Their core distinction lies in RRBS's use of restriction enzymes (e.g., MspI) to selectively digest and enrich CpG islands — enabling focused interrogation of gene promoters and regulatory elements — whereas WGBS interrogates methylation signatures across the entire genome without enrichment [34].

Furthermore, methylation sequencing methods have been developed that do not require bisulfite conversion, leveraging the binding affinity of methylcytosine and the sensitivity of restriction enzymes to methylcytosine. MBD-seq and MeDIP-seq are representative methods using affinity-based approaches. The utilization of affinity-based methodologies proves to be disadvantageous in the context of single-cell sequencing due to their tendency to generate average DNA methylation profiles, which are derived from DNA fragments. As a consequence, these methods fail to discern discrepancies in DNA methylation patterns among individual cells. Therefore, scRRBS proposed by the team in 2013 is still based on the bisulfite conversion method [35].

Histone modifications are often thought of as molecular switches in gene expression, mediating reversible and heritable regulation controlled by enzymes to maintain cellular homeostasis. This perturbation of homeostasis can influence the onset and progression of disease [36]. To explore histone modification information, it is often necessary to combine chromatin immunoprecipitation with next-generation sequencing, and efficiently detect DNA sequences that interact with histones and transcription factors on a genome-wide scale. Weitz's team first proposed a single-cell ChIP-seq technology, Drop-ChIP [37]. It combines microfluidics, DNA barcoding and high-throughput sequencing to generate H3K4me3 and H3K4me2 chromatin profiles at single-cell resolution in mouse embryonic stem cells, embryonic fibroblasts and hematopoietic progenitor cells. Subsequently, in 2019, three research teams published articles on single-cell ChIP-seq methods, CoBATCH, CUT&Tag and ACT-seq [38–40]. These are the three main single-cell ChIP-seq methods commonly used in the laboratory. The core technologies all use concanavalant-conjugated magnetic beads and protein A-Tn5 fusion proteins. Technically, all three methods have been improved, but there are still some limitations, such as high thresholds, high labor costs and cumbersome operation. At the same time, scCUT&TAG-pro is a multimodal extension of scCUT&TAG that can analyze protein-DNA interactions and single-cell surface protein abundance [41].

## 9.3 Integrating Single-Cell Transcriptomics and Computational Algorithms for Cellular Heterogeneity Analysis

Transcriptomics is the scientific study of all RNA molecules present in a cell at a specific moment and under particular conditions. This includes messenger RNA (mRNA), non-coding RNA (such as small RNA and long non-coding RNA), and other RNA categories. Transcriptomic analysis is a scientific approach that aims to reveal patterns and levels of gene expression. By studying the expression levels of genes, researchers can gain a deeper understanding of the functions and characteristics of cells in specific physiological or pathological states. This analysis can also reveal insights into the processes related to life development, disease advancement, and the effects of pharmaceutical interventions.

Transcriptomic analysis provides fundamental insights into gene expression research. In recent years, a significant advancement in the field of molecular biology has been the development of a technique known as bulk RNA-seq, which stands for "whole RNA sequencing." This method has been instrumental in elucidating the biological functions of mixed cell populations from a transcriptomic perspective [42]. However, it should be noted that this measurement merely reflects the mean of the numerous cells within the tissue sample and is therefore representative of the characteristics of the larger population of cells. Furthermore, it has been demonstrated that bulk RNA-seq is incapable of revealing alterations at the single-cell level. Additionally, this method does not accurately reflect the expression levels of infrequent cells [43].

The development of next-generation sequencing technology in 2009 led to the proposal of the first scRNA-seq technique [44] (Figure 9.4). Islam *et al.* created the first multiple scRNA-seq library using mouse embryos [45]. Until 2012, scRNA-seq technology enabled gene expression analysis with unprecedented detail. However, its effective implementation in single-cell transcript research is constrained by the limited amount

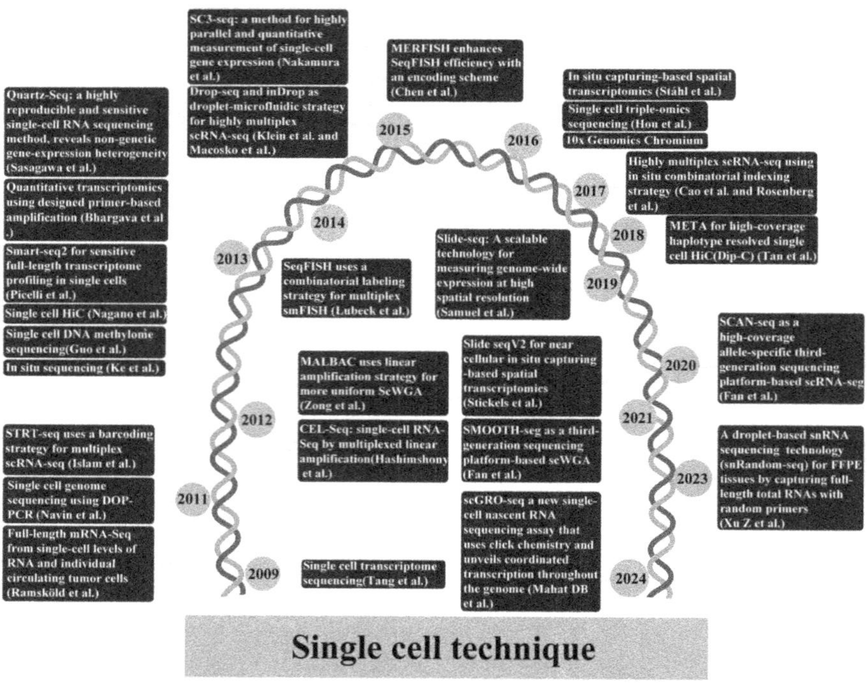


**Figure 9.4** Timeline of milestones in the development of single-cell sequencing technologies.

of RNA available for initial processing. The aforementioned problem was resolved with the advent of CEL-seq, a technique that utilizes barcoding and the amalgamation of samples to achieve linear amplification and sequencing [46]. In 2014, the advent of single-cell sequencing technology and the maturation of separation technology precipitated the commercialization of sequencing, thereby rendering it accessible to the general public [47]. A novel technique, known as Drop-seq, was subsequently developed and applied. This technique demonstrated superior accuracy in the identification of single-cell transcriptome sequencing [48]. In a 2016 study, Tirosh and colleagues explored the phenotypic relationships of thousands of cells from multiple melanoma samples with different genotypes by conducting single-cell sequencing analysis [49]. Concurrently, the analysis of individual cells from tissue samples can ascertain diverse cell states or cell types at the single-cell level. To illustrate, the examination of a solitary murine epidermis identified 25 distinct types of epidermal cell subclusters [50]. In a similar vein, a subsequent investigation sought to elucidate the correlation between particular genes, which have been identified as the causative agents of certain diseases, and the progression of said diseases. This investigation was undertaken through the utilization of a sophisticated molecular biology technique known as "sequencing analysis of single-cell transcripts" [51].

Furthermore, recent advancements in single-cell sequencing technology, SCOPE-seq (which integrates optical technology), have enabled the *in vivo* analysis of single-cell sequencing. The utilization of diverse technological approaches has facilitated the identification of a range of tumor tissues [52] .

Since then, the field of single-cell sequencing has grown rapidly and is mainly divided into microfluidics-based transcriptomics and microplate-based transcriptomics [53, 54]. Over the past decade, a variety of single-cell sequencing technologies have emerged, including titer platforms [46, 55]. For example, 10x Genomics' Chromium and Bio-Rad Laboratories' ddSEQThe isotiter platform is now a wet-lab scRNA-seq reagent. The titer instrument under consideration is distinctive in its design, wherein each minute dividing unit is equipped with all the necessary reagents for the execution of cell lysis, inverse transcription, and molecular labeling. This method enables the encapsulation of cells within these units, obviating the necessity for flow cytometry or microdissection. This approach allows researchers to perform RNA-seq analysis on thousands of cells, although specialized hardware is required to use the titer effectively [56].

From bulk RNA-seq to scRNA-seq, in addition to changes in technology, algorithms and analysis strategies based on transcriptome data have also emerged. The three most commonly used R packages, DESeq2 [57], edgeR [58] and limma [59], are commonly used for variance analysis and enrichment analysis using databases such as GO and KEGG. Several representative algorithms based on the gene enrichment algorithm GSEA [60] include ESTIMATE [61], xCell [62] and MCP-counter [63]. Based on gene expression features, the ESTIMATE algorithm uses the single-sample GSEA method to provide immune scores and stromal scores representing the proportion and distribution of immune cells and stromal cells. xCell is an alternative single-sample GSEA-based method that employs gene sets from various RNA sequencing and microarray data sources to characterize distinct cell types, thereby enhancing its resilience to noise interference. The WGCNA algorithm is used to identify co-expression patterns between genes, build gene co-expression networks and explore the relationship between genes and phenotypes or traits [64]. Algorithms such as consensus clustering have been widely used in the field of tumors and other diseases.

At the single-cell level, the most influential package is Seurat [65], which has established a relatively well-developed pipeline for single-cell analysis. In addition, Python-based packages such as Scanpy are also widely used [66]. Representative single-cell data analysis algorithms include Monocle [67], RNA velocity [68], CytoTRACE [69], CellChat [70], etc.

Monocle is an advanced algorithm designed for facilitating pseudo-temporal inference analysis. It capitalizes on the high variability of gene expression levels, a feature that sets it apart from other algorithms in this field. The latest version of Monocle3 uses UMAP for trajectory inference. Entropy-based pseudo-temporal analysis is also a method that exploits the negative correlation between entropy and the state of cell differentiation. A higher entropy value indicates that the cell is in a more primitive and undifferentiated state.

RNA velocity is a commonly used technique in scRNA-seq analysis based on the principle that unspliced (nascent) mRNA always precedes spliced (mature) mRNA in dynamic regulation. By assessing the abundance of unspliced and spliced mRNAs, it is possible to reveal the dynamics of the transcriptome over time.

CytoTRACE reconstructs cell trajectories through gene counting and expression, allowing the relative differentiation status of individual cells to be predicted from single-cell RNA expression data, without relying on specific time scales or data from successive developmental processes. In addition, CytoTRACE is tissue type-, species- and platform-independent and can be used to predict differentiation status in scRNA-seq data without any prior information.

CellChat is an algorithm for analyzing cell-to-cell communication and is particularly suited to scRNA-seq data. It helps researchers understand how cells communicate through secreted signaling molecules, such as cytokines and ligands, to identify and quantify cell-to-cell signaling.

In addition, tools such as InferCNV and CopKat can be used to infer and visualize copy number variation in scRNA-seq data. This helps researchers to identify chromosomal structural changes in cells by analyzing single-cell gene expression data, which is particularly important in tumor research. In addition, there is an algorithm to identify scRNA-seq based on bulk RNA-seq data. The most important aspect in single-cell data analysis is cell identity. singleR [71] has built-in transcripome data of various cells of multiple species, and the algorithm can automatically identify the type of single cell, greatly promoting the development of single-cell data analysis (Figure 9.5). In addition, due to the high cost of single cells and the small number of samples, it is difficult to conduct batch analysis of data based on phenotype. Similar to Scissor algorithm [72], bulk RNA-seq samples with clinical information can be identified at the single-cell level, which greatly improves the availability of single-cell data. Of course, in order to integrate public data, a variety of single-cell algorithms to eliminate batch effect have emerged in an endless stream, such as Conos, BBKNN, MNN, Seurat CCA, etc. Among them, Harmony is the most balanced in all aspects and has the highest acceptance at present [73].

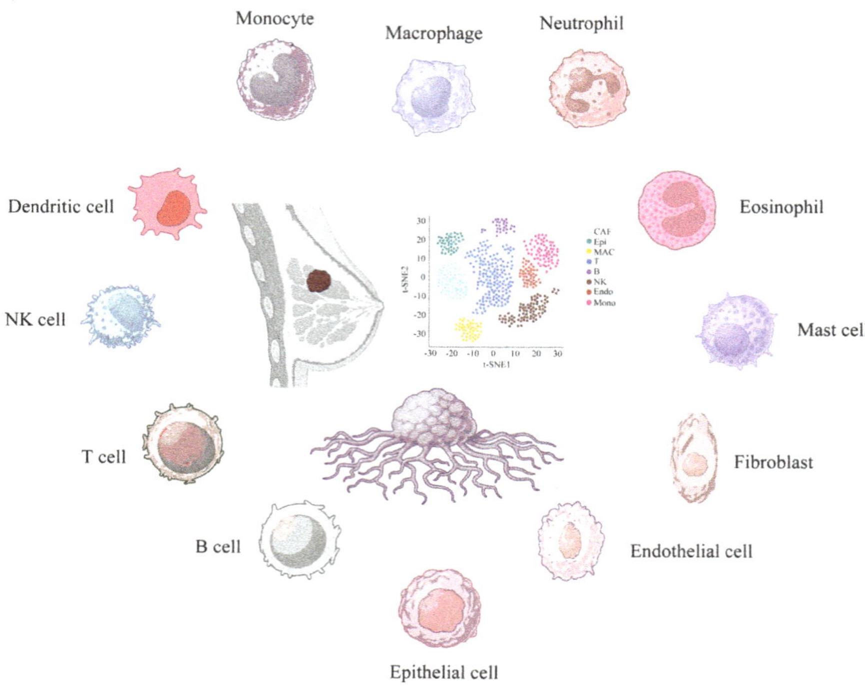


**Figure 9.5** Schematic diagram of a breast tumor microenvironment revealed using single-cell sequencing methods. In the center is a drawing of breast tissue with a tumor, and next to it is a scatter plot of cellular populations from the analysis. Around the periphery, a variety of cells are arranged in a circular pattern, including immune cells (such as monocytes, macrophages, and neutrophils), as well as fibroblasts, endothelial cells, and epithelial cells. This provides a visual representation of the cell types in the breast tumor microenvironment.

## 9.4 Dilemma of the Single-cell Proteome

Proteins are major macromolecules in cells that play important roles in providing structure, replicating genetic information, regulating gene expression, controlling signal transduction, catalyzing metabolic reactions and molecular trafficking. Proteomics is the discipline of comprehensive analysis of all proteins in cells, tissues or entire organisms [75].

In recent years, studies on single-cell transcription have revealed the heterogeneity within the same cell population, proving that there is a significant difference in the state of the same type of cell population. This phenomenon helps to explain that biotransformation is a continuous process rather than a discrete collection of steps, and may also have important implications for understanding and treating disease. However, transcriptomic descriptions lack an understanding of post-transcriptional regulation, which leads to changes in functional proteins that are not always fully positively correlated with mRNA expression [76].

The year 1994 marked a significant milestone in the field of molecular biology with the advent of green fluorescent protein (GFP) technology, which pioneered a novel method for the dynamic tracking of protein levels within individual cells [77]. This technique shows that even proteins expressed from the same promoter can have unexpected fluctuations in abundance within a single cell. In a multitude of instances, the prevalence of proteins within a singular cell is indicative of the cell's condition, thereby yielding particular outcomes. For example, during the mitotic cycle of MCF10A cells, levels of the cyclin-dependent kinase 2 inhibitor p21 determine whether the cells proliferate or enter a quiescent state [78]. In other cases, the levels of endogenous proteins can provide a hierarchical response to stress at the population level, allowing a small subset of cells to survive certain stressful events. For example, in the apoptotic response of MCF10A and HeLa cells to tumor necrosis factor-associated apoptosis-inducing ligand, although most cells died at an exponential rate, a small fraction survived due to the expression levels of five intracellular proteins that regulate apoptosis [79]. The observed phenomena indicate that fluctuations in protein expression may potentially function as regulatory mechanisms within the cell. This underscores the necessity for the development of sophisticated tools for single-cell protein analysis, which are essential for conducting comprehensive quantifications of the diverse protein forms encoded by a single gene, a process referred to as "protein morphology". This has great potential for the development of cell biology and clinical medicine, and the technology of single-cell proteomics is therefore of great importance to research [80].

As the main carriers of life's functions, the study of proteins started early, from the concept proposed in 1938, to the amino acid sequence of bovine insulin first measured in 1949, to the introduction of proteomics in 1994, to single-cell proteomics today [81]. Compared to other omics (e.g., genomics, transcriptomics), the development of proteomics has been relatively slow [82]. This delay is in stark contrast to the rapid iteration of sequencing technology, where the number of proteins is much higher due to sequence variation and subsequent processing, even though the human genome contains approximately 20,000 genes encoding proteins. In addition, proteins vary greatly in size, from small monomeric proteins to large macroscopic molecular complexes, which are clearly not consistent with nucleic acid sequences [83]. Nucleic acid sequencing technology is a unified technology that can be used to measure multiple parameters, such as mRNA, genome sequence, genomic accessibility, epigenetic markers, and others. It possesses the capacity to measure hundreds of millions of parameters with a high degree of precision and can be used to multiplex different measurements. In multiplexing, different measurements are labeled by specific DNA sequences. Proteomics, on the other hand, does not have a similar unified technique, and each method has its specific uses and limitations [84].

Single-cell proteomics currently lacks a universal, well-defined, advanced method that can be applied to all research questions [85]. Nevertheless, a number of techniques have been developed for high-throughput proteomics, and the most commonly used methods are as follows (Figure 9.6):

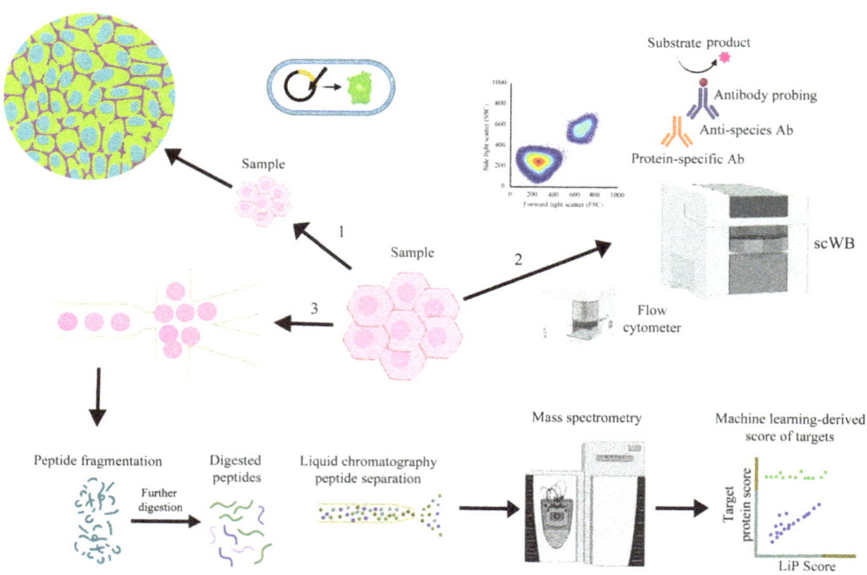


**Figure 9.6** Schematic diagram of a common process for single-cell proteome analysis. Reproduced with permission from [85].

1. Genetically encoded fluorescent proteins coupled with high-resolution imaging;
2. Antibody-based strategies in conjunction with flow cytometry, mass spectrometry, or microfluidics;
3. Direct mass spectrometry analysis.

Fundamental cell functions are subject to regulation by dynamic signaling mechanisms that are contingent not solely on protein abundance, but also on the spatiotemporal distribution of proteins within living cells. Genetically encoded fluorescent proteins can be tracked using high-resolution microscopy to precisely follow spatiotemporal changes in proteins [86]. Since the discovery and cloning of GFP, many fluorescent proteins have been engineered to improve their biophysical properties, such as folding and maturation, spectral range, fluorescence output and resistance to photobleaching. Due to their superior biocompatibility, fluorescent proteins have been widely used for single-cell protein analysis by gene transfection technology [87]. In this process, the expression of the fluorescent protein is linked to that of the target protein gene, forming a fusion protein comprising the fluorescent protein and the target gene after transcription. A number of mutants of wild-type GFP have been generated, providing novel spectral properties. In addition, several engineered fluorescent proteins, such as mEos27 and Dendra28, can be activated by UV irradiation and undergo irreversible photoconversion, changing from one luminescent state to another [88].

The analytical method of fluorescent protein fusion libraries is subject to limitations arising from the number of reads, the spectral overlap of fluorescent dyes, and the configuration of the linker between the fluorescent protein and the host protein. Inadequate flexibility of the linker can result in interference with the native protein's functionality. Secondly, the design and engineering of fluorescent proteins is a time- and effort-consuming process. Furthermore, the utilization of these proteins in systems where genetic engineering is not feasible, such as clinical samples, is constrained. Once the photobleaching threshold is attained, the application of these proteins is also restricted, thereby impeding their use in prolonged experimental studies.

Antibody-based single-cell protein detection methods can be integrated with a variety of techniques, including microscopy, flow cytometry, mass spectrometry, and microfluidic platforms, to generate extensive data sets. Microscopy techniques such as immunocytochemistry and immunohistochemistry are the simplest methods for single-cell protein detection, providing spatial information on protein localization at single-cell resolution [89].

Routine antibody-based protein quantification is a well-established technique that is typically used at the microliter scale. When a protein is diluted to this volume in a single cell, its concentration is below the detection limit [90]. The immediate solution to increase sensitivity is miniaturization. Consequently, microfluidic technology has emerged as the pivotal enabling technology for single-cell protein quantification. Microfluidic devices have been demonstrated to exhibit the capability of precisely regulating the flow of liquids through micron-scale laminar flow and automated equipment. These reactions can be performed at the nanoscale in microfluidic chips and micropores or in microdroplets. Each method of single-cell protein quantification is characterized by miniaturization, with the primary distinction lying in the manner in which the quantification method is integrated with a small-scale approach. In each case, the device has been designed to minimize the reaction volume, to control the chemical environment of the cell, or to combine protein measurements with other measurements in the same cell. Advancements in miniaturization have precipitated the development of single-cell Western blotting [91]. Microfluidic devices are used to create micron-scale polyacrylamide channels to quantify very small amounts of protein. This technique isolates individual cells by combining microplates, ultimately allowing single-cell measurements. In addition, flow cytometry-based fluorescence-activated cell sorting and mass Cytometry by Time of Flight, which combine flow cytometry and mass spectrometry, have become common analytical methods [92–94].

Mass spectrometry, as the most comprehensive technique, provides insight into the composition, structure, function and regulation of the proteome and is particularly suited to the study of post-translational modifications of proteins, as these changes result in significant mass changes that can be identified at the resolution of a single amino acid [95]. The successful application of mass spectrometry in proteomics is due to its inherent specificity and high sensitivity, theoretically allowing the detection of single ions. Traditional tandem mass spectrometry breaks down proteins into peptides based on enzymatic hydrolysis and predicts the sequence of the parent protein through a bottom-up proteomics workflow. However, it remains a challenge to identify many proteins, especially when proteins have the same peptide sequence. Currently, mass spectrometry is a widely used method for protein analysis, although it still suffers from insufficient sensitivity and limited cell throughput. However, with continued improvements in sampling efficiency, ion accumulation, automation, data processing and interpretation methods, the sensitivity, accuracy, and depth of mass spectrometry at the single-cell level are expected to continue to improve [96].

## 9.5 Multi-Omics Combination Techniques in Single-Cell Analysis

The rapid development of molecular analysis strategies and techniques, particularly based on high-throughput sequencing and mass spectrometry technologies, has led to the generation of large multi-omics datasets, mainly from three types of omics, namely genomics, transcriptomics and proteomics, based on the central principles of molecular biology [97].

With the advent of single-cell technology, multi-omics technology has reached new heights. With the recognition of cellular identity through the transcriptome, we have for the first time truly understood the microscopic world within tissues, the cellular composition of the microenvironment, the exploration of genomes in combination with organoids, cellular processes in organ development and the refinement of cellular functions through the proteome. Not only do we have data on a larger scale, but we also face the challenge of data integration. Unlike the integration of single-omics data, which only needs to take batch effects into account, multi-omics integration requires more considerations.

Today's multi-omics studies typically focus on the transcriptome, combined with other omics, to unbiasedly investigate the association between gene expression and various diseases or other biological phenotypes.

### 9.5.1 *Integrating Genome and Transcriptome Analysis*

Parallel analysis of the genome and transcriptome of the same single cell can reflect the transcriptional state of the genome. However, RNA-seq methods alone do not provide coverage of key mutations or genome-transcriptome correlation at the cellular level, ultimately making it difficult to discover novel gene expression programs in disease [98, 99].

In 2014, single-cell genome and transcriptome amplification and sequencing using microfluidics was first reported. This technique uses microvalves to control channels to capture individual cells, selectively lyse and isolate cytoplasmic and nuclear contents, and then perform microarray amplification to enable multiplex genomic measurements [100].

In the following year, genome and transcriptome sequencing (G&T-seq) [101] and gDNA-mRNA sequencing (DR-seq) [102] were successively introduced.

In G&T-seq, full-length mRNA is isolated from 220 individual cells using oligomeric magnetic bead-coated technology which, combined with a modified Smart-seq2 protocol, isolates and lyses cells to release genomic DNA and mRNA for genomic and whole transcriptome analysis, respectively [103].

DR-seq is a low-throughput method primarily associated with G&T; The difference between DR-seq and T-seq is the amplification step. It amplifies DNA and RNA prior to isolation, reducing contamination and RNA loss. This method is similar to G&T-seq in that DNA and RNA must be physically separated, which can lead to loss of genetic material, reduced sensitivity or amplification bias, limiting the ability to reliably detect small pathogenic variants.

In 2019, TARGET-seq proposed a plate-based technique capable of analyzing 5,000 single cells per session with a reduced reaction volume. By using a mixture of barcodes and libraries and a protein digestion method, mutation coverage is increased and the release of DNA and RNA during cell lysis is improved. This distinguishes it from the previous approach [104].

Another microplate-based method, called SIDR, isolates genomic DNA and total RNA simultaneously. In this method, single cells are incubated with antibody-coupled magnetic beads, sorted by microplate and selectively lysed by permeability to obtain a separate supernatant and precipitation solution to distinguish DNA from total RNA [105]. The development of these methods has enabled the combined analysis of the genome and transcriptome of single cells, allowing more sophisticated and comprehensive intracellular gene expression and variant detection.

### 9.5.2 *Integrating Transcriptomics and Epigenomics*

Although traditional combined genomic and transcriptomic analyses can provide a wealth of information, even the same DNA sequences can have different expression patterns in different cells, leading to the joint analysis of epigenomics.

Based on whole genome methylation sequencing, a variety of multi-omics co-analysis methods have been developed. For example, in combination with transcriptome sequencing [106], G&T-seq [101] and scBS-seq [107] technologies allow the simultaneous measurement of DNA methylation heterogeneity in single cells, and combined with Smart-seq2 technology to generate transcriptome data and genome-wide methylation data. Similarly, scRMT-seq [108] performs scRNA-seq by manually isolating the cytoplasm (containing mRNA), and the nuclear fraction (containing DNA) is used for scRRBS [109] methylome analysis. Subsequent technological developments, such as single-cell triomics sequencing (scTrio-seq), combine scRRBS and whole-genome sequencing to analyze the genome, methylome and transcriptome of individual cancer cells [110]. For example, scTrio-seq2 combines scTrio-seq and scBS-seq to analyze mRNA methylation and copy number variation. scNOMe-seq [111] is uniquely read to distinguish inaccessible chromatin regions and characterize nucleosome localization, chromatin accessibility and DNA methylation.

### 9.5.3 *Integrating Transcriptomics and Proteomics*

Proteins are at the core of all cellular processes and functions, as they not only form the cellular structure but also carry out biochemical processes through enzymatic reactions. It is therefore necessary to characterize proteins at the single-cell level through post-translational modifications and protein-protein interactions [112]. Many multi-omics studies (simultaneous analysis of proteins and mRNA) rely on the use of pre-determined combinations of antibodies to produce a single cell phenotype, which may miss new, unanticipated proteomic information.

For example, the RNA Proximity Linking Analysis (PLAYR) technique, developed in 2016, allows the simultaneous quantification of more than 40 target mRNAs and proteins from multiple cell types. PLAYR uses metal isotope-labeled antibodies to label proteins, while RNA transcripts are bound to isotope-labeled probes and measured by mass spectrometry flow cytometry. Another approach is to use an affinity proximity assay (PEA), which detects approximately 100 protein targets in a single cell lysate by ligating matching oligonucleotide-antibody conjugated pairs to the target antigen [113], while co-detecting RNA by real-time PCR. In 2016, a combined RNA and protein assay was developed using PEA and target-specific amplification technology to detect RNA and protein from the same single cell in a single chamber on the Fluidigm C1 platform [114].

In 2017, the development of cellular labeling technology for transcriptome and surface proteins (CITE-seq) enabled significant advances in combined transcriptome and proteome analysis [115]. This method enables unbiased analysis of the transcriptome of thousands of individual cells by labeling cell surface proteins with antibodies conjugated to PCR probe-compatible oligonucleotides, combined with drop-seq and a 10x Genomics microfluidic system. Once the mRNA and oligonucleotide-labeled antibodies are released from the lysed single cells, they bind to the beads for isolation and quantification by next-generation sequencing. RNA Expression and Protein Sequencing (REAP-seq) demonstrates how to quantify surface proteins with 82 antibodies and perform genome-wide mRNA analysis in a single workflow [116]. Unlike CITE-seq, the DNA barcode in REAP-seq binds to the antibody through a small stable covalent bond, whereas the barcode in CITE-seq is attached to the antibody via streptavidin. Subsequently, SCITO-seq was developed using a panel of spliced oligonucleotides from barcoded antibodies to simultaneously analyze single-cell RNA expression and more than 150 surface proteins. The combination of sample multiplexing and droplet- or microwell-based platforms such as 10x Genomics or BD Rhapsody greatly increases the throughput for co-analysis of mRNA and proteins [117].

In single-cell proteomics methods, antibody-independent techniques allow a more comprehensive analysis of cellular proteomic characteristics as they are not limited to antigen-specific reagents and are able to analyze thousands of proteins in a single cell.

SCoPE-MS [118] and SCoPE2 [119] are examples of methods using mass spectrometry, but there are no options for integration with other omics, so further development is needed.

Phage-atac74 is a newly developed method for demonstrating PHAGE epitope recognition based on nanobodies, as opposed to methods using fluorescent or oligonucleotide-conjugated antibodies [120]. In particular, the gene sequence encoded by the hypervariant complementarity determinant region 3 (CDR3) of the nanobody acts as an antigen detector, but can also be identified by downstream sequencing as a unique genetic barcode. This multi-omics approach can reliably detect cell surface proteins, mitochondrial DNA genotypes and epigenomic modifications while analyzing thousands of individual cells.

Intracellular post-translational modifications, such as those that regulate signaling pathways and metabolic activity, are essential for single-cell proteomics. Techniques that enable the analysis of proteins inside and outside cells can better elucidate the signaling pathways that regulate single cell function [121].

RNA and Immunoassay (RAID) is an immunoassay for the analysis of intracellular or phosphorylated proteins and mRNA, allowing association analysis of environmental stimuli and heterogeneous cellular responses [122].

More recently, ASAP-seq (ATAC-seq for Selective Antigen Analysis) and DOGMA-seq (Proteomic Analysis by Sequencing) have shown how reagents and protocols similar to mtscATAC-seq, CITE-seq and scATAC-seq can be used to simultaneously analyze chromatin accessibility, gene expression and protein expression [31, 123]. In particular, ASAP-seq supports the use of existing antibody conjugates through molecular bridging, making it a user-friendly and widely available technique. NEAT-seq combines more models to analyze the abundance of nuclear protein epitopes, chromatin accessibility and transcriptome data in single cells. NEAT-seq improves the signal-to-noise ratio by using *Escherichia coli* single-stranded DNA to block the charge of the antibody-oligonucleotide conjugate [124]. Nucleoproteins play an important role in gene regulation, and gene regulatory mechanisms can be effectively studied by studying their association with the epigenetic and transcriptional states of cells.

Finally, extended CRISPR-compatible CITE-seq (ECCITE-seq) expands the field of proteomics to include CRISPR-compatible transcriptomes, immune repertoires and proteome indices, and enables clonotyping and CRISPR-directed perturbations with high sensitivity and single-cell resolution [125]. Thus, multi-omics techniques enable the measurement of the effects of cellular perturbations and signaling pathways on single cell states. The analysis of proteins and other patterns in cells or secretions has led some companies to commercialize these technologies.

### 9.5.4 *Other Multi-Omics Models*

To understand cellular heterogeneity and its intrinsic complexity, it is essential to be able to characterize as many cellular functions as possible simultaneously. By using emerging omics methods to capture multiple layers of cellular information, we can obtain more specific data and thus gain a clearer understanding of cellular function.

For example, RNA sequencing can be combined with CRISPR screens to analyze the relationship between CRISPR-Cas9-mediated genetic perturbations and transcriptome phenotypes. Perturb-seq is an approach that provides rich data by analyzing thousands of CRISPR-mediated perturbations and mRNA profiles in 200,000 cells.

CROP-seq is another CRISPR-based genetic screening method that combines single-cell transcriptomics to directly link the expression of a single guide RNA (sgRNA) to transcriptomic responses in thousands of single cells. The sgRNA expression vector has been redesigned to embed the sgRNA into a polyadenylated mRNA transcript, allowing it to be easily integrated into most RNA sequencing platforms.

In 2016, a CRISPR-seq approach elucidated the function of multiple regulators by capturing mRNA and genomic perturbations from CRISPR hybridization screens [126].

In addition, Mosaic-seq is used to systematically perturb enhancers and measure their endogenous activity while simultaneously measuring the transcriptome at single-cell resolution. CRISPR screens are also combined with other methods, such as scATAC-seq, allowing researchers to characterize the epigenetic status of more than 100,000 single cells and analyze more than 400 CRISPR perturbations.

Other multi-omics models include complex genomic libraries to characterize T-cell receptors and B-cell receptors. These are key components of adaptive immunity. These data can provide important information for understanding an individual's immune lineage and how different receptor configurations contribute to adaptive immune responses, autoimmunity and tumor growth. There are several ways to pair T-cell receptor sequences with gene expression data from single cells to further explore the relationship between the transcriptome, clonal composition and antigen receptor characteristics such as its CDR3 length and specific sequences [127].

The V(D)J region is the first 500 nucleotides of the rearranged T- and B-cell receptor mRNA, and the short reads of scRNA-seq are not always sufficient to address the genomic complexity of these isoforms while maintaining accurate quantification of transcriptional gene expression. As a result, most technologies capable of capturing T- and B-cell receptor isoform sequences while preserving whole-cell transcriptome information have been commercialized using 5' RNA amplification and have been introduced by companies such as 10x Genomics. The technique also extends to proteomics (ECCITE-seq) and chromatin accessibility analysis (T-ATAC-seq) [128]. 10x Genomics and Oxford Nanopore recently announced a collaboration to co-sequence full-length transcripts in single cells. These techniques allow antigen receptor sequences and transcriptomes to be characterized with high precision and sensitivity. Sequencing of the immune repertoire, combined with technological advances and integration with other omics models, enables a deeper understanding of how T and B cell clonality and specificity affect immune responses.

## 9.6 Decoding Complexity: Organoids Meet Single-Cell Multi-Omics for Disease Modeling and Translation

### 9.6.1 *Multi-Omics-Driven Characterization of Organoid Models*

Organoids and multi-omics are forming cross-validation in advancing biomedical research. Organoids, 3D miniature models derived from stem cells, retain much of the complexity and heterogeneity of *in vivo* tissues. Compared to traditional 2D cell cultures, they offer greater plasticity. Significant advancements have been made in developing organoid models for various organs such as the liver, brain [129], skin [130], bone, and kidney. These models can help alleviate the substantial sample demands of multi-omics studies. Organoids may also more accurately represent human diseases compared to traditional animal models [131]. This intrinsic advantage positions organoids as valuable platforms for understanding the dynamics of tumorigenesis, tissue regeneration, and other complex biological processes.

Multi-omics provides critical quantitative frameworks for assessing organoid models, enabling standardization and validation of their *in vivo*-like functionality amid expanding diversity. For instance, in Velasco *et al.*'s study, nine brain organoid models were constructed, and through single-cell sequencing, the diversity of cortical cells was assessed over time. The analysis revealed that some models lacked representative cell types, leading to the selection of models more closely aligned with *in vivo* conditions [129]. Furthermore, the impact of long-term passage, cryopreservation, recovery, and re-cultivation of organoids on molecular characteristics remains unclear. In Yan *et al.*'s study, the mutational differences between early- and late-stage colorectal cancer organoids (cultured for more than six months) and their primary tissues were compared through omics analysis. The results showed that gene mutation drift was less than 20% in short-term passage organoids, while it could reach up to 50% in long-term passages. Such findings highlight the need for genomic approaches to track and integrate changes, making them a key method for evaluating organoid quality [132].

### 9.6.2 *Challenges in Multi-Omics Integration and the Need for Advanced Computational Tools*

In recent years, numerous algorithms, tools, and machine learning models have been developed to integrate multi-omics data. However, most of these tools focus on combining a limited number of omics layers, such as genomics and transcriptomics, and integrating large-scale multi-omics datasets remains a significant challenge. The complexity of biological systems and the heterogeneity of data across different omics layers make extracting actionable insights from multi-omics analyses a difficult task.

A major obstacle is the lack of standardized platforms that can integrate various omics data types, such as genomics, transcriptomics, proteomics, metabolomics, and epigenomics, into a unified framework. As multi-omics continue to evolve, it is clear that developing comprehensive computational platforms is crucial. These platforms should enable researchers to effectively manage, analyze, and visualize complex, multidimensional data. The absence of large-scale integration algorithms is one of the primary barriers to the widespread adoption of multi-omics in organoid-based research.

Differential technological advances in omics also exacerbate these challenges. For example, proteomics lags behind genomics and transcriptomics in terms of technological development and standardization. While next-generation sequencing technologies have made significant strides in genomics and transcriptomics, proteomics and metabolomics analyses still face high technical demands, including issues with sensitivity, dynamic range, and reproducibility. Overcoming these limitations requires introducing new chemical or physical principles, technologies, or methods to advance proteomics and other underdeveloped omics fields.

Moreover, integrating multi-omics data often necessitates powerful computational resources and complex machine learning models. These tools must handle the high dimensionality and heterogeneity of omics data while accounting for the intricate biological interactions that govern disease processes. By leveraging artificial intelligence and deep learning techniques, patterns and correlations across different omics layers can be identified, some of which may not be immediately apparent through traditional statistical methods. This integrated approach will provide a more comprehensive understanding of disease biology and pave the way for more precise and targeted interventions.

There is also a critical need for unified standards and consensus across the industry for multi-omics integration. Currently, the lack of standardization in data processing, analysis, and interpretation makes it difficult to compare results across different studies. Establishing robust, widely accepted protocols and platforms for multi-omics data integration will not only improve reproducibility but also foster greater collaboration within the research community.

### 9.6.3 *Standardization and Reproducibility in Organoid Research*

Standardization in organoid research is crucial for ensuring the reproducibility and reliability of experimental results. Although organoid models offer significant advantages over traditional 2D cultures, they present unique challenges in terms of consistency and scalability. Variability in growth conditions, differentiation protocols, and stem cell source selection can lead to differences in organoid morphology, function, and gene expression. These variations can impact the interpretation of experimental data, especially when integrating multiple omics layers [133].

To address these challenges, it is essential to develop standardized protocols for generating, maintaining, and analyzing organoids. Such protocols should encompass factors like cell source selection, culture conditions, and differentiation schemes to ensure that organoid models remain consistent and reproducible across different laboratories. Additionally, the standardization of methods for collecting and processing omics data from organoids will allow for more reliable comparisons between studies and facilitate multi-omics integration.

Standardization efforts should also extend to the analysis of omics data. Integrating large, heterogeneous datasets often requires complex computational pipelines. Standardizing methods for data preprocessing, normalization, and quality control will ensure that results are comparable and reproducible across different research groups. As organoid-based models become increasingly prominent in preclinical drug discovery and personalized medicine, the importance of this standardization will only grow.

### 9.6.4 *Addressing Cost and Scalability Issues in Organoid and Multi-Omics Research*

Despite the promising potential of organoid models and multi-omics technologies in advancing biomedical research, their application in large-scale drug development and clinical settings is currently hindered by cost and scalability issues. Organoid culture systems remain relatively expensive, requiring specialized equipment and expertise. Similarly, multi-omics technologies such as high-throughput sequencing, mass spectrometry, and metabolomics are resource-intensive, limiting their routine use in large-scale applications.

To facilitate the broader adoption of organoids in drug discovery, clinical research, and personalized medicine, cost-effective platforms and protocols must be developed.

Advances in high-throughput culture systems, automation, and bioreactor technologies can help reduce the cost of organoid production, making these models more accessible for large-scale research. Furthermore, the development of more affordable and efficient multi-omics technologies will promote their widespread use in organoid research, enabling the integration of genomic, transcriptomic, proteomic, and metabolomic data in a cost-effective manner.

Scalability is another key consideration. In preclinical drug development, using organoid models for large-scale screening of drug candidates is crucial for evaluating efficacy and toxicity. However, scaling up organoid culture systems while maintaining reproducibility and relevance to human diseases presents a significant challenge. Addressing this issue will require the development of scalable organoid culture platforms that can produce large quantities of consistent and functional organoids in a cost-efficient manner.

The integration of multi-omics and organoid research has the potential to revolutionize drug discovery, biomarker identification, and the development of personalized therapies. However, overcoming the challenges related to cost, scalability, and integration requires concerted efforts from researchers, clinicians, and industry leaders. By addressing these challenges, organoid-based models coupled with multi-omics technologies will become powerful tools in advancing biomedical research and clinical applications.

## 9.7 Conclusion

The integration of multi-omics with organoid research represents a transformative approach for elucidating human disease mechanisms — particularly in cancer — and accelerating personalized therapeutics. This chapter delineates fundamental principles and advances in multi-omics technologies, highlighting their synergistic potential to revolutionize biomedical research through characterization of organoid models. Single-cell techniques resolve cellular heterogeneity at unprecedented resolution, capturing genomic alterations, transcriptomic dynamics, and proteomic fluctuations, while organoids provide physiologically relevant 3D systems that recapitulate tissue complexity. This convergence overcomes limitations of traditional models by enabling precise investigation of tumor evolution, drug responses, and developmental processes. However, key challenges persist: proteomic profiling trails genomic/transcriptomic methods due to sensitivity constraints; multi-omics data integration requires sophisticated computational frameworks; and organoid standardization remains underdeveloped. Future progress depends on overcoming technical barriers (e.g., high-throughput proteomics), establishing unified analytical pipelines, and cost reduction. Collectively, these technologies form a powerful paradigm for decoding disease pathogenesis and advancing precision medicine, though realizing their full potential demands cross-disciplinary innovation in experimental methodologies and artificial intelligence-driven data synthesis.

## Key Opinion Points

1. The continuous development of single-cell multi-omics technology has met the basic conditions for constructing and screening organoids in terms of accuracy. This technology has promoted the development of organoids by exploring minor changes in their organizational structure from a multi-omics perspective with single-cell resolution.
2. The establishment of reproducible industry standards is imperative for the efficient operation of industrial organoid technology. The application of omics technology has the potential to improve the microscopic, cell-level framework of the organoid industry, facilitating integration and communication. This technology is expected to evolve into a unifying metric for evaluation and supervision in the future.
3. Using organoid models has become a key solution for overcoming sample procurement challenges in medical research. Using organoid models in large-scale drug target screening through single-cell multi-omics has been shown to be significant in developing sophisticated data models.
4. In preclinical trials, single-cell multi-omics can assist in constructing organoids *in vitro*, maximizing the reduction of the *in vivo* environment and simulating the clinical effect.
5. In the future, combining a large amount of existing single-cell multi-omics data with artificial intelligence to create a cloud platform that guides organoid construction will be a promising approach in the fields of personalized medicine and fully automated biological products.

# References

1. Baysoy A, *et al.* The technological landscape and applications of single-cell multi-omics. Nat Rev Mol Cell Biol. 2023;24(10):695–713.
2. Manolio TA, *et al.* Finding the missing heritability of complex diseases. Nature. 2009;461(7265):747–53.
3. Goodwin S, McPherson JD, McCombie WR. Coming of age: ten years of next-generation sequencing technologies. Nat Rev Genet. 2016;17(6):333–51.
4. Abecasis GR, *et al.* A map of human genome variation from population-scale sequencing. Nature. 2010;467(7319):1061–73.
5. Meyts I, *et al.* Exome and genome sequencing for inborn errors of immunity. J Allergy Clin Immunol. 2016;138(4):957–969.
6. Mardis ER. Next-generation sequencing platforms. Annu Rev Anal Chem (Palo Alto Calif). 2013;6:287–303.
7. Cirulli ET, Goldstein DB. Uncovering the roles of rare variants in common disease through whole-genome sequencing. Nat Rev Genet. 2010;11(6):415–25.
8. Wang Y, *et al.* Nanopore sequencing technology, bioinformatics and applications. Nat Biotechnol. 2021;39(11):1348–1365.
9. Youk J, *et al.* Dissecting single-cell genomes through the clonal organoid technique. Exp Mol Med. 2021;53(10):1503–1511.
10. Park S, *et al.* Clonal dynamics in early human embryogenesis inferred from somatic mutation. Nature. 2021;597(7876):393–397.
11. Loveless TB, *et al.* Open-ended molecular recording of sequential cellular events into DNA. Nat Chem Biol. 2024.
12. Mullikin JC, *et al.* An SNP map of human chromosome 22. Nature. 2000; 407(6803):516–20.
13. Ju YS, *et al.* Somatic mutations reveal asymmetric cellular dynamics in the early human embryo. Nature. 2017;543(7647):714–718.
14. McCarroll SA, Altshuler DM. Copy-number variation and association studies of human disease. Nat Genet. 2007;39(7 Suppl):S37–42.
15. Martincorena I, Campbell PJ. Somatic mutation in cancer and normal cells. Science. 2015;349(6255):1483–9.
16. Szilard L. On the nature of the aging process. Proc Natl Acad Sci U S A. 1959;45(1):30–45.
17. Lee JH. Somatic mutations in disorders with disrupted brain connectivity. Exp Mol Med. 2016;48(6):e239.
18. Pan-cancer analysis of whole genomes. Nature. 2020;578(7793):82–93.

19. Tate JG, *et al.* COSMIC: the Catalogue Of Somatic Mutations In Cancer. Nucleic Acids Res. 2019;47(D1):D941-D947.
20. Lee JK, *et al.* Clonal history and genetic predictors of transformation into small-cell carcinomas from lung adenocarcinomas. J Clin Oncol. 2017;35(26):3065–3074.
21. Coorens THH, *et al.* Extensive phylogenies of human development inferred from somatic mutations. Nature. 2021;597(7876):387–392.
22. van de Wetering M, *et al.* Prospective derivation of a living organoid biobank of colorectal cancer patients. Cell. 2015;161(4):933–45.
23. Nanki K, *et al.* Somatic inflammatory gene mutations in human ulcerative colitis epithelium. Nature. 2020;577(7789):254–259.
24. Alexandrov LB, *et al.* Clock-like mutational processes in human somatic cells. Nat Genet. 2015;47(12):1402–7.
25. Klemm SL, Shipony Z, Greenleaf WJ. Chromatin accessibility and the regulatory epigenome. Nat Rev Genet. 2019;20(4):207–220.
26. Mattei AL, Bailly N, Meissner A. DNA methylation: a historical perspective. Trends Genet. 2022;38(7):676–707.
27. Park J, *et al.* The role of histone modifications: from neurodevelopment to neurodiseases. Signal Transduct Target Ther. 2022;7(1):217.
28. Buenrostro JD, *et al.* ATAC-seq: A Method for Assaying Chromatin Accessibility Genome-Wide. Curr Protoc Mol Biol. 2015;109:21.29.1-21.29.9.
29. Lareau CA, *et al.* Droplet-based combinatorial indexing for massive-scale single-cell chromatin accessibility. Nat Biotechnol. 2019;37(8):916–924.
30. Mimitou EP, *et al.* Scalable, multimodal profiling of chromatin accessibility, gene expression and protein levels in single cells. Nat Biotechnol. 2021;39(10):1246–1258.
31. Buenrostro JD, *et al.* Single-cell chromatin accessibility reveals principles of regulatory variation. Nature. 2015;523(7561):486–90.
32. Gong T, *et al.* Analysis and Performance Assessment of the Whole Genome Bisulfite Sequencing Data Workflow: Currently Available Tools and a Practical Guide to Advance DNA Methylation Studies. Small Methods. 2022;6(3):e2101251.
33. Stevens M, *et al.* Estimating absolute methylation levels at single-CpG resolution from methylation enrichment and restriction enzyme sequencing methods. Genome Res. 2013;23(9):1541–53.
34. Gu H, *et al.* Preparation of reduced representation bisulfite sequencing libraries for genome-scale DNA methylation profiling. Nat Protoc. 2011;6(4):468–81.
35. Zeng X, *et al.* Digital-scRRBS: A Cost-Effective, Highly Sensitive, and Automated Single-Cell Methylome Analysis Platform via Digital Microfluidics. Anal Chem. 2023;95(35):13313–13321.

36. Audia JE, Campbell RM. Histone Modifications and Cancer. Cold Spring Harb Perspect Biol. 2016;8(4):a019521.
37. Rotem A, *et al.* Single-cell ChIP-seq reveals cell subpopulations defined by chromatin state. Nat Biotechnol. 2015;33(11):1165–72.
38. Wang Q, *et al.* CoBATCH for High-Throughput Single-Cell Epigenomic Profiling. Mol Cell. 2019;76(1):206–216.e7.
39. Kaya-Okur HS, *et al.* CUT&Tag for efficient epigenomic profiling of small samples and single cells. Nat Commun. 2019;10(1):1930.
40. Carter B, *et al.* Mapping histone modifications in low cell number and single cells using antibody-guided chromatin tagmentation (ACT-seq). Nat Commun. 2019; 10(1):3747.
41. Zhang B, *et al.* Characterizing cellular heterogeneity in chromatin state with scCUT&Tag-pro. Nat Biotechnol. 2022;40(8):1220–1230.
42. Hwang B, Lee JH, Bang D. Single-cell RNA sequencing technologies and bioinformatics pipelines. Exp Mol Med. 2018;50(8):1–14.
43. Ahmed R, *et al.* Single-Cell RNA Sequencing with Spatial Transcriptomics of Cancer Tissues. Int J Mol Sci. 2022;23(6).
44. Tang F, *et al.* mRNA-Seq whole-transcriptome analysis of a single cell. Nat Methods. 2009;6(5):377–82.
45. Islam S, *et al.* Characterization of the single-cell transcriptional landscape by highly multiplex RNA-seq. Genome Res. 2011;21(7):1160–7.
46. Hashimshony T, *et al.* CEL-Seq: single-cell RNA-Seq by multiplexed linear amplification. Cell Rep. 2012;2(3):666–73.
47. Jaitin DA, *et al.* Massively parallel single-cell RNA-seq for marker-free decomposition of tissues into cell types. Science. 2014;343(6172):776–9.
48. Klein AM, *et al.* Droplet barcoding for single-cell transcriptomics applied to embryonic stem cells. Cell. 2015;161(5):1187–1201.
49. Tirosh I, *et al.* Dissecting the multicellular ecosystem of metastatic melanoma by single-cell RNA-seq. Science. 2016;352(6282):189–96.
50. Joost S, *et al.* Single-Cell Transcriptomics Reveals that Differentiation and Spatial Signatures Shape Epidermal and Hair Follicle Heterogeneity. Cell Syst. 2016;3(3):221–37.
51. Zheng GX, *et al.* Massively parallel digital transcriptional profiling of single cells. Nat Commun. 2017;8(1):14049.
52. Stoeckius M, *et al.* Simultaneous epitope and transcriptome measurement in single cells. Nat Methods. 2017;14(9):865–868.
53. Lareau CA, *et al.* Comprehensive single-cell analysis of immune cell transcriptome and open chromatin. Nat Biotechnol. 2019;37(12):1452–1463.

54. Stoeckius M, *et al.* Cell Hashing with barcoded antibodies enables multiplexing and doublet detection for single cell genomics. Genome Biol. 2018;19(1):224.
55. Wu AR, *et al.* Quantitative assessment of single-cell RNA-sequencing methods. Nat Methods. 2014;11(1):41–6.
56. Ziegenhain C, *et al.* Comparative analysis of single-cell RNA sequencing methods. Mol Cell. 2017;65(4):631–643.e4.
57. Cao J, *et al.* The single-cell transcriptional landscape of mammalian organogenesis. Nature. 2019;566(7745):496–502.
58. Deng Q, Ramskold D, Reinius B, Sandberg R. Single-cell RNA-seq reveals dynamic, random monoallelic gene expression in mammalian cells. Science. 2014;343(6167): 193–6.
59. Fincher CT, *et al.* Cell type transcriptome atlas for the planarian Schmidtea mediterranea. Science. 2018;360(6391).
60. Han X, *et al.* Mapping the Mouse Cell Atlas by Microwell-Seq. Cell. 2018;172(5): 1091–1107.e17.
61. van den Brink SC, *et al.* Single-cell sequencing reveals dissociation-induced gene expression in tissue subpopulations. Nat Methods. 2017;14(10):935–936.
62. Vieira Braga FA, *et al.* A cellular census of human lungs identifies novel cell states in health and asthma. Nat Med. 2019;25(7):1153–1163.
63. Denisenko E, *et al.* Systematic assessment of tissue dissociation and storage biases in single-cell and single-nucleus RNA-seq workflows. Genome Biol. 2020;21(1):130.
64. Wu AR, *et al.* Single-cell analysis reveals dosage compensation in human preimplantation embryos. Dev Cell. 2018;44(4):364–376.e4.
65. MacParland SA, *et al.* Single cell RNA sequencing of human liver reveals distinct intrahepatic macrophage populations. Nat Commun. 2018;9(1):4383.
66. Grun D, *et al.* Single-cell messenger RNA sequencing reveals rare intestinal cell types. Nature. 2015;525(7568):251–5.
67. Tanay A, Regev A. Scaling single-cell genomics from phenomenology to mechanism. Nature. 2017;541(7637):331–338.
68. Zhu C, *et al.* Single-cell multimodal omics: the power of many. Nat Methods. 2020;17(1):11–14.
69. Stuart T, Satija R. Integrative single-cell analysis. Nat Rev Genet. 2019;20(5):257–272.
70. Traag VA, Waltman L, van Eck NJ. From Louvain to Leiden: guaranteeing well-connected communities. Sci Rep. 2019;9(1):5233.
71. McInnes L, Healy J, Melville J. UMAP: Uniform Manifold Approximation and Projection for Dimension Reduction. arXiv. 2018.

72. Hao Y, *et al.* Integrated analysis of multimodal single-cell data. Cell. 2021;184(13):3573–3587.e29.
73. Hafemeister C, Satija R. Normalization and variance stabilization of single-cell RNA-seq data using regularized negative binomial regression. Genome Biol. 2019;20(1):296.
74. Kiselev VY, *et al.* SC3: consensus clustering of single-cell RNA-seq data. Nat Methods. 2017;14(5):483–486.
75. Traag VA, Waltman L, van Eck NJ. From Louvain to Leiden: guaranteeing well-connected communities. Sci Rep. 2019;9(1):5233.
76. Luecken MD, Theis FJ. Current best practices in single-cell RNA-seq analysis: a tutorial. Mol Syst Biol. 2019;15(6):e8746.
77. Cao Y, *et al.* Single-cell multi-omics integration: a review of computational methods and challenges. Comput Struct Biotechnol J. 2022;20:2143–2153.
78. Huang M, *et al.* SAVER: gene expression recovery for single-cell RNA sequencing. Nat Methods. 2018;15(7):539–42.
79. Lopez R, *et al.* Deep generative modeling for single-cell transcriptomics. Nat Methods. 2018;15(12):1053–1058.
80. Eraslan G, *et al.* Single-cell RNA-seq denoising using a deep count autoencoder. Nat Commun. 2019;10(1):390.
81. Stuart T, *et al.* Comprehensive integration of single-cell data. Cell. 2019;177(7):1888–1902.e21.
82. Welch JD, *et al.* Single-cell multi-omic integration compares and contrasts features of brain cell identity. Cell. 2019;177(7):1873–1887.e17.
83. Bues J, *et al.* Single-cell chromatin accessibility analysis reveals human hematopoietic cell fate commitment. Nat Commun. 2022;13(1):581.
84. Hughes JR, *et al.* Analysis of hundreds of cis-regulatory landscapes at high resolution in a single, high-throughput experiment. Nat Genet. 2014;46(2):205–12.
85. Buenrostro JD, *et al.* Integrated single-cell analysis maps the continuous regulatory landscape of human hematopoietic differentiation. Cell. 2018;173(6):1535–1548.e16.
86. Mimitou EP, *et al.* Multiplexed detection of proteins, transcriptomes, clonotypes and CRISPR perturbations in single cells. Nat Methods. 2019;16(5):409–412.
87. Xiong L, *et al.* SCALE method for single-cell ATAC-seq analysis via latent feature extraction. Nat Commun. 2019;10(1):4576.
88. Specht AT, *et al.* Single-cell proteomic and transcriptomic analysis reveals the impact of chronic lymphocytic leukemia on T cell populations. Nat Commun. 2021;12(1):3644.
89. Stoeckius M, *et al.* Cell Hashing with barcoded antibodies enables multiplexing and doublet detection for single cell genomics. Genome Biol. 2018;19(1):224.
90. Stuart T, Satija R. Integrative single-cell analysis. Nat Rev Genet. 2019;20(5):257–272.

91. Trapnell C. Defining cell types and states with single-cell genomics. Genome Res. 2015;25(10):1491–8.
92. Cusanovich DA, *et al.* A single-cell atlas of in vivo mammalian chromatin accessibility. Cell. 2018;174(5):1309–1324.e18.
93. Yost KE, *et al.* Clonal replacement of tumor-specific T cells following PD-1 blockade. Nat Med. 2019;25(8):1251–1259.
94. Satpathy AT, *et al.* Massively parallel single-cell chromatin landscapes of human immune cell development and intratumoral T cell exhaustion. Nat Biotechnol. 2019;37(8):925–936.
95. Chung W, *et al.* Single-cell RNA-seq enables comprehensive tumour and immune cell profiling in primary breast cancer. Nat Commun. 2017;8(1):15081.
96. Azizi E, *et al.* Single-cell map of diverse immune phenotypes in the breast tumor microenvironment. Cell. 2018;174(5):1293–1308.e36.
97. Patel AP, *et al.* Single-cell RNA-seq highlights intratumoral heterogeneity in primary glioblastoma. Science. 2014;344(6190):1396–401.
98. Puram SV, *et al.* Single-cell transcriptomic analysis of primary and metastatic tumor ecosystems in head and neck cancer. Cell. 2017;171(7):1611–1624.e24.
99. Kim KT, *et al.* Single-cell mRNA sequencing identifies subclonal heterogeneity in anti-cancer drug responses of lung adenocarcinoma cells. Genome Biol. 2015;16:127.
100. Tirosh I, *et al.* Single-cell RNA-seq supports a developmental hierarchy in human oligodendroglioma. Nature. 2016;539(7628):309–13.
101. Patel AP, *et al.* Single-cell RNA-seq highlights intratumoral heterogeneity in primary glioblastoma. Science. 2014;344(6190):1396–401.
102. Puram SV, *et al.* Single-cell transcriptomic analysis of primary and metastatic tumor ecosystems in head and neck cancer. Cell. 2017;171(7):1611–1624.e24.
103. Kim KT, *et al.* Single-cell mRNA sequencing identifies subclonal heterogeneity in anti-cancer drug responses of lung adenocarcinoma cells. Genome Biol. 2015;16:127.
104. Tirosh I, *et al.* Single-cell RNA-seq supports a developmental hierarchy in human oligodendroglioma. Nature. 2016;539(7628):309–13.
105. Gaiti F, *et al.* Epigenetic evolution and lineage histories of chronic lymphocytic leukemia. Nature. 2019;569(7757):576–580.
106. Stuart T, *et al.* Comprehensive integration of single-cell data. Cell. 2019;177(7):1888–1902.e21.
107. Welch JD, *et al.* Single-cell multi-omic integration compares and contrasts features of brain cell identity. Cell. 2019;177(7):1873–1887.e17.
108. Mimitou EP, *et al.* Multiplexed detection of proteins, transcriptomes, clonotypes and CRISPR perturbations in single cells. Nat Methods. 2019;16(5):409–412.

109. Luecken MD, Theis FJ. Current best practices in single-cell RNA-seq analysis: a tutorial. Mol Syst Biol. 2019;15(6):e8746.
110. Cao Y, *et al.* Single-cell multi-omics integration: a review of computational methods and challenges. Comput Struct Biotechnol J. 2022;20:2143–2153.
111. Huang M, *et al.* SAVER: gene expression recovery for single-cell RNA sequencing. Nat Methods. 2018;15(7):539–42.
112. Lopez R, *et al.* Deep generative modeling for single-cell transcriptomics. Nat Methods. 2018;15(12):1053–1058.
113. Eraslan G, *et al.* Single-cell RNA-seq denoising using a deep count autoencoder. Nat Commun. 2019;10(1):390.
114. Stuart T, Satija R. Integrative single-cell analysis. Nat Rev Genet. 2019;20(5):257–272.
115. Traag VA, Waltman L, van Eck NJ. From Louvain to Leiden: guaranteeing well-connected communities. Sci Rep. 2019;9(1):5233.
116. McInnes L, Healy J, Melville J. UMAP: Uniform Manifold Approximation and Projection for Dimension Reduction. arXiv. 2018.
117. Hafemeister C, Satija R. Normalization and variance stabilization of single-cell RNA-seq data using regularized negative binomial regression. Genome Biol. 2019;20(1):296.
118. Kiselev VY, *et al.* SC3: consensus clustering of single-cell RNA-seq data. Nat Methods. 2017;14(5):483–486.
119. Bues J, *et al.* Single-cell chromatin accessibility analysis reveals human hematopoietic cell fate commitment. Nat Commun. 2022;13(1):581.
120. Hughes JR, *et al.* Analysis of hundreds of cis-regulatory landscapes at high resolution in a single, high-throughput experiment. Nat Genet. 2014;46(2):205–12.
121. Buenrostro JD, *et al.* Integrated single-cell analysis maps the continuous regulatory landscape of human hematopoietic differentiation. Cell. 2018;173(6):1535–1548.e16.
122. Xiong L, *et al.* SCALE method for single-cell ATAC-seq analysis via latent feature extraction. Nat Commun. 2019;10(1):4576.
123. Specht AT, *et al.* Single-cell proteomic and transcriptomic analysis reveals the impact of chronic lymphocytic leukemia on T cell populations. Nat Commun. 2021;12(1):3644.
124. Yost KE, *et al.* Clonal replacement of tumor-specific T cells following PD-1 blockade. Nat Med. 2019;25(8):1251–1259.
125. Satpathy AT, *et al.* Massively parallel single-cell chromatin landscapes of human immune cell development and intratumoral T cell exhaustion. Nat Biotechnol. 2019;37(8):925–936.
126. Chung W, *et al.* Single-cell RNA-seq enables comprehensive tumour and immune cell profiling in primary breast cancer. Nat Commun. 2017;8(1):15081.

127. Azizi E, *et al.* Single-cell map of diverse immune phenotypes in the breast tumor microenvironment. Cell. 2018;174(5):1293–1308.e36.
128. Patel AP, *et al.* Single-cell RNA-seq highlights intratumoral heterogeneity in primary glioblastoma. Science. 2014;344(6190):1396–401.
129. Puram SV, *et al.* Single-cell transcriptomic analysis of primary and metastatic tumor ecosystems in head and neck cancer. Cell. 2017;171(7):1611–1624.e24.
130. Kim KT, *et al.* Single-cell mRNA sequencing identifies subclonal heterogeneity in anti-cancer drug responses of lung adenocarcinoma cells. Genome Biol. 2015;16:127.
131. Tirosh I, *et al.* Single-cell RNA-seq supports a developmental hierarchy in human oligodendroglioma. Nature. 2016;539(7628):309–13.
132. Gaiti F, *et al.* Epigenetic evolution and lineage histories of chronic lymphocytic leukemia. Nature. 2019;569(7757):576–580.
133. Stuart T, *et al.* Comprehensive integration of single-cell data. Cell. 2019;177(7):1888–1902.e21.

https://doi.org/10.1142/9789819817597_0010

Chapter 10

# Artificial Intelligence and Machine Learning in Organoid Technology

Hong Kai Lee[1,*], Min Qiu[1], Yijun Chen[2]

[1]*Department of Digital Medicine, Hangzhou AimingMed Technologies Co., Ltd, Hangzhou 310000, China*

[2]*China Pharmaceutical University, Nanjing 210009, China*

**Abstract:** The convergence of artificial intelligence (AI) and organoid technology presents a paradigm shift in biomedical research, impacting drug discovery and precision medicine. Organoids, 3D cell cultures mimicking human organs, provide unprecedented physiological relevance, including patient-derived organoids (PDOs) that capture individual disease characteristics. AI offers powerful tools for analyzing the complex, high-dimensional imaging, omics, and functional data generated from these models. This chapter explores the synergy between these fields, focusing on advancements since 2022. In drug discovery, AI enhances organoid-based platforms by automating high-throughput screening, improving prediction of drug efficacy and toxicity, identifying novel therapeutic targets, and accelerating drug repurposing, thereby addressing key industry challenges. For precision medicine, AI combined with PDOs enable personalized healthcare. By analyzing individual PDO responses and integrating multi-omics data, AI models predict patient-specific treatment outcomes, guiding therapy selection and optimization, particularly in oncology. Despite immense potential, significant challenges persist. These include inherent organoid variability and biological limitations (fidelity, maturity, lack of components), data quality and standardization issues, the need for interpretable AI (explainable AI or XAI), computational demands, and complex ethical considerations surrounding consent, data privacy, and advanced brain organoids. Future directions should focus on developing more sophisticated organoid and AI models, increasing automation, pursuing rigorous clinical validation toward regulatory acceptance (building on FDA Modernization Act 2.0), exploring concepts like

*Corresponding author. Email: leehongkai@gmail.com

organoid intelligence and digital twins, and fostering interdisciplinary collaboration. Addressing these hurdles is crucial to fully translate the transformative potential of AI-enabled organoids into tangible benefits for human health.

**Keywords:** organoids, artificial intelligence, machine learning, drug discovery, personalized medicine, predictive modeling, image analysis

## Key Points

1. The convergence of artificial intelligence/machine learning and organoid technology, particularly patient-derived organoids, offers transformative potential for both drug discovery and personalized medicine by combining physiologically relevant models with powerful data analysis.
2. Artificial intelligence is crucial for overcoming challenges in using organoids for drug discovery, enabling automated high-throughput screening, improving predictions of drug efficacy and toxicity, identifying novel targets, and facilitating drug repurposing efforts.
3. Artificial intelligence analysis of patient-derived organoid responses and integrated multi-omics data allows for personalized treatment strategies, predicting individual patient responses to therapies, guiding therapy selection, and informing clinical decision-making, especially in oncology.
4. Significant hurdles remain, including inherent organoid variability and biological limitations (e.g., lack of vascularization, incomplete maturation, cellular stress), data quality and standardization issues, the need for interpretable artificial intelligence models, computational resource demands, and complex ethical/regulatory considerations.
5. The field is advancing towards improved predictive accuracy through better models and validation, enhanced automation and standardization, integration with technologies like digital twins, and focused efforts on clinical translation and regulatory acceptance, requiring continued interdisciplinary collaboration.

## 10.1 Introduction

The convergence of artificial intelligence (AI) and organoid technology is revolutionizing drug discovery and precision medicine. Organoids, which are 3D cell cultures derived from stem cells, mimic the architecture and functionality of human organs. These miniature organ replicas have rapidly become indispensable tools across diverse biomedical domains, including developmental biology, disease modeling, drug discovery, personalized medicine, and regenerative therapies [1]. For instance, patient-derived organoids (PDOs) have shown high concordance with patient tumors in terms of molecular profiles and drug responses, suggesting their potential in personalized medicine [2–5]. This chapter explores how AI and machine learning (ML) are enhancing predictive modeling in drug discovery and facilitating personalized medicine and precision health.

AI and its subdiscipline ML have witnessed explosive growth. AI encompasses the development of computer systems capable of performing tasks that typically require human intelligence, while ML focuses on algorithms that enable systems to learn from and make decisions based on data without explicit programming [6]. These computational tools excel at identifying complex patterns, extracting meaningful features, and making predictions from the large, high-dimensional datasets that increasingly characterize modern biological research [1]. The application of AI/ML is revolutionizing data analysis across genomics, imaging, clinical records, and drug development pipelines [7].

## 10.2 Transformative Potential in Drug Discovery and Precision Medicine

In drug discovery, the high cost, lengthy timelines, and alarmingly high failure rates of bringing new therapeutics to market represent major hurdles [8]. AI-enabled organoid platforms offer a path to mitigate these challenges by providing more predictive preclinical models [1]. AI can accelerate screening processes, improve the prediction of drug efficacy and toxicity early in the pipeline, identify novel therapeutic targets, and facilitate drug repurposing efforts [1].

The pursuit of precision medicine — tailoring medical treatments to the individual characteristics of each patient — stands to benefit enormously from this technological marriage [1]. PDOs, generated directly from an individual's cells, capture patient-specific genetics and disease phenotypes. When coupled with AI analysis, PDOs can serve as personalized avatars for testing potential therapies, predicting individual drug responses, optimizing treatment regimens, and ultimately guiding clinical decision-making [1, 9].

Significantly, this technological convergence aligns with evolving regulatory landscapes. The U.S. Food and Drug Administration (FDA) Modernization Act 2.0, enacted in late 2022, formally recognized the potential of non-animal testing methods, including microphysiological systems like organoids, for preclinical research [6]. This regulatory shift creates a timely and fertile ground for AI-enabled organoid systems (Figure 10.1). The maturation of AI tools capable of extracting robust, predictive insights from these complex biological models provides the necessary analytical power to establish organoids as viable, human-relevant alternatives in drug development pipelines, potentially accelerating the translation of safer and more effective therapies [10].

Given the rapid pace of innovation in both organoid technology and AI/ML methodologies, particularly highlighted by developments like advanced large language models emerging since late 2022 [6], this chapter focuses primarily on advancements reported from 2022 onwards. It aims to provide a comprehensive overview of the current state-of-the-art at the intersection of these fields. The subsequent sections will delve into the specific applications of AI/ML in predictive modeling for drug discovery (Section 10.3) and its role in advancing personalized medicine using patient-specific organoids (Section 10.4). We will then critically examine the key challenges and limitations hindering progress (Section 10.5) before exploring the exciting future directions and emerging trends poised to shape the field (Section 10.6).

## 10.3 Predictive Modeling and Drug Discovery

### 10.3.1 *The Role of Organoids in Drug Discovery*

Organoids, self-organizing 3D structures grown from stem cells or tissues, have emerged as a revolutionary tool in biomedical research and drug discovery. These "mini-organs" possess the remarkable ability to replicate the intricate architecture of human organs and maintain the histology, gene expression, and cellular interactions of the original tissues, making them a more physiologically relevant model compared to conventional 2D cell cultures and animal models for studying disease mechanisms and drug responses [3, 5, 11, 12].

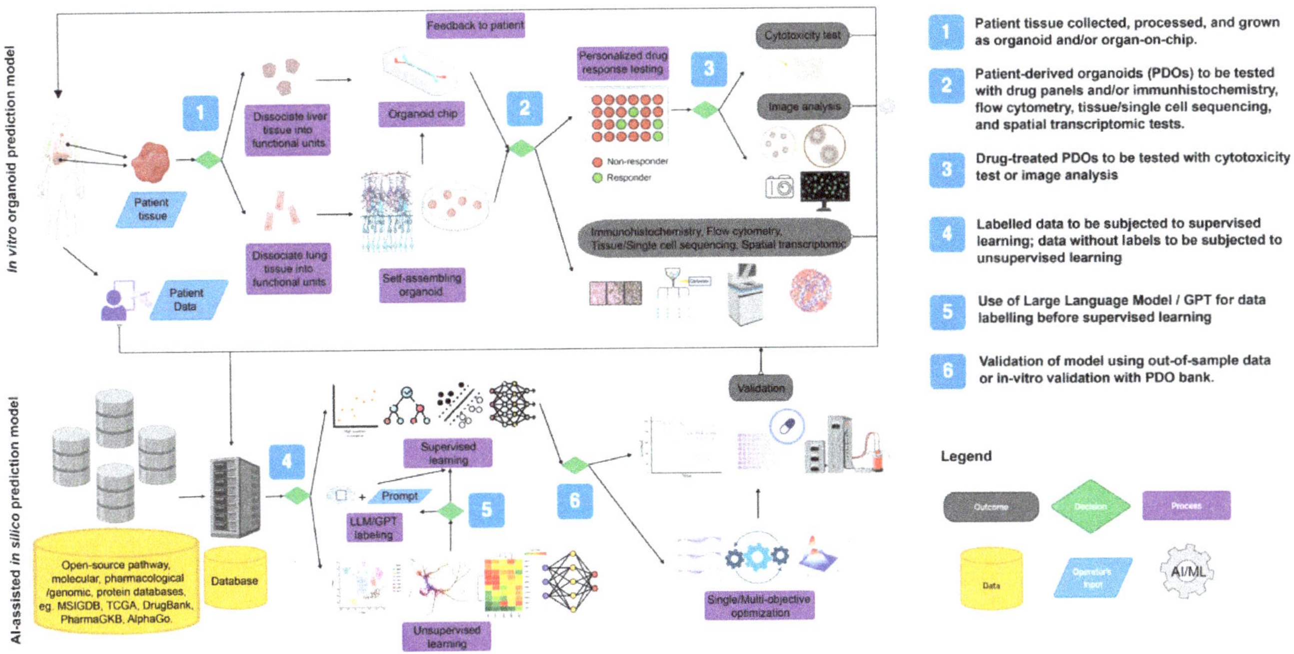


**Figure 10.1** The landscape of combining AI and organoid technologies. Some of the figure components were reproduced from NIH BioArt (public domain), and some created via BioRender by the authors.

An *in vitro* drug treatment outcome predicted from PDOs is a critical aspect of their utility in drug discovery. Studies have demonstrated that organoids can recapitulate patient responses to drugs, thereby serving as a reliable platform for drug screening and development outside of the human body [2, 4, 5, 13]. For instance, a study on various surgically resected lung cancer types showed that PDOs could predict clinical outcomes on drug sensitivity with 100% accuracy and specificity within a week, highlighting their potential for informing timely personalized treatment strategies [5]. Similarly, pancreatic cancer-derived organoids have been used to establish a drug testing platform that accurately predicts *in vivo* responses [4]. Moreover, multi-organ chips incorporating PDOs are now available, allowing for the simultaneous assessment of drug efficacy on target tissues (e.g., lung cancer and chronic lung disease) and potential side effects on non-target tissues (e.g., liver) [14, 15]. This technology, by providing high amount of reliable patient surrogates for *ex vivo* drug testing, allows researchers to screen a wider range of drug candidates on a single patient sample. This generates a wealth of data that can be used to train ML algorithms to identify meaningful molecular features of drugs and disease characteristics within specific patient populations. Consequently, this enables the development of more accurate *in silico* predictive models for drug efficacy and toxicity, leading to more efficient drug discovery pipelines.

## 10.3.2 *Artificial Intelligence-Enhanced Drug Screening and Development with Organoids*

### 10.3.2.1 *High-Throughput Screening and Automation*

Organoids present challenges for traditional high-throughput screening due to their complexity, variability, and often demanding culture requirements. However, AI is proving instrumental in overcoming these hurdles and enabling the use of organoids in larger-scale screening campaigns. AI-powered image analysis software, often integrated with automated microscopy and liquid handling systems, allows for the automated quantification of complex morphological features, viability metrics, and phenotypic changes across thousands of organoid cultures. This automation not only increases throughput but also enhances objectivity and reproducibility by minimizing manual intervention and bias from subjective judgement by a human operator. Platforms leveraging AI can analyze vast quantities of imaging data generated during screens, making intuitive decisions within workflows, such as optimizing feeding schedules or identifying ideal time points for assays. This capability is crucial for making organoid-based high-throughput screening feasible, effectively managing the inherent "snowflake effect" — the variability observed even between organoids derived from the same source under identical conditions — and extracting meaningful data despite this complexity [16]. Thus, AI is not merely analyzing high-throughput screening data but actively enabling the use of complex organoid models in high-throughput settings.

#### 10.3.2.2 *Predicting Drug Efficacy and Toxicity*

A primary goal in preclinical drug development is to accurately predict how a compound will perform in humans. Organoids offer superior physiological relevance compared to traditional 2D cell cultures. AI algorithms are adept at analyzing the multifaceted responses of organoids to drug exposure — including changes in morphology, size, growth rate, cell death, functional outputs (e.g., electrophysiology, barrier integrity), and molecular profiles (omics data) — to predict drug efficacy [1]. ML models can be trained on data from organoid drug screens to predict metrics like half-maximal-inhibitory-concentration (IC50)/area-under-the dose-response-curve (AUC) values or classify compounds as effective or ineffective [17]. A similar cell line-derived prediction model based on genetic mutations and expressions has shown possibility to predict the drug response in pre-clinical settings [18].

Equally important is the early identification of potential toxicity. AI analysis of organoid responses can predict adverse effects, such as cardiotoxicity [19], neurotoxicity [1], or hepatotoxicity [20]. For example, a liver-on-a-chip system incorporating hepatic organoids correctly predicted the toxicity of an antiretroviral drug combination that had previously escaped detection until phase 2 trials [20]. By leveraging the human-relevant biology of organoids [1] and the predictive capacity of AI, this approach aims to improve the translation of preclinical findings to the clinic and reduce the high attrition rates caused by unforeseen efficacy or safety issues in human trials [20]. This combination offers a potential paradigm shift, enabling better candidate selection before expensive and time-consuming clinical testing begins.

#### 10.3.2.3 *Target Identification and Validation*

Identifying novel drug targets and validating their roles in disease remain critical bottlenecks. AI algorithms can mine complex datasets generated from organoid models, particularly multi-omics data, to uncover previously unknown molecular pathways or dependencies that could serve as therapeutic targets. By perturbing potential targets (e.g., using gene editing) within the organoid system and observing the downstream effects on cellular phenotype or function through AI-assisted analysis, researchers can validate targets in a context that better reflect human physiology [1].

#### 10.3.2.4 *Drug Repurposing Applications*

AI can accelerate the identification of new uses for existing drugs (drug repurposing), a strategy that significantly reduces development timelines and costs by leveraging compounds with established safety profiles [17]. AI algorithms can computationally screen libraries of approved drugs against disease-specific organoid models (including PDOs) by analyzing structural similarities, predicted interactions, or actual experimental responses measured via imaging or omics [19]. This allows for the rapid identification of candidates with potential efficacy in new indications.

### 10.3.3 *Analyzing Organoid and Drug Data: Modalities and Artificial Intelligence/Machine Learning Techniques*

The effectiveness of AI in organoid-based drug discovery hinges on its ability to process and interpret the diverse and complex data generated from these models.

#### 10.3.3.1 *Key Data Types*

1. **High-Content Imaging:** This is a cornerstone of organoid analysis. Various microscopy techniques (brightfield, phase-contrast, fluorescence, confocal, light-sheet) capture rich visual information about organoid morphology (size, shape, complexity), internal structure, spatial organization of different cell types, cell viability, and dynamic processes over time [1]. Techniques like cell painting, which uses multiple fluorescent dyes to label different cellular compartments, generate detailed morphological profiles amenable to AI analysis for phenotypic screening and mechanism-of-action studies [21]. AI is essential for extracting quantitative metrics from these often complex and heterogeneous 3D images.
2. **Omics Data:** Molecular profiling provides deep insights into the state of organoids. This includes genomics (identifying mutations or copy number variations,

especially in PDOs), transcriptomics (bulk or single-cell RNA sequencing to measure gene expression profiles and identify cell types/states), proteomics (quantifying protein expression and modifications), metabolomics (measuring small molecule metabolites), and epigenomics (analyzing DNA methylation or histone modifications) [1]. Integrating these multi-omics layers offers a comprehensive molecular snapshot but presents significant analytical challenges that AI is well-suited to address [19, 22].

3. **Functional Assays:** Beyond structure and molecules, assessing organoid function is crucial. This involves diverse assays depending on the organoid type, such as electrophysiological recordings (e.g., multi-electrode arrays for neural organoids), calcium imaging (tracking $Ca^{2+}$ transients in cardiac or neural organoids), contractility measurements (for muscle or cardiac organoids), barrier function tests (e.g., transepithelial electrical resistance in intestinal organoids), and assays measuring the secretion of hormones or other factors [19]. AI can analyze the often complex and dynamic data streams from these functional readouts.
4. **Drug molecular features and descriptors:** In drug discovery, predictive modeling often relies on the accurate representation of drug molecules using molecular features and descriptors. These features capture the physicochemical properties, structural characteristics, and biological activities of drugs, enabling the development of ML models for various outcomes [23, 24].

#### 10.3.3.2 *Toolkit: A Range of Artificial Intelligence and Machine Learning Techniques Employed to Analyze these Data Modalities*

1. Deep Learning for Image Analysis: Deep learning, particularly convolutional neural networks (CNNs), has revolutionized organoid image analysis [25]. Various CNN architectures, including U-Net (for segmentation), ResNet, DenseNet, EfficientNet, and more recently Vision Transformers, and single-stage object detection training framework, You Only Look Once family of models from the Ultralytics, are used for tasks such as:
   a. **Segmentation:** Automatically delineating organoid boundaries and internal structures.
   b. **Classification:** Categorizing organoids based on type, quality, developmental stage, or treatment response [19].
   c. **Object Detection:** Identifying and counting organoids within images [26].

d. **Feature Extraction:** Quantifying morphological parameters (size, shape, texture) for phenotypic analysis [26].
e. **Tracking:** Monitoring organoid growth, movement, or cell dynamics over time in time-lapse sequences [26].
f. **Quality Assessment:** Predicting organoid viability or developmental potential from label-free images [27]. Specific platforms like OrganoID leverage modified U-Nets for robust, label-free analysis [16], while commercial systems like IN Carta incorporate AI for workflow automation and analysis [28].

2. ML for Omics/Functional Data: For analyzing omics data and quantitative functional readouts, classical ML algorithms like random forests, support vector machines, k-nearest neighbors, logistic regression, and various regression techniques (e.g., ridge regression) are widely used for tasks such as:
   a. **Classification:** Assigning samples to predefined categories (e.g., responder vs. non-responder, disease vs. healthy) [19].
   b. **Regression:** Predicting continuous values (e.g., drug IC50, functional parameters) [29].
   c. **Clustering:** Identifying subgroups within data based on similarity (e.g., discovering novel cell subtypes in single cell RNA sequencing data) [19].
   d. **Biomarker Discovery:** Identifying features (genes, proteins, metabolites) that are predictive of a specific outcome [30].
   e. **Deep Learning:** Multi-layer perceptrons and potentially recurrent neural networks for time-series data can capture complex, non-linear relationships within omics or functional datasets [31].
   f. **Dimensionality Reduction:** Techniques like principal component analysis, uniform manifold approximation, and projection and t-distributed stochastic neighbor embedding are often used, sometimes in conjunction with ML, for visualizing high-dimensional omics or functional data [19].
   g. **Data Integration:** Specialized ML frameworks and network-based approaches are developed to integrate multi-omics data, aiming to provide a more holistic view of the biological system [1]. Tools like Brain and Organoid Manifold Alignment (BOMA) align transcriptomic data [19], while OmicsFootPrint uses deep neural networks to visualize integrated multi-omics profiles [32]. Network-based ML leverages protein-protein interaction networks to contextualize omics data for biomarker discovery [29].

The interplay between these data types and analytical techniques is crucial (Table 10.1). For instance, AI analysis of imaging data might identify morphological changes upon drug treatment, which can then be correlated with transcriptomic changes identified by ML analysis of single cell RNA sequencing data from the same organoids, providing deeper mechanistic insights.

**Table 10.1** Selected AI/ML techniques for organoid data analysis.

| Data Type | Analysis Task(s) | AI/ML Technique(s) | Example Application [Reference] |
|---|---|---|---|
| Brightfield/ phase image | Segmentation, tracking, morphology analysis | U-Net CNN (modified) | OrganoID platform for label-free analysis of various organoid types [16] |
| Brightfield image | Quality prediction/ developmental assessment | EfficientNetV2-S, vision transformer (ensemble) | Predicting hypothalamic-pituitary organoid quality (RAX expression proxy) from early images [27] |
| Fluorescence image | Neuronal network classification | Random forest | Automated classification of control vs. treated neural organoids [19] |
| Fluorescence image | Cardiomyocyte structural change detection | CNNs | Detecting drug-induced changes from captured image indicative of cardiotoxicity [19] |
| Fluorescence image | Retinal pigment epithelium segmentation | U-Net CNN | Detecting/segmenting retinal pigment epithelium cell boundaries in large-scale imaging [19] |
| Single cell RNA sequencing | Cell type classification/ annotation transfer | Random forest, k-nearest neighbors | Identifying cell types in heart organoids; comparing brain organoids to tissue [19] |
| Single cell RNA sequencing | Transcriptomic data alignment | Manifold learning (k-nearest neighbors-based, e.g., BOMA) | Aligning brain and organoid transcriptomics to map developmental trajectories [19] |
| Bulk RNA sequencing/ microarray | Drug response biomarker ID (pathway-based) | Ridge regression (network-informed) | Identifying predictive pathway biomarkers from colorectal/bladder organoid pharmacogenomics data [29] |

*(Continued)*

**Table 10.1** (*Continued*)

| Data Type | Analysis Task(s) | AI/ML Technique(s) | Example Application [Reference] |
|---|---|---|---|
| Calcium imaging | Cardiac function assessment/disease class | Support vector machine, k-nearest neighbors, random forest classifiers | Classifying $Ca^{2+}$ transient signals to detect genetic cardiac diseases (CPVT, LQT1, HCM) [19] |
| Action potential data | Arrhythmia detection/ quantification | CNNs | Detecting/quantifying arrhythmic waveforms in cardiac organoids for cardiotoxicity testing [19] |
| Multi-omics data | Data integration, visualization, prediction | Deep neural networks (e.g., OmicsFootPrint), ML models | Integrating multi-omics for drug response prediction, cancer subtyping [32]; predicting neurotoxicity [1] |
| Microscopy images | Automated workflow decisions | AI-powered image analysis software (e.g., IN Carta) | Optimizing cell culture feeding/ passaging; high-throughput screening analysis [28] |

### 10.3.4 *Recent Case Studies in Artificial Intelligence-Driven Drug Discovery (2022–Present)*

Several recent studies exemplify the application of AI/ML in organoid-based drug discovery:

1. **Network-based ML for Biomarker Discovery:** While the initial publication predates 2022, the framework by Kong *et al.* remains highly relevant and influential [29]. They demonstrated a systematic approach using pharmacogenomic data from colorectal and bladder cancer organoids. By integrating gene expression data of pathways proximal to known drug targets within a protein-protein interaction network, they trained ridge regression models to predict drug sensitivity (5-fluorouracil and cisplatin). The pathways identified as having high predictive weight in the organoid models (e.g., "activation of BH3-only proteins" for 5-fluorouracil) subsequently served as robust biomarkers capable of predicting overall survival in corresponding patient cohorts from The Cancer Genome Atlas. This work provides a blueprint for leveraging organoid data and network biology through ML to bridge the gap between preclinical models and patient outcomes.

2. **Deep Learning for Automated Organoid Phenotyping (OrganoID):** Addressing the need for automated, label-free image analysis, the OrganoID platform was developed around 2022 [16]. Utilizing a modified U-Net CNN architecture, OrganoID accurately segments and tracks individual organoids in standard brightfield or phase-contrast microscopy images across various cancer types (pancreatic, lung, colon, adenoid cystic carcinoma). Its performance showed excellent agreement with manual measurements (95–97% for count and size) and robust tracking accuracy (>89% over four days). Crucially, the platform was applied to analyze morphological changes (circularity, solidity, eccentricity) in pancreatic cancer organoids during a chemotherapy dose-response experiment, automatically identifying significant drug effects. This demonstrates the power of deep learning to enable high-throughput phenotypic drug screening without complex labeling procedures.
3. **AI for Predicting Organoid Quality and Development:** A significant challenge in organoid research is ensuring quality and predicting successful differentiation. A recent study (reported Dec 2024) tackled this using deep learning [27]. Researchers trained an ensemble model combining EfficientNetV2-S and Vision Transformer architectures on brightfield images of developing hypothalamic-pituitary organoids. The model learned to predict the quality of the organoids at an early stage (day 30), based on visual features correlating with the expression of the RAX protein (a marker linked to later ACTH hormone secretion). The AI model achieved 70% accuracy in classifying organoid quality, significantly outperforming experienced researchers (<60% accuracy) and doing so much faster. This highlights AI's potential to streamline organoid production by enabling early selection of high-quality batches, saving considerable time and resources.

These case studies illustrate the diverse ways AI is being applied — from extracting deep biological insights and biomarkers to automating laborious analysis tasks and optimizing the organoid generation process itself. There appears to be a dynamic interplay where AI analysis of organoid data not only yields predictive insights but also reveals limitations in current organoid models (such as stress responses or incomplete differentiation [33]). This feedback drives bioengineering efforts to create more sophisticated organoids (e.g., incorporating vascular or immune components [6]), which in turn generate higher-fidelity data, fueling the development of more accurate and reliable AI models in a continuous cycle of improvement.

## 10.4 Personalized Medicine and Precision Health

The ultimate goal of precision medicine is to tailor healthcare interventions to the unique biological characteristics of each individual. The combination of PDOs and AI/ML offers a powerful platform to realize this vision, particularly in complex diseases like cancer.

### 10.4.1 *Tailoring Treatments with Artificial Intelligence and Patient-Derived Organoids*

PDOs are generated directly from a patient's tissue sample, typically a biopsy or surgical resection of a tumor, but also potentially from healthy tissue. These models serve as personalized *ex vivo* avatars, capturing the specific genetic landscape, epigenetic state, cellular heterogeneity, and phenotypic characteristics of the individual's own tissue or disease [34]. This high degree of personalization makes PDOs exceptionally valuable preclinical models for predicting how an individual patient might respond to different therapies [35].

AI and ML algorithms are critical for unlocking the predictive potential of PDOs [1]. By analyzing the response of a patient's PDOs to a panel of drugs in the lab — assessed through imaging, viability assays, or omics profiling — AI models can be trained to predict the likelihood of clinical benefit for that specific patient. This approach is gaining significant traction in oncology, where inter-patient heterogeneity dramatically influences treatment outcomes [30]. AI-PDO systems have the potential to:

1. **Guide Therapy Selection:** Predict which available drug or combination therapy is most likely to be effective for a given patient, moving beyond population-level statistics [35].
2. **Optimize Dosages:** Inform decisions about appropriate drug concentrations.
3. **Predict Resistance:** Identify potential mechanisms of drug resistance before they manifest clinically, allowing for proactive adjustments to treatment strategies [35].
4. **Inform Clinical Decision-Making:** Provide oncologists with objective, patient-specific data to support treatment planning, potentially within clinically relevant timeframes [36].

The establishment of PDO biobanks, containing collections of organoids from diverse patient populations, further enhances these possibilities by providing larger datasets for training more robust AI models and enabling broader research into disease subtypes and treatment responses [37]. While the correlation between PDO drug response and actual patient outcomes is increasingly supported by evidence [35], it is the sophisticated analytical capabilities of AI that are essential for translating this correlation into actionable clinical predictions. Handling the complexity of multi-drug regimens, integrating diverse data types (imaging, omics, clinical history), and delivering predictions rapidly requires computational power far beyond manual interpretation [30].

### 10.4.2 *Artificial Intelligence-Powered Multi-Omics Integration for Deeper Insights*

A single data modality rarely captures the full complexity of biological systems. Precision medicine increasingly relies on integrating multiple layers of information, including genomics, transcriptomics, proteomics, metabolomics, epigenomics, alongside clinical data and imaging to build a holistic understanding of an individual's health or disease state [1]. Analyzing and integrating these high-dimensional, heterogeneous datasets is a significant challenge [31].

AI and ML techniques are particularly well-suited for this task [19]. Applied to multi-omics data generated from PDOs, AI algorithms can:

1. **Uncover Complex Patterns:** Identify subtle correlations and interactions between different molecular layers (e.g., how specific mutations influence gene expression patterns and protein levels) that are associated with disease characteristics or drug response [19].
2. **Identify Patient-Specific Signatures:** Discover unique molecular fingerprints within a patient's PDO data that predict sensitivity or resistance to particular therapies [30].
3. **Develop Predictive Biomarkers:** Identify robust biomarkers from integrated multi-omics data that can be used for companion diagnostics (predicting who will benefit from a targeted therapy), stratifying patients for clinical trials, or monitoring treatment efficacy over time [30].

Tools like OmicsFootPrint exemplify this potential, using deep neural networks to transform complex multi-omics data into intuitive visual maps that correlate with drug response and disease subtypes, demonstrating superior performance compared to traditional models even with limited data [32]. Network-based ML approaches also show promise by integrating omics data within the context of known biological networks to identify functionally relevant predictive signatures [29].

However, the predictive accuracy of AI models in this context is fundamentally dependent on the quality and biological fidelity of the PDOs themselves. If a PDO fails to fully recapitulate critical aspects of the patient's *in vivo* tumor microenvironment (e.g., lacking relevant immune cell interactions or vascularization) or exhibits significant culture-induced artifacts like cellular stress, the data fed into the AI algorithm will be inherently limited [33, 38]. This can lead to inaccurate or biased predictions for the individual patient, highlighting the critical interdependence between advancements in organoid technology and AI model reliability for personalized medicine.

Furthermore, the generation and analysis of PDOs using AI raise unique ethical considerations. These living models, derived from a patient's own cells, contain a wealth of deeply personal biological information [28]. AI analysis extracts highly predictive insights from this data [35]. This raises complex questions regarding informed consent for potentially broad or unforeseen future analyses, data ownership, robust security measures for combined biological and computational data, and ensuring equitable access to these advanced technologies [6]. The specific case of brain organoids introduces further profound ethical questions about potential consciousness or sentience in advanced models [39].

### 10.4.3 *Recent Case Studies in Artificial Intelligence-Powered Personalized Medicine (2022–Present)*

While the field is rapidly evolving, several recent studies showcase the potential of using PDOs, often implicitly or explicitly involving advanced computational analysis, to predict individual patient responses:

1. **Individualized Patient Tumor Organoid (IPTO) Model for Brain Tumors:** Peng *et al.* developed the IPTO model by culturing patient brain tumor explants

within induced pluripotent stem cell-derived cerebral organoids, enabling the study of a wide range of central nervous system tumors [35]. Comprehensive multi-omics analyses (genomics, epigenomics, single cell RNA sequencing), which typically rely on sophisticated computational pipelines potentially involving ML, confirmed that the IPTOs faithfully recapitulated the cellular heterogeneity and molecular features of the original patient tumors. Crucially, in a prospective patient cohort, the drug responses observed in the IPTO models predicted the actual clinical responses of the patients, including identifying resistance mechanisms. This study provides compelling evidence for the predictive power of complex, patient-specific organoid models for personalized therapy guidance in brain cancer.

2. **Lung Cancer Organoid Drug Sensitivity Testing:** A real-world study published in early 2023 focused on generating lung cancer organoids (LCOs), primarily from malignant serous effusions, from over 100 patients [40]. Drug sensitivity testing (DST) was performed on these LCOs for both chemotherapy and targeted therapies. The results from the LCO-DST accurately predicted the clinical response (or lack thereof) observed in the corresponding patients with advanced lung cancer. While the study abstract does not explicitly detail the use of AI for analyzing the DST results, correlating multi-drug response data with clinical outcomes often benefits from computational modeling. This work highlights the feasibility and predictive potential of PDO-based assays in a clinical setting for lung cancer.
3. **Large-Scale Sarcoma PDO Biobank:** Researchers at UCLA recently reported the creation of the largest sarcoma PDO biobank to date, derived from 126 patients representing 25 different subtypes [37]. Extensive analyses confirmed that the organoids retained key characteristics of the original tumors. Importantly, for a subset of cases, the drug responses observed in the lab-grown organoids matched the clinical outcomes of the patients. Although AI analysis was not explicitly mentioned in the initial report (published September 2024), the generation of such a large, diverse dataset strongly implies the future application of AI/ML for deeper analysis and prediction. The team plans a larger clinical trial to validate the organoid-based approach for predicting treatment response, which will likely leverage AI to analyze the resulting data.

4. **AI-Driven Multi-Omics Analysis (OmicsFootPrint):** As previously mentioned, the OmicsFootPrint tool demonstrates how AI can directly contribute to personalized medicine insights [32]. By using deep neural networks to integrate and visualize multi-omics data from cancer patients, it achieved superior performance in predicting drug response (median AUC 0.74 across benchmarks) and classifying cancer subtypes with high accuracy (e.g., >95% for lung cancer subtypes, 87% for breast cancer subtypes) compared to existing models. Its ability to perform well even with reduced datasets suggests potential for clinical utility where patient data may be limited.

These examples, along with numerous ongoing clinical trials utilizing PDOs (summarized in Table 10.2), underscore the trajectory towards integrating PDOs and AI into personalized cancer care. While many trials are currently focused on feasibility or prognosis, the ultimate aim is to use these systems to actively guide patient-specific treatment decisions.

**Table 10.2** Selected clinical trials utilizing patient-derived organoids (potential for AI integration).

| Disease Area | Application | Phase | Trial Identifier(s) (Example) | Brief Description/Goal | Mention of AI/ Computational Analysis |
|---|---|---|---|---|---|
| Brain cancer | Feasibility | NA | NCT05772767 | Assess feasibility of generating PDOs from brain tumors. | Unspecified |
| Brain cancer | Treatment guidance | Early phase 1 | NCT05432518 | Use PDO drug sensitivity to guide therapy selection. | Unspecified |
| Breast cancer | Feasibility | Early phase 1 | NCT04727632 | Establish PDOs from breast cancer samples. | Unspecified |
| Breast cancer | Prognostic | NA | NCT04531696 | Correlate PDO characteristics/ response with patient outcomes. | Unspecified |
| Breast cancer | Treatment guidance | Phase 1 | NCT05177432 | Prospective trial using PDOs to guide treatment for metastatic breast cancer. | Quadratic phenotypic optimization platform [9] |
| Rectal cancer | Feasibility | NA | NCT04371198 | Feasibility of PDO generation and drug screening for rectal cancers. | Unspecified |

Table 10.2 (*Continued*)

| Disease Area | Application | Phase | Trial Identifier(s) (Example) | Brief Description/Goal | Mention of AI/ Computational Analysis |
|---|---|---|---|---|---|
| Rectal cancer | Treatment guidance | NA | NCT05352165 | Use PDO testing to personalize therapy for advanced colorectal cancer. | Unspecified |
| Liver cancer | Treatment guidance | NA | NCT05644743 | PDO-guided therapy selection for hepatocellular carcinoma. | Likely multi-omics data to predict drug resistance |
| Lung cancer | Treatment guidance | NA | Real-world study [40] | LCO-DST accurately predicted clinical response to chemo/targeted therapy. | Likely computational analysis, not specified AI |
| Sarcoma | Treatment guidance | NA | Planned trial [37] | Validate PDO approach for predicting treatment response in osteosarcoma. | (Likely AI analysis planned for larger trial) |
| Multiple cancers | Treatment guidance | Phase 1/2 | Review on clinical trials [41] | List of multiple trials across cancer types using PDOs to inform therapy choices. | Unspecified |

## 10.5 Overcoming Hurdles: Challenges and Limitations

Despite the immense potential, the integration of AI and organoid technology faces significant hurdles that must be addressed to realize its full promise in drug discovery and precision medicine. These challenges span data generation, organoid model fidelity, AI model characteristics, computational resources, and ethical considerations.

### 10.5.1 *Data-Related Challenges*

1. **Quality, Quantity, and Standardization:** A major bottleneck is the difficulty in generating large, high-quality, and standardized datasets from organoid experiments [1]. Organoids exhibit inherent biological variability due to factors like stem cell source, differentiation protocols, culture conditions, and stochastic self-organization processes [10]. This leads to the "fingerprint effect" (variability between patients) and the "snowflake effect" (variability even within the same patient line) [10]. Lack of standardized protocols across labs for culture, imaging, and data processing further exacerbates inconsistencies. This variability

complicates AI model training, reduces reproducibility, and hinders the ability to compare results across studies [19]. Generating sufficient quantities of high-quality data for training robust AI models remains a challenge.

2. **Heterogeneity:** Both inter-organoid (between different organoids in a batch) and intra-organoid (within a single organoid, e.g., core vs. periphery) heterogeneity pose analytical challenges [30]. AI algorithms must be sophisticated enough to either account for this heterogeneity or require sufficiently large sample sizes to overcome the noise it introduces.
3. **Data Integration:** Effectively integrating multi-modal data (imaging, multi-omics, functional assays, clinical information) remains complex [30]. Developing AI frameworks that can meaningfully combine these diverse data types to yield synergistic insights is an active area of research.

### 10.5.2 *Organoid Model Limitations*

1. **Fidelity and Complexity:** While organoids are advanced models, they do not yet fully replicate the complexity of native human organs [38]. Common limitations include the lack of a functional vascular network (leading to hypoxic cores and necrosis [33]), absence of immune cell components (critical for studying immunotherapy [38]), lack of innervation, and incomplete representation of the stromal microenvironment [33]. These missing elements can significantly impact organoid physiology and drug responses, thereby limiting the predictive accuracy of AI models trained on data from these systems.
2. **Maturation and Cell Types:** Many organoid protocols yield models representing fetal or early developmental stages, with limited capacity for full maturation to adult-like states [33]. Furthermore, cell type specification can be incomplete, with some cell subtypes missing or exhibiting atypical gene expression profiles [33]. Organoids also frequently display markers of cellular stress (e.g., metabolic or endoplasmic reticulum stress) not typical of healthy *in vivo* tissue, which could confound experimental results and AI analysis [33].

### 10.5.3 *Artificial Intelligence Model Challenges*

1. **Interpretability and Explainable AI (XAI):** Many powerful AI models, especially deep learning networks, function as "black boxes," making it difficult to

understand how they arrive at a specific prediction [19]. This lack of transparency hinders trust, makes it difficult to identify potential biases or failure modes, complicates troubleshooting, and poses significant barriers to clinical adoption and regulatory approval [42]. There is a critical need for robust XAI methods tailored for biological data that can provide meaningful insights into the model's decision-making process [42]. Developing and validating such XAI techniques is itself challenging [43]. However, the potential benefit extends beyond trust; XAI applied to organoid data could potentially illuminate the biological features (e.g., morphological patterns, gene signatures) driving predictions, thereby generating new, testable hypotheses about organoid biology or drug mechanisms [42].

2. **Generalizability and Bias:** AI models trained on data from one specific organoid type, protocol, or patient cohort may not perform well when applied to new, unseen data (poor generalizability). Biases present in the training data (e.g., stemming from specific patient demographics or experimental artifacts) can be learned and amplified by the AI model, leading to unreliable or inequitable predictions [19]. Ensuring models are robust and fair requires careful dataset curation, bias detection methods, and validation across diverse conditions.

### 10.5.4 *Computational and Resource Requirements*

Training state-of-the-art AI models, particularly deep learning networks, on large, high-resolution imaging or omics datasets demands significant computational resources, including powerful graphics processing units and substantial data storage capacity. Furthermore, developing and applying these models requires specialized expertise in both computational science and biology, necessitating interdisciplinary teams [1].

### 10.5.5 *Ethical and Regulatory Considerations*

The use of AI with organoids, especially PDOs, raises significant ethical questions [6]. Key issues include:

1. **Informed Consent:** Ensuring patients fully understand how their derived organoids and associated data (potentially vast and highly predictive) will be used, stored, and potentially shared, including for future research unforeseen at the time of consent [6].

2. **Data Privacy and Security:** Protecting sensitive biological and computational data generated from PDOs and AI analysis is paramount [38].
3. **Equity and Access:** Ensuring that the benefits of these advanced and potentially expensive technologies do not exacerbate existing healthcare disparities [38].
4. **Brain Organoids:** Advanced brain organoid research introduces unique and profound ethical dilemmas concerning the potential for emergent consciousness, sentience, or the capacity to experience suffering *in vitro* [39]. These questions about moral status and the limits of research require careful, proactive ethical deliberation and potentially specific governance frameworks to maintain public trust [39]. Addressing these fundamental ethical concerns is crucial, as they could represent a significant bottleneck to progress, distinct from purely technical challenges.

Navigating the evolving regulatory landscape for both AI-driven medical devices and organoid-based testing platforms is also critical [6]. Establishing clear validation strategies, demonstrating safety and efficacy, and achieving regulatory approval are necessary steps for clinical translation [31].

These challenges are often interconnected. For example, poor data standardization directly impacts model generalizability, while the biological limitations of current organoids constrain the ultimate clinical relevance of AI predictions derived from them. The lack of model interpretability hinders efforts to diagnose and correct for biases stemming from either flawed data or inherent model limitations. Addressing these multifaceted challenges requires a concerted, interdisciplinary effort involving biologists, engineers, data scientists, clinicians, ethicists, and regulators.

## 10.6 Horizon Scanning: Future Directions and Emerging Trends

The intersection of AI and organoid science is a rapidly evolving frontier with exciting prospects for transforming biomedical research and clinical practice. Several key trends and future directions are emerging as outlined below.

### 10.6.1 *Improving Predictive Accuracy and Model Robustness*

A major focus is on enhancing the accuracy, reliability, and generalizability of AI models used for analyzing organoid data [44]. This involves developing more sophisticated algorithms capable of capturing subtle biological signals and handling the inherent variability of organoid systems. Efforts are underway to train models on larger, more diverse datasets encompassing multiple organoid types, genetic backgrounds, and experimental conditions [27]. Crucially, rigorous validation strategies are paramount. This includes not only retrospective validation on existing data but also prospective studies that test AI-organoid predictions against real-world clinical outcomes in patient cohorts [45]. Such clinical validation is essential for building confidence and demonstrating the translational value of these approaches.

### 10.6.2 *Enhanced Automation and Standardization*

The field is moving towards greater automation and standardization to improve reproducibility and scalability. Future workflows envision fully automated systems integrating robotic liquid handling, environmental control, high-content imaging, and real-time AI-driven analysis for organoid culture, monitoring, and screening [28]. This will minimize manual variability, increase throughput, and potentially reduce costs [27]. Parallel efforts focus on establishing standardized protocols for organoid generation, characterization, data acquisition, and data reporting formats [19]. These standardization initiatives are critical for generating the high-quality, comparable data needed for training robust and generalizable AI models.

### 10.6.3 *Integration with Advanced Technologies*

The synergy between AI and organoids is expected to deepen through integration with other cutting-edge technologies:

1. **Organoid Intelligence Brainoware:** This nascent and ambitious field explores the potential of using brain organoids, interfaced with computational hardware and AI, as biological computing units [38, 46]. Early experiments have shown brain organoid cultures learning rudimentary tasks, like playing Pong or recognizing speech patterns, driven by their inherent neuroplasticity [46]. Proponents suggest potential advantages over silicon-based computing in terms of energy efficiency and capacity for complex learning [38]. However, significant technical hurdles remain, including scaling up organoid size and complexity, developing stable interfaces, and addressing profound ethical concerns [38]. Organoid intelligence represents a long-term vision distinct from using AI to analyze organoids.

2. **Digital Twins:** The concept of a "digital twin" — a dynamic, virtual replica of a physical entity, continuously updated with real-time data — is gaining traction in healthcare [47, 48]. A patient's digital twin could integrate diverse data streams (genomics, imaging, wearables, clinical records) to simulate physiological processes, predict disease progression, and optimize treatments [47]. Data derived from AI analysis of a patient's own organoids could serve as a crucial input for building more accurate and personalized digital twins, particularly for modeling tissue-level responses or complex diseases like cancer. While still largely in preclinical development [49], the integration of AI-interpreted organoid data into patient digital twins offers a powerful paradigm for future personalized medicine.

This integration highlights a crucial aspect of the future: the co-evolution of AI and organoid technology. As bioengineers develop more complex and physiologically faithful organoids (e.g., incorporating vascular networks, immune cells, or forming multi-organoid "assembloids" [6]), the data generated will become richer but also vastly more complex. This necessitates the development of even more powerful and sophisticated AI algorithms capable of extracting meaningful information from these next-generation models [1]. Conversely, insights gleaned from AI analysis of current organoid limitations (e.g., identifying specific missing cell interactions or aberrant signaling pathways [33]) will directly inform and guide the rational design and engineering of improved organoid systems. This reciprocal relationship will likely accelerate progress in both fields.

### 10.6.4 *Bridging the Gap to Clinical Translation and Regulatory Acceptance*

Ultimately, the success of AI-enabled organoids will be measured by their impact on patient care. Bridging the gap from laboratory research to routine clinical use requires several critical steps [1, 31]. As mentioned, robust clinical validation through well-designed prospective studies is non-negotiable [31]. Furthermore, practical integration into existing clinical workflows needs careful consideration. Gaining regulatory acceptance from bodies like the FDA is essential [10]. The FDA Modernization Act 2.0 provides a supportive framework, but specific guidance for AI-driven analyses of organoid data will likely be needed [10].

A crucial factor for clinical adoption is trust. Clinicians must be able to understand and trust the predictions generated by AI-organoid systems to confidently base treatment decisions upon them. This underscores the critical importance of developing effective XAI methods specifically tailored for clinical users [42]. These methods need to provide explanations that are not just technically accurate but also clinically meaningful and actionable. Achieving successful translation will necessitate strong, ongoing collaboration between fundamental researchers, AI experts, engineers, clinicians, patient advocates, ethicists, and regulatory agencies [1].

## 10.7 Conclusion

The convergence of AI and organoid technology marks a significant inflection point in biomedical research and development. AI and ML are rapidly transforming the organoid field, moving beyond simple data analysis to actively enhancing model generation, enabling high-throughput experimentation, and extracting deep biological insights from complex datasets. The synergy between the enhanced physiological relevance of organoids and the predictive power of AI offer unprecedented opportunities to accelerate the discovery and development of more effective and safer therapeutics, addressing the longstanding challenges of high costs and failure rates in the pharmaceutical industry.

Furthermore, the combination of AI with PDOs is paving the way towards true precision medicine. By creating personalized *ex vivo* models that capture individual patient biology and leveraging AI to predict treatment responses, this approach promises to revolutionize clinical decision-making, particularly in heterogeneous diseases like cancer, leading to more tailored and effective therapies.

However, the path forward is not without significant challenges. Issues related to data quality and standardization, the biological limitations of current organoid models, the need for interpretable and robust AI algorithms, substantial resource requirements, and complex ethical and regulatory considerations must be proactively addressed. Overcoming these hurdles will require sustained innovation and collaboration across disciplines.

Looking ahead, continued efforts in automation, standardization, rigorous clinical validation, and the development of clinician-focused XAI are crucial for translating these powerful technologies into tangible benefits for human health. By fostering interdisciplinary collaboration and maintaining a strong commitment to ethical diligence and scientific rigor, the field of AI-enabled organoids is poised to make transformative contributions to our understanding of biology, the treatment of disease, and the future of personalized healthcare.

## Key Opinion Points

1. **AI and Organoids Offer Unprecedented Predictive Power:** The convergence of AI/ML with organoid technology, especially PDOs, represents a significant leap forward. Organoids provide superior physiological relevance compared to traditional models, while AI delivers the analytical power needed to interpret complex data (imaging, multi-omics, functional assays). This synergy is creating more predictive preclinical models, crucial for accelerating drug discovery, improving efficacy/toxicity prediction, and reducing the high attrition rates in clinical trials. The FDA Modernization Act 2.0 further validates this approach, recognizing the potential of these systems as alternatives to animal testing.
2. **AI is Essential for Realizing Personalized Medicine with PDOs:** PDOs capture individual tumor heterogeneity and characteristics, serving as personalized avatars for testing therapies. However, translating the complex responses of these PDOs into actionable clinical insights requires sophisticated AI/ML algorithms. AI enables the prediction of patient-specific drug responses, guides therapy selection beyond population averages, identifies potential resistance mechanisms, and integrates multi-omics data for deeper understanding, paving the way for truly personalized treatment strategies, particularly in oncology.
3. **Addressing Key Hurdles (Interpretability, Fidelity, Ethics) is Critical for Translation:** Despite the promise, significant challenges must be overcome for widespread clinical adoption. These include standardizing protocols to manage organoid variability ("snowflake effect"), improving organoid fidelity (e.g., vascularization, immune components, maturation, reducing stress artifacts), ensuring AI model robustness and generalizability, and developing XAI to build trust and facilitate regulatory approval. Furthermore, navigating complex ethical considerations, particularly regarding data privacy, consent, and the unique issues surrounding brain organoids, is paramount for responsible innovation and public acceptance.

## References

1. Bai L, Wu Y, Li G, Zhang W, Zhang H, Su J. AI-enabled organoids: Construction, analysis, and application. Bioact Mater. 2024;31:525–548.
2. Vlachogiannis G, Hedayat S, Vatsiou A, Jamin Y, Fernández-Mateos J, Khan K, *et al.* Patient-derived organoids model treatment response of metastatic gastrointestinal cancers. Science. 2018;359:920–926.
3. Rae C, Amato F, Braconi C. Patient-Derived Organoids as a Model for Cancer Drug Discovery. Int J Mol Sci. 2021;22:3483.
4. Frappart P, Walter K, Gout J, Beutel AK, Morawe M, Arnold F, *et al.* Pancreatic cancer-derived organoids — a disease modeling tool to predict drug response. United European Gastroenterol J. 2020;8:594–606.
5. Hu Y, Sui X, Song F, Li Y, Li K, Chen Z, *et al.* Lung cancer organoids analyzed on microwell arrays predict drug responses of patients within a week. Nat Commun. 2021;12:2581.
6. Wang H, Li X, You X, Zhao G. Harnessing the power of artificial intelligence for human living organoid research. Bioact Mater. 2024;42:140–164.
7. Howell HJ, McGale JP, Choucair A, Shirini D, Aide N, Postow MA, *et al.* Artificial Intelligence for Drug Discovery: An Update and Future Prospects. Semin Nucl Med. 2025;55:406–422.
8. Sun D, Gao W, Hu H, Zhou S. Why 90% of clinical drug development fails and how to improve it? Acta Pharm Sin B. 2022;12:3049–3062.
9. Rashid MBMA, Toh TB, Hooi L, Silva A, Zhang Y, Tan PF, *et al.* Optimizing drug combinations against multiple myeloma using a quadratic phenotypic optimization platform (QPOP). Sci Transl Med. 2018;10. doi:10.1126/scitranslmed.aan0941.
10. Annelies KO, Courtney T, Pradipta G. Organoids, Beyond the Hype. https://www.technologynetworks.com/cell-science/articles/organoids-beyond-the-hype-395924.
11. Struzyna LA, Watt ML. The Emerging Role of Neuronal Organoid Models in Drug Discovery: Potential Applications and Hurdles to Implementation. Mol Pharmacol. 2021; 99:256–265.
12. Xu H, Jiao Y, Qin S, Zhao W, Chu Q, Wu K. Organoid technology in disease modelling, drug development, personalized treatment and regeneration medicine. Exp Hematol Oncol. 2018;7:30.
13. Millard M, Williams NA, Elrod AK, DesRochers TM. Abstract 3086: Organoids standardized to a clinically validated drug response assay for truly predictive in vitro drug response profiling. Cancer Res. 2022;82:3086–3086.
14. Bovard D, Sandoz A, Luettich K, Frentzel S, Iskandar A, Marescotti D, *et al.* A lung/liver-on-a-chip platform for acute and chronic toxicity studies. Lab Chip. 2018;18:3814–3829.

15. Zheng L, Wang B, Sun Y, Dai B, Fu Y, Zhang Y, *et al.* An Oxygen-Concentration-Controllable Multiorgan Microfluidic Platform for Studying Hypoxia-Induced Lung Cancer-Liver Metastasis and Screening Drugs. ACS Sens. 2021;6:823–832.
16. Matthews JM, Schuster B, Kashaf SS, Liu P, Ben-Yishay R, Ishay-Ronen D, *et al.* OrganoID: A versatile deep learning platform for tracking and analysis of single-organoid dynamics. PLoS Comput Biol. 2022;18:e1010584.
17. Wan Z, Sun X, Li Y, Chu T, Hao X, Cao Y, *et al.* Applications of Artificial Intelligence in Drug Repurposing. Advanced Science. 2025;12. doi:10.1002/advs.202411325.
18. Barretina J, Caponigro G, Stransky N, Venkatesan K, Margolin AA, Kim S, *et al.* The Cancer Cell Line Encyclopedia enables predictive modelling of anticancer drug sensitivity. Nature. 2012;483:603–607.
19. Maramraju S, Kowalczewski A, Kaza A, Liu X, Singaraju JP, Albert MV, *et al.* AI-organoid integrated systems for biomedical studies and applications. Bioeng Transl Med. 2024;9. doi:10.1002/btm2.10641.
20. Zhang CJ, Meyer SR, O'Meara MJ, Huang S, Capeling MM, Ferrer-Torres D, *et al.* A human liver organoid screening platform for DILI risk prediction. J Hepatol. 2023; 78:998–1006.
21. Nikki Carter. Innovations in Multimodal Image Analysis Help Improve Biopharma Productivity. https://www.labcompare.com/10-Featured-Articles/616679-Innovations-in-Multimodal-Image-Analysis-Help-Improve-Biopharma-Productivity/.
22. Dai J, Xu H, Chen T, Huang T, Liang W, Zhang R, *et al.* Artificial intelligence for medicine 2025: Navigating the endless frontier. The Innovation Medicine. 2025;3:100120.
23. Cheng T, Li Q, Zhou Z, Wang Y, Bryant SH. Structure-Based Virtual Screening for Drug Discovery: a Problem-Centric Review. AAPS J. 2012;14:133–141.
24. Lavecchia A, Giovanni C. Virtual Screening Strategies in Drug Discovery: A Critical Review. Curr Med Chem. 2013;20:2839–2860.
25. Mienye ID, Swart TG, Obaido G, Jordan M, Ilono P. Deep Convolutional Neural Networks in Medical Image Analysis: A Review. Information. 2025;16:195.
26. Ulhaq A. Organoid Computer Vision: A Survey and Outlook. 2024. doi:10.31224/3883.
27. Asano T, Suga H, Niioka H, Yukawa H, Sakakibara M, Taga S, *et al.* A deep learning approach to predict differentiation outcomes in hypothalamic-pituitary organoids. Commun Biol. 2024;7:1468.
28. Molecular Devices. The drug discovery landscape is changing. https://www.moleculardevices.com/lab-notes/3d-biology/3d-biology-paradigm-shift-for-next-gen-drug-discovery.
29. Kong J, Lee H, Kim D, Han SK, Ha D, Shin K, *et al.* Network-based machine learning in colorectal and bladder organoid models predicts anti-cancer drug efficacy in patients. Nat Commun. 2020;11:5485.

30. Yang Q, Li M, Xiao Z, Feng Y, Lei L, Li S. A New Perspective on Precision Medicine: The Power of Digital Organoids. Biomater Res. 2025;29. doi:10.34133/bmr.0171.
31. Herráiz-Gil S, Nygren-Jiménez E, Acosta-Alonso DN, León C, Guerrero-Aspizua S. Artificial Intelligence-Based Methods for Drug Repurposing and Development in Cancer. Applied Sciences. 2025;15:2798.
32. Tang X, Prodduturi N, Thompson KJ, Weinshilboum R, O'Sullivan CC, Boughey JC, *et al.* OmicsFootPrint: a framework to integrate and interpret multi-omics data using circular images and deep neural networks. Nucleic Acids Res. 2024;52:e99.
33. Andrews MG, Kriegstein AR. Challenges of Organoid Research. Annu Rev Neurosci. 2022;45:23–39.
34. Abbasian MH, Sobhani N, Sisakht MM, D'Angelo A, Sirico M, Roudi R. Patient-Derived Organoids: A Game-Changer in Personalized Cancer Medicine. Stem Cell Rev Rep. 2025;21:211–225.
35. Peng T, Ma X, Hua W, Wang C, Chu Y, Sun M, *et al.* Individualized patient tumor organoids faithfully preserve human brain tumor ecosystems and predict patient response to therapy. Cell Stem Cell. 2025;32:652–669.e11.
36. Li Y, Wu W, Yao J, Wang S, Wu X, Yan J. Patient-Derived Tumor Organoids: A Platform for Precision Therapy of Colorectal Cancer. Cell Transplant. 2025;34. doi:10.1177/09636897251314645.
37. University of California — Los Angeles Health Sciences. Unlocking the potential of patient-derived organoids for personalized sarcoma treatment. www.sciencedaily.com/releases/2024/09/240920122203.htm.
38. Miroslav M. Diving into Organoid Intelligence. https://www.wevolver.com/article/diving-into-organoid-intelligence.
39. Morales Pantoja IE, Smirnova L, Muotri AR, Wahlin KJ, Kahn J, Boyd JL, *et al.* First Organoid Intelligence (OI) workshop to form an OI community. Front Artif Intell. 2023;6. doi:10.3389/frai.2023.1116870.
40. Wang H-M, Zhang C-Y, Peng K-C, Chen Z-X, Su J-W, Li Y-F, *et al.* Using patient-derived organoids to predict locally advanced or metastatic lung cancer tumor response: A real-world study. Cell Rep Med. 2023;4:100911.
41. Soto-Gamez A, Gunawan JP, Barazzuol L, Pringle S, Coppes RP. Organoid-based personalized medicine: from tumor outcome prediction to autologous transplantation. Stem Cells. 2024;42:499–508.
42. Alizadehsani R, Oyelere SS, Hussain S, Jagatheesaperumal SK, Calixto RR, Rahouti M, *et al.* Explainable Artificial Intelligence for Drug Discovery and Development: A Comprehensive Survey. IEEE Access. 2024;12:35796–35812.

43. Kim J, Maathuis H, Sent D. Human-centered evaluation of explainable AI applications: a systematic review. Front Artif Intell. 2024;7. doi:10.3389/frai.2024.1456486.
44. Momoli C, Costa B, Lenti L, Tubertini M, Parenti M, Martella E, *et al.* The Evolution of Anticancer 3D In Vitro Models: The Potential Role of Machine Learning and AI in the Next Generation of Animal-Free Experiments. Cancers (Basel). 2025;17:700.
45. Conte L, Caruso G, Philip AK, Cucci F, De Nunzio G, Cascio D, *et al.* Artificial Intelligence-Assisted Drug and Biomarker Discovery for Glioblastoma: A Scoping Review of the Literature. Cancers (Basel). 2025;17:571.
46. Adithi I. Is OI the New AI? Questions Surrounding "Brainoware". https://petrieflom.law.harvard.edu/2024/03/13/is-oi-the-new-ai-questions-surrounding-brainoware/.
47. Nagaraj D, Khandelwal P, Steyaert S, Gevaert O. Augmenting digital twins with federated learning in medicine. Lancet Digit Health. 2023;5:e251-e253.
48. Björnsson B, Borrebaeck C, Elander N, Gasslander T, Gawel DR, Gustafsson M, *et al.* Digital twins to personalize medicine. Genome Med. 2020;12:4.
49. Shen S, Qi W, Liu X, Zeng J, Li S, Zhu X, *et al.* From virtual to reality: innovative practices of digital twins in tumor therapy. J Transl Med. 2025;23:348.

https://doi.org/10.1142/9789819817597_0011

Chapter 11

# Ethical and Regulatory Considerations

Khatri Simran[1,#], Win Lwin Thuya[1,#], Cao Yang[1,2,#], Yifeng Ren[3,#], Malia Alexandra Foo[4,*], Fengming You[3]

[1]*Cancer Science Institute of Singapore, National University of Singapore, Singapore 117599*

[2]*Department of Laboratory Medicine, Lequn Brance, The First Hospital of Jilin University, Changchun, Jilin 130031, China*

[3]*TCM Regulating Metabolic Diseases Key Laboratory of Sichuan Province, Hospital of Chengdu University of Traditional Chinese Medicine, Chengdu 610072, Sichuan Province, China*

[4]*Singapore MOHH, 1 N Buona Vista Link, #09-01 Elementum, Singapore 139691, Singapore*

**Abstract:** Organoids — 3D multicellular constructs mimicking human organ structure/function — revolutionize biomedical research by enabling physiologically relevant disease modeling, drug screening, and personalized medicine. Derived from pluripotent or tissue-specific adult stem cells, they offer patient-specific platforms for predicting therapeutic responses and reducing animal testing. However, rapid advancement necessitates robust ethical frameworks. In this chapter, progress of the ethical and regulatory considerations has been summarized and some concerns have also been discussed in terms of informed consent, biobanking and ownership, moral status, and clinical translation.

**Keywords:** organoids, drug screening, personalized medicine, ethics, regulatory considerations

*Corresponding author. Email: malia.foo@mohh.com.sg
#Contributed equally.

## Key Points

1. Ethical challenges on the use of organoids.
2. Moral status and sensitive research, e.g., synthetic embryoids, challenge definitions of human embryos.
3. Governance needs due to lack of international standards for brain organoids or biobanking.

## 11.1 Introduction

Organoids — 3D multicellular constructs that recapitulate key structural and functional aspects of human organs — have revolutionized biomedical research by serving as physiologically relevant *in vitro* models for drug testing and personalized medicine. These autonomously assembling structures mimic the cellular and functional complexity of human organs, offering a high-fidelity platform for studying disease pathophysiology, therapeutic responses, and toxicological effects. Organoid platforms can be integrated into multi-organ-on-a-chip systems, allowing for inter-organ communication studies. For example, a drug may exhibit beneficial effects in diseased tissue but simultaneously pose cardiotoxic risks, necessitating thorough preclinical evaluation. Using such platforms, researchers can assess these risks at an early stage of drug discovery, thereby reducing reliance on animal models. Organoid technology enables personalized medicine by generating individual-specific 3D tissue models derived from patient's tumors or tissue, allowing researchers to test drug responses and tailor treatments to their unique genetic and disease profile. This approach enhances precision therapy, minimizes adverse effects, and improves clinical outcomes by predicting patient-specific reactions before actual treatment. Despite their transformative potential, the rapid advancement of organoid technology necessitates careful consideration of ethical and regulatory frameworks to ensure responsible clinical application.

Key ethical concerns encompass multiple dimensions, including the ethical sourcing of stem cells, ensuring robust informed consent processes for donors, and addressing the potential emergence of human-like characteristics, particularly in cerebral organoids that mimic aspects of brain functionality. Additionally, commercialization and profit-driven motives raise concerns about equitable access to organoid-based therapies, as patenting and proprietary interests may limit affordability and availability. Furthermore, the integration of organoids into personalized medicine must be approached with a commitment to clinical translation that prioritizes equity, ensuring that advancements benefit diverse

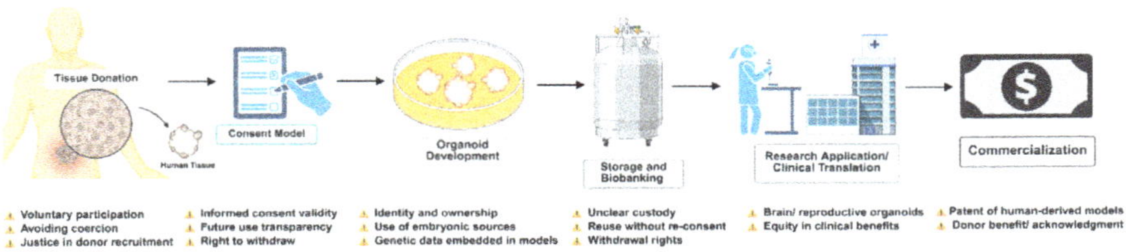


**Figure 11.1** Ethical pathway of human organoid research: from tissue to therapy. This schematic illustrates the sequential stages of human organoid research, highlighting key ethical considerations at each step. Beginning with tissue donation, the pathway proceeds through consent model selection, organoid development, biobanking, research application, and eventual commercialization. Each stage is accompanied by specific ethical challenges, including donor autonomy, privacy, re-consent, the moral status of advanced organoids, and benefit sharing in commercial settings. This life cycle framework emphasizes the need for ethically grounded oversight across the translational pipeline.

patient populations while striving to bridge existing healthcare disparities (Figure 11.1). Addressing these challenges within a well-defined framework is imperative for the responsible development and application of organoid technologies in clinical research and therapeutic innovation. This chapter explores the evolving ethical considerations and regulatory frameworks governing organoid research, ensuring that this groundbreaking technology is implemented in a socially responsible and clinically effective manner.

## 11.2 Source of Organoids

Organoids can be obtained from embryonic stem cells (ESCs) found in early-stage embryos typically from blastocysts, or from induced pluripotent stem cells (iPSCs), which are generated by reprogramming somatic adult cells. ESCs and iPSCs have the ability to differentiate into any cell type needed for organoid development (e.g., neurons for brain organoids and hepatocytes for liver organoids). Both serve as excellent *in vitro* models for developmental biology; however, iPSCs raise fewer ethical concerns than ESCs because they can be generated from patient-specific cells (e.g., skin or blood cells) using Yamanaka factors. This avoids the ethical dilemmas (Figure 11.2) surrounding embryo destruction and allows for patient-matched organoid development, reducing the risk of immune rejection in potential therapies such as organoid transplantation. Additionally, iPSC technology enables researchers to study human diseases and develop personalized treatments without relying on embryonic sources, making it a more widely accepted approach in regenerative medicine and organoid research. While iPSCs and ESCs have indefinite differentiative potential, adult stem cells (ASCs) also play a role in organoid research, though their capabilities are more limited. Unlike iPSCs and ESCs, which can give rise to any cell type, ASCs are tissue-specific and primarily generate cell types corresponding to their tissue of origin. For example, intestinal stem cells can develop into intestinal organoids, while neural stem cells can generate brain organoids. Additionally, ASCs have a restricted ability to proliferate and expand compared to pluripotent stem cells, which limits their use for large-scale or highly diverse organoid applications. However, they remain valuable for studying tissue regeneration, disease modeling, and patient-specific therapies, particularly when ethical considerations favor their use over pluripotent alternatives. ASCs avoid concerns related to embryo destruction, genetic privacy, and regulatory restrictions, making them a viable option when pluripotent cells face ethical or legal constraints.

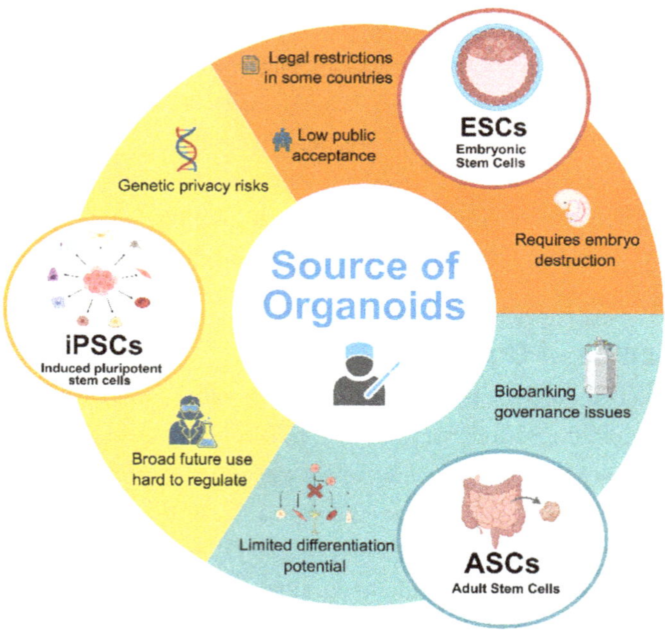


**Figure 11.2** Ethical concerns across different stem cell sources for organoid research. This diagram illustrates the three primary sources of stem cells used to generate organoids: embryonic stem cells (ESCs), induced pluripotent stem cells (iPSCs), and adult stem cells (ASCs). Each source presents distinct ethical challenges. ESCs, derived from human embryos, face controversies related to embryo destruction and legal restrictions. iPSCs, reprogrammed from adult somatic cells, raise issues surrounding genetic privacy and long-term governance of use. ASCs, harvested from tissue-specific organs, pose fewer ethical concerns but are limited by their differentiation capacity and biobanking oversight. Understanding these source-specific concerns is essential to guiding ethically responsible organoid research and clinical applications.

### 11.2.1 *Informed Consent*

Informed consent is the process by which individuals voluntarily agree to participate in research or medical procedures after receiving comprehensive information about the risks, benefits, and purpose of the study. It ensures that participants understand their rights, potential implications, and the ability to withdraw at any time, promoting ethical transparency and autonomy.

The source of organoids significantly influences the ethical framework surrounding informed consent. ASC-derived organoids, originating from tissue-specific stem cells, require standard tissue donation consent, as their differentiation potential is limited to specific cell types. In contrast, organoids derived from iPSCs, which can differentiate into any cell type, necessitate a more extensive consent process. Because iPSCs retain the donor's genetic material, their use raises concerns regarding broad consent, genetic privacy, and potential unintended applications in research. ESC-derived organoids, while less common due to ethical and legal constraints, require explicit donor consent as their source (human embryo) carries significant ethical considerations. Thus, the informed consent process must be tailored to the specific stem cell source, ensuring transparency and ethical integrity in organoid research and applications.

Informed consent in relation to organoid research remains a complicated subject as there is a lack of clear boundary about what the exact purpose and end point of the research will be; donors should be informed if their tissues will be used for development of a therapy, disease modelling, drug discovery, etc. It is natural for donors to have a different decision based on the objective of the research being carried out. If the organoid is patient-derived, patients should be informed whether they will have early access to any treatment or therapy that may potentially be developed from their tissue. However, it is important to note that any unclear purpose of use of human tissue for organoid research is not acceptable for any sort of informed consent documentation.

### 11.2.2 *Concept of Anonymization*

Tissue donors typically have the option to either provide explicit consent for sample use or opt for de-identification [1]. De-identification is considered to serve as a protective measure to uphold donor privacy and mitigate ethical concerns related to data security and misuse. Through the elimination of personally identifiable data, researchers can utilize organoids without direct traceability to individual donors, thereby reducing risks associated with unauthorized data exposure and genetic exploitation. This approach enhances ethical integrity in biomedical research while fostering broader scientific advancements in organoid applications. However, with recent advancements in genomic technologies, including high-throughput sequencing and bioinformatics, it has become increasingly difficult to achieve complete de-identification of biological samples. Genetic data, by its very nature, contains unique identifiers and mutations that can potentially link samples back to their donors, even in the absence of explicit personal information [2, 3]. Additionally, de-identification has drawbacks, as it limits follow-up studies and hinders advancements in personalized medicine [4, 5]. Furthermore, an ethical concern against anonymization is that donors lose control over their samples, including the ability to withdraw consent, which is particularly relevant when their tissues are used to create controversial organoids like brain organoids or early embryonic models.

Given that anonymization is sometimes impossible to achieve, it is best to follow a standardized informed consent protocol. Various informed consent models have been developed, including specific, tiered, broad, blanket, opt-in, opt-out, governance, and dynamic consent [6]. These models differ in the extent of donor control over future use of their biological samples.

In organoid research, the choice of consent model is crucial in balancing donor autonomy, ethical transparency, and scientific progress. Specific consent ensures that donated biological material is used solely for a predefined research project, providing donors with clear control over the intended purpose of their samples. While this model strengthens ethical clarity, it significantly limits future research applications, as any new study involving the organoid requires additional donor approval, creating logistical and administrative burdens that can slow innovation. On the other hand, blanket consent allows for unrestricted future use of organoids across multiple areas of research, facilitating large-scale scientific advancements without the need for re-consent. However, this model reduces donor oversight and raises ethical concerns, as individuals may not be fully aware of how their samples will be used, including in potential commercial applications or in development of controversial brain organoids.

An alternative approach, the opt-out model, automatically includes donated samples in organoid research unless the donor actively withdraws. While this method increases research participation and ensures a diverse pool of biological material, it risks compromising informed consent if donors are not adequately informed about their right to opt out. A more balanced model is broad consent, which permits the use of organoids within a general field of research, such as neurological or cancer studies, while still maintaining some level of donor oversight. This model reduces the need for repeated re-consent while ensuring ethical transparency and regulatory compliance.

The selection of a consent framework has far-reaching ethical and practical consequences. Specific consent prioritizes donor control but limits research flexibility, whereas blanket and opt-out models enhance scientific progress but reduce individual oversight. Regulatory bodies, such as institutional review boards and ethics committees, play a key role in ensuring that consent procedures protect donor rights while enabling responsible organoid research. As the field continues to advance, a hybrid approach that incorporates elements of transparency, ethical stewardship, and research efficiency may be the most sustainable solution. Key ideas behind donor involvement and research flexibility are summarized in Table 11.1.

**Table 11.1** Comparative analysis of donor consent models used in organoid research. Models are categorized by the degree of donor involvement and the level of flexibility they provide for future scientific reuse [13].

| Consent Model | Donor Involvement | Research Flexibility |
|---|---|---|
| Specific and Re-consent | Donors are re-contacted for every new study involving their tissue. | Low – Each reuse requires fresh consent, limiting efficiency. |
| Tiered | Donors choose from a list of approved research uses at the time of consent. | Moderate – Use is limited to selected categories. |
| Broad | One-time consent for future research, even if specific details are unknown. | High – Allows flexible reuse without re-contacting donors. |
| Blanket | Consent given for any type of future research without restrictions. | Very High – No limitations on tissue use. |
| Opt-in | Donors explicitly agree to research use before samples are stored. | Moderate – Use limited to initial terms of consent. |
| Opt-out | Consent is presumed unless the donor refuses beforehand. | High – Enables broad use unless opted out. |
| Governance-based | Donors contribute to oversight mechanisms but do not select specific studies. | Moderate – Use governed by ethical boards or committees. |
| Dynamic | Ongoing interaction via digital platforms allows donor feedback over time. | Moderate – Enables continuous donor input and updates. |

Specific consent confines the utilization of samples to a designated research project, thus providing clarity to donors while limiting potential future applications. In contrast, blanket consent and opt-out models facilitate unrestricted future use of donated tissue, necessitating minimal additional approvals. Broad consent serves as an intermediary approach, allowing for the use of organoids within a general category of research, such as disease-specific studies, while still preserving a degree of donor oversight.

### 11.2.3 *Biobanking and Long-term Data Use*

A biobank is a systematically organized repository that collects, stores, and manages biological specimens (e.g., blood, tissues, DNA, and other biomolecules) along with associated clinical and demographic data. Their operation involves standardized protocols for sample processing, storage, and ethical considerations such as informed consent and data privacy. Biobanking of organoids has tremendous potential to advance biomedicine in terms of study of diseases — drug discovery and personalised medicine. Organoids can be stored in living biobanks as mini-organs, viable cells or tissues [7]. Patient-derived organoids are stored in biobanks with their genetic signature that might resemble future patients with similar cancer types and thus similar drug sensitivity, and various treatment therapies can be tested on the organoid models and a predictive *in clinic* response can be established. This paves the way for personalized medicine for cancer patients and saves them from side effects of ineffective drugs.

Despite these promising advancements, ethical issues relevant to organoid biobanking persist. The long-term storage of organoids in biobanks introduces ethical challenges related to governance, ownership, and donor consent. Questions arise about who has the right to access and use stored organoids, especially if their intended purpose evolves over time. Additionally, maintaining privacy and safeguarding data linked to biobanked organoids must be prioritized to prevent breaches or misuse.

Currently, no set rules or guidelines have been established that regulate the role and responsibilities of donors and biobankers. While general ethical frameworks for biobanking exist, they may not fully address the unique challenges posed by organoids. Neither can organoids be categorized as any well-defined biological material-like tissue, cell or gametes that are legally regulated [7]. Seemingly, the rapid advancement of organoid technology has outpaced the development of specific ethical guidelines and regulations, leading to a gap in governance.

Organoid biobanks differ from ordinary biobanks in many ways, one being the clinical relevance as biobanks are usually seen as a means of storing scientifically relevant material to advance research and knowledge. However, organoid biobanks can be used to predict drug response for patients, indicating a clear shift in purpose and prospect which should effectively be seen in regulatory guidelines that should be established for organoid biobanking [8].

Nevertheless, it is of utmost importance that the roles and responsibilities of the key stakeholders involved in organoid biobanking are defined formally, especially when organoids are derived from human sources. Four guiding points that have been discussed by O'Brien [9] on the ownership and custodianship of Human Biological Material repositories can be considered in the case of organoid biobanking and technology:

1) Promoting openness and scientific inquiry to maximize full potential of donor tissue and contributing to better healthcare.
2) Prioritizing and guaranteeing the privacy of donors and including provisions for the unforeseen use of their tissue in the informed consent.
3) Acknowledgement for investigators' intellectual input in the development of technology and associated treatment.
4) Safeguarding ownership details while addressing the concerns of funding agencies in specimen distribution.

In summary, while specific regulations for organoid biobanking are still under development, existing ethical guidelines and legal frameworks for human tissue research provide a foundational basis. Ongoing discussions aim to adapt these frameworks to address the unique considerations associated with organoid research and biobanking.

## 11.3 Organoids in Personalized Medicine

To date, many attempts have been made in biomedical science to tailor treatments to individual patients, such as genome sequencing to predict adverse reactions linked to specific mutations or gene combinations. Nevertheless, organoid technology holds the most promising future in this domain. This is demonstrated by a growing number of applications, ranging from multi-drug screening to the repurposing of FDA-approved therapeutics. For instance, in a study on biliary tract carcinoma, Saito *et al.* identified 22 compounds, including antifungals, HMG-CoA reductase inhibitors, and dopamine D2 receptor agonists, that effectively suppressed organoid growth [10]. Similarly, De Poel *et al.* employed intestinal organoids to repurpose existing drugs for rare cystic fibrosis genotypes [11], showcasing the translational potential of this technology. In today's healthcare landscape, patient-derived organoids are increasingly used to guide therapeutic decisions *in vitro*, offering tangible benefits such as reduced exposure to costly or ineffective treatments, minimization of adverse drug reactions, and increased patient trust in therapeutic outcomes. A striking example is the use of patient-derived gut organoids to determine cystic fibrosis patients' eligibility for treatment with ivacaftor, a high-cost therapy administered upon a favorable organoid-based response [12].

Beyond one-time drug testing, patient-derived organoids can also serve as dynamic models to monitor treatment responses, track the emergence of drug resistance, and evaluate the evolution of disease pathology over time. This provides clinicians with continuous feedback and enables timely, precise adjustments to therapy. To overcome limitations such as the lack of systemic context or inter-organ interactions in single-organoid models, advances such as organoids-on-a-chip have emerged. These platforms integrate multiple organoids through microfluidic systems, offering a more physiologically relevant representation of the human body.

Yet, as organoid technology rapidly progresses, it brings with it a constellation of ethical, legal, and social challenges. Each novel application, whether testing drugs, modeling long-term disease progression, or integrating organoids into chip-based systems, raises distinct ethical questions about privacy, access, clinical translation, and regulatory oversight. Even more futuristic developments, such as organoid intelligence, where neural organoids are interfaced with computing systems, begin to stretch the boundaries of traditional bioethics. While the promise of organoids in personalized medicine is immense, it is critical to reflect on the accompanying ethical concerns to ensure that innovation remains aligned with patient rights, societal values, and responsible research practice.

### 11.3.1 *Ethical and Practical Challenges in Personalized Organoid-Based Drug Testing*

While patient-derived organoids hold significant potential in the advancement of personalized medicine, their clinical application is accompanied by a range of ethical, practical, and regulatory challenges [13]. Ensuring the ability to return clinically relevant findings requires maintaining a link between the patient and their organoid sample, which introduces important concerns related to privacy and data protection. In addition, the time, expertise, and financial cost required to develop individualized organoids limit the widespread use of this technology, making it accessible only to a subset of patients. Although organoids closely resemble the biological characteristics of the tissue from which they are derived, they do not account for whole-body physiology, which limits their capacity to accurately predict how a patient will respond to a drug in a real-world clinical setting.

Establishing the clinical validity of organoid-based drug screening is particularly complex in rare diseases, where large clinical trials are often unfeasible. One proposed solution is the use of n-of-1 trials, in which an individual patient undergoes a personalized, crossover-style clinical protocol to generate case-specific evidence on drug safety and efficacy. This type of data may support informed treatment decisions and provide a basis for reimbursement when broader trials are not practical.

Furthermore, organoid-based drug testing represents a shift from the conventional translational pipeline, where safety and efficacy are validated through large-scale clinical trials. Without this broader context, important safety signals may go undetected. Furthermore, even when promising results are achieved, patients may not receive access to therapies developed using their own organoids. This is due in part to variations in national reimbursement policies and the limited clinical implementation of laboratory-based tests. Such limitations are ethically concerning, especially given that many patients participate in organoid research with the expectation that they will receive personal therapeutic benefits, an outcome that is still uncertain and cannot yet be guaranteed.

The growing use of organoids in both experimental research and clinical care creates an overlap between two domains that are typically governed by separate ethical and legal standards. This overlap can create uncertainty for clinicians and researchers regarding their responsibilities and obligations. As newer applications emerge, such as the use of neural organoids in computational models, the need for clearly defined regulatory and ethical frameworks becomes even more urgent. Finally, while organoid technologies can improve clinical decision-making and enable more tailored therapies, they also raise important concerns related to incidental findings, privacy, and potential harm. These challenges highlight the importance of establishing robust, transparent, and ethically grounded policies to support the responsible use of organoids in personalized medicine [13].

### 11.3.2 *Organoid Transplantation: Therapeutic Promise and Emerging Ethical Considerations*

The use of laboratory-grown organoids in transplantation therapies is increasingly seen as a transformative step in regenerative medicine. Unlike conventional transplantation, which relies on the availability of organs or tissues from living or deceased donors, organoid-based therapies offer the potential to generate functional, patient-specific tissues in a controlled laboratory setting. When derived from a patient's own cells, organoids may present a lower risk of immune rejection and reduce the need for lifelong immunosuppressive therapy. Furthermore, advances in genetic modification allow researchers to correct disease-causing mutations before the organoid is implanted, opening possibilities for offering better quality of life to patients with genetic defects.

One of the most significant advantages of organoid transplantation lies in its availability. Organoids can be manufactured more rapidly and on-demand compared to traditional donor organs, potentially easing the burden of organ shortages and long waitlists. A key promise of this innovation could be the use of liver organoids to restore liver function in patients with metabolic liver disease [8, 14, 15].

Despite these clinical benefits, the transplantation of organoids raises important ethical concerns. These range from questions of safety, use of genetically modified material, equitable access, long-term physical and psychological integration into host body to implications for the society that will start to perceive organ failures differently with the advent of this technology.

#### 11.3.2.1 *Ethics in First-in-Human Studies*

Although organoid transplantation remains largely experimental, recent developments have marked important clinical milestones. In 2022, Tokyo Medical and Dental University team successfully transplanted patient-derived intestinal organoids into an individual with ulcerative colitis, demonstrating initial safety and feasibility [16]. A similar step was taken in ophthalmology, where retinal organoids derived from iPSCs were used in patients with retinitis pigmentosa to investigate vision restoration [17]. While these pioneering trials illustrate the therapeutic potential of organoid-based interventions, they also raise pressing ethical considerations around trial design and risk justification.

Building upon one of the first known established ethical principles outlined in the Nuremberg Code, that included the foundational idea of first, do no harm, the transition of organoid-based therapies into first-in-human clinical trials demands careful ethical scrutiny and assurance of minimal risk to patients. This imperative is especially critical because organoid transplantation differs fundamentally from traditional drug testing. Unlike oral or intravenous drugs, organoid transplantation is invasive, involving the implantation of living tissue into the human body, which introduces additional risks that demands careful oversight.

One safety concern arises from the possibility of organoid cells migrating to unintended locations in the body, such as the lungs, heart or brain [15]. Such translocation events raise serious questions regarding safety, particularly the risk of unwanted tumor formation. Secondly, since each organ system has distinct structural and functional characteristics, it is essential to develop tailored protocols for different types of organoid transplants and medical conditions that allow for their use. These protocols must also consider vulnerable populations, such as pediatric patients with congenital disorders like metabolic liver diseases, where ethical justification must be even more rigorous.

Beyond minimizing harm, ethical clinical research must also aim to maximize potential medical benefit to the participant [8]. However, determining this benefit in first-in-human trials is challenging. Current preclinical evidence is largely derived from animal models, which may not reliably predict outcomes in humans. This gap underscores the ethical tension in early human experimentation, where the promise of innovation must be balanced against the uncertainty of risk and benefit.

## 11.4 Moral Status of Organoids

The moral status of organoids has long been argued to be different from mere objects since specialized organoids like brain organoids may offer potential to gain consciousness. Organoids can be considered objects based on several principles as highlighted by Boers *et al.* [5].

- **Organoids as Models:** They are models developed in lab using living samples through biotechnological transformations.
- **Organoids as Technology:** Organoids are not just biological samples but complex technologies involving interactions between people, lab systems, and non-human components.
- **Functional Models:** They serve as tools to replicate the structure and function of human tissues, supporting scientific, clinical, and commercial research.
- **Commercial Value:** Organoids are gaining economic significance, especially with the rise of organoid biobanks used in personalized medicine.
- **Intellectual Property:** There is a growing number of patents related to organoid technologies, reflecting increasing industrial and commercial interest.

## 11.5 Discussion: Grey Areas in Organoid Use and Potential Solutions

As the field of organoid science advances rapidly, it increasingly intersects with domains of ethical uncertainty. While some applications, such as drug screening or disease modeling, are relatively uncontroversial, others dwell in grey areas where traditional ethical frameworks offer limited guidance. These ambiguities pose a significant challenge to researchers, ethics committees, and policymakers seeking to balance innovation with responsibility.

### 11.5.1 *Consent and Ownership*

Organoids are derived from human tissue yet manipulated, propagated, and potentially commercialized by institutions and industry. This blurring of personal biological origin and institutional custodianship challenges traditional bioethical frameworks, demanding new models for participant protection, justice, and accountability [28].

Informed consent is the ethical cornerstone of human tissue donation. It ensures that participants voluntarily agree to the use of their biological material with a full understanding of its purpose, risks, and potential future applications. In the context of organoid research, standard consent procedures — originally developed for static tissue samples — are increasingly inadequate due to the long-term, scalable, and multifunctional nature of organoids [28].

Consent for organoid research faces several key challenges. Organoids may be used far beyond their original purpose, maintained indefinitely, and potentially commercialized, all of which raise concerns about how fully informed and ethically valid consent truly is — especially when research involves morally sensitive areas like brain or reproductive models [28]. Traditional models such as specific consent offer ethical clarity but limit research flexibility, while broad consent allows wider use but may lack donor understanding for ethically complex applications.

Unlike static biospecimens, organoids can be cultured indefinitely, manipulated, and reused across multiple research contexts and over long timeframes. This complicates the adequacy of single-point consent. Dynamic consent, a digital, ongoing model of engagement, offers a promising solution by allowing donors to adjust preferences over time [29].

In most jurisdictions, individuals who donate biological tissue relinquish legal ownership of their samples at the point of donation. However, as organoids — particularly those replicating sentient or reproductive functions — are derived from a person's genome and can closely model human biological identity, they raise ethical questions about moral ownership and the donor's ongoing right to influence how their biological material is used. A landmark case, Moore v. Regents of the University of California (1990), held that a patient did not retain proprietary rights over his excised cells, even when they led to a profitable patented cell line. This case continues to serve as a focal point in debates over tissue rights and commercialization, and its implications are being revisited in the era of organoid research. As organoids grow more complex, scholars such as Hyun argue that the moral significance of person-derived organoids — especially in ethically sensitive domains like cerebral or reproductive studies — warrants a reconsideration of donor agency, suggesting that individuals should retain some degree of influence over morally consequential downstream applications, even in the absence of legal ownership [30].

### 11.5.2 *Commercialization and Equity*

The commercialization of organoid technologies — ranging from personalized drug testing platforms to organoid-based therapeutics — has brought significant attention to issues of equity and fairness in biomedical research. While donors provide the foundational biological material, they typically receive no compensation or recognition when their samples contribute to profitable innovations. This disparity raises ethical concerns about benefit-sharing, particularly when tissue is sourced from vulnerable or underserved populations who may not ultimately have access to the resulting therapies. For instance, the commercial licensing of organoid-based drug screening platforms by entities such as Hubrecht Organoid Technology has sparked debate over donor recognition and justice. As Blasimme and Vayena argue, "the commodification of human-derived organoids without reciprocal benefit undermines social trust and raises distributive justice concerns" [31]. To mitigate these concerns, ethicists have proposed non-monetary benefit-sharing strategies, including community health investments, transparency reports, and the public recognition of donor contributions in scientific outputs [32]. Without deliberate governance, the commercialization of organoid-based products may deepen the gap between those who contribute to research and those who benefit from it, undermining public trust and the ethical legitimacy of precision medicine.

### 11.5.3 *Identity and Humanity*

#### 11.5.3.1 *Brain Organoids*

This subject-like status of organoids gets into scrutiny when ethical concerns arise from the use of brain/cerebral organoids as they are associated with establishing neural networks and exhibiting spontaneous electrical activity *in vitro* and thereby gaining 'consciousness' [18]. In that case, these specialized lab models should no longer be treated as samples and should be considered of a higher moral status potentially capable of responding to signals like light [19], having interests and experiencing pain. This complicated scenario calls for the need of ethical oversight on their use since they should be perceived differently from other organoids and some forms of experimentation may be deemed unethical [13].

Whether or not brain organoids can develop human-like consciousness remains a debatable issue to date. A heavily discussed study in literature by Muotri *et al.* describes electroencephalogram patterns of brain organoids as comparable to brains of premature babies [20]. To date, these specialized brain models have not only proved their revolutionary potential in so-far unsolvable neuroscience research questions [21, 22] but also have enabled development of techniques where interactions with external environments are explored by connecting brain organoids to tractable robotics [23] and muscles [24].

Keeping in mind the ethical implications of potential consciousness in brain organoids, a key issue that arises is the question of donor consent. If a brain organoid were ever to attain consciousness, some argue that the donor should retain the right to withdraw consent, given the deeply personal nature of constructing what could be viewed as a "brain clone" [25, 26]. To prevent such scenarios, a range of solutions has been proposed. These include genetically manipulated brain organoids to inhibit consciousness-related development [27] or developing novel objective and non-invasive tests to detect signs of consciousness in brain models or using known tools like the Perturbational Complexity Index [13].

It is a recurring theme that special ethical oversight and rules should be developed for researchers dealing with brain organoids like establishing special ethical committees for such research and the requirement for following the 3R's of animal research and especially reducing the total number of brain organoids used in research [26].

While scientists generally emphasize that it is currently very unlikely that brain organoids could achieve human-like consciousness, the rapid pace of research calls for proactive ethical governance. These should include protocols that govern permissible procedures, such as genetic engineering, clinical applications like transplantation, guidelines for organoid destruction after experimentation, and importantly, policymakers and bioethicists must collaborate from the earliest stages of development to identify emerging ethical issues and guide research responsibly [13]. See Koplin and Savulescu [27] for a comprehensive ethical model suggesting firm limitations on the use of brain organoids. Despite the growing volume of literature on these concerns, comprehensive international guidelines for brain organoid research and clinical use remain urgently needed.

As brain organoids advance in complexity — exhibiting region-specific architecture, synaptic activity, and even electroencephalogram-like patterns — questions about identity and humanity emerge with increasing urgency [20, 38]. Particularly in cerebral models, which aim to simulate aspects of human cognition, there exists a theoretical possibility that organoids may develop rudimentary forms of consciousness or sentience, challenging long-held assumptions about the moral status of biological models [18]. This becomes ethically charged in contexts like human-animal chimerism, where integration into the host brain may enhance the animal's cognitive abilities or blur species boundaries [34]. The concept of a "detached consciousness" — an *in vitro* neural network capable of independent experiential processing — complicates notions of personhood and raises concerns over whether such entities merit rights or protections. Scholars like Hoppe *et al.* propose a shift from binary thinking toward a moral continuum, wherein more complex organoids are subject to increased ethical scrutiny [35]. Tools like the Perturbational Complexity Index have been suggested to monitor emergent neural integration and potential markers of consciousness [18, 33]. Preventive ethical strategies include limiting transplantation into non-human primates, adopting international classification frameworks for organoid maturity, and embedding neurorights — such as mental integrity and cognitive liberty — into governance policies [36, 37]. To ensure responsible innovation, researchers must also foster interdisciplinary collaboration and engage public stakeholders in shaping the ethical landscape surrounding organoid identity and humanity. As brain organoids inch closer to mimicking core features of human cognition, ethical frameworks must evolve to address the grey zone between model and mind. Adopting tiered protections, standardizing consciousness assessment, and fostering international dialogue are essential steps toward safeguarding both human dignity and scientific responsibility.

#### 11.5.3.2 *Use in Reproductive and Genetic Research*

Organoid technologies have enabled significant advancements in reproductive and genetic research, including the development of endometrial, testicular, and ovarian organoids for studying fertility, implantation, and early human development [41, 43]. More recently, synthetic embryo models — or embryoids — derived from stem cells have been used to mimic pre-implantation development, raising profound ethical concerns about embryo equivalency and human identity [42]. These models challenge existing regulatory frameworks, as they fall outside traditional definitions of human

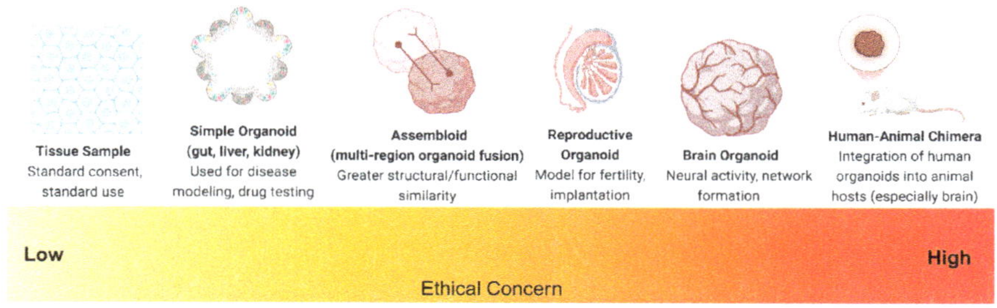


**Figure 11.3** Ethical continuum of organoid models. The moral and regulatory significance of organoids increases with their biological complexity and functional resemblance to human systems. Simple tissue-derived organoids raise minimal ethical concerns, while more advanced models such as assembloids, reproductive organoids, brain organoids, and human-animal chimeras present escalating challenges. These range from donor consent and governance to questions of identity, potential consciousness, and species boundaries. Ethical oversight must therefore be proportionate to model complexity and application.

embryos but may replicate key developmental features. Genetic editing in organoids, particularly when applied to germline or reproductive tissues, introduces additional risks related to heritable changes and societal inequity [39]. Scholars have called for the development of international regulatory frameworks to define ethical boundaries, such as limiting embryo-like research to pre-gastrulation stages and prohibiting reproductive use of organoid-derived gametes [36, 40]. To ensure ethical integrity, dynamic consent processes and multidisciplinary oversight are recommended to navigate this ethically complex and rapidly evolving field [6] (Figure 11.3).

#### 11.5.3.3 *Biobanking and Data Privacy*

Biobanking in organoid research raises complex ethical issues surrounding data privacy, consent, and equitable governance. Traditional de-identification methods are increasingly vulnerable, as genomic data can be re-identified through cross-referencing, compromising donor anonymity [44]. Moreover, the use of broad consent — where donors permit unspecified future research — may not align with individual values, especially in morally sensitive domains such as brain or reproductive organoid research [6]. In response, dynamic consent models have been proposed, enabling continuous digital engagement with donors, allowing them to update preferences and fostering greater transparency [29]. Ethical frameworks like “consent for governance” further suggest donors be informed upfront about oversight processes and potential commercial use, promoting trust and fair benefit-sharing [6]. As organoid complexity grows — especially cerebral organoids — emerging neuroethical frameworks like neurorights emphasize safeguarding mental privacy and identity [37]. Together, these strategies aim to uphold participant dignity while enabling responsible scientific advancement.

#### 11.5.3.4 *Animal Alternatives vs. Organoids*

The ethical concerns surrounding the large-scale manipulation of human tissue and the creation of "living models" such as organoids are significant and multifaceted. Central to the debate is the moral unease associated with engineering complex, semi-autonomous biological systems that increasingly mimic human development and function. As organoids — especially cerebral or reproductive ones — achieve greater structural and functional sophistication, the distinction between experimental models and entities with potential moral significance becomes less clear [18]. This ambiguity raises concerns about the commodification of human biological materials, where tissues donated under altruistic premises may be transformed into commercial assets without donor engagement or benefit-sharing frameworks [5]. Furthermore, the scaling of organoid technologies for high-throughput screening and personalized medicine introduces a risk of eroding informed consent processes, turning donors into depersonalized sources within the biotechnology value chain. These issues are exacerbated by the emerging possibility that brain organoids could develop rudimentary forms of sentience or pain perception, which calls into question the moral and legal status of such models [30, 49].

In parallel, organoids are being heralded as ethically preferable and scientifically superior alternatives to animal models in many areas of biomedical research. They offer more human-relevant physiological and pathological insights, particularly in modeling complex organ systems like the brain, gut, and liver [45, 48]. Compared to animal models, which often suffer from translational limitations due to interspecies differences, human organoids derived from pluripotent stem cells provide more predictive platforms for testing drug efficacy, toxicity, and disease progression [46]. This aligns with the 3Rs framework — Replacement, Reduction, and Refinement — by reducing reliance on animal testing while enhancing research accuracy [47]. However, organoids still lack systemic features such as vascularization, immune components, and complex inter-organ interactions, limiting their current applicability in whole-organism studies [50]. To address these limitations, researchers are developing sophisticated constructs like assembloids (multi-region organoid fusions), organoids-on-chips with microfluidics, and immunocompetent organoid systems to better simulate *in vivo* complexity [51]. Although full replacement of animal models may not yet be feasible for regulatory or pharmacokinetic studies, ongoing innovations are rapidly closing this gap, offering a future in which ethical imperatives and scientific goals are more closely aligned.

## Key Opinion Points

1. Ethical Challenges in Organoid Sourcing and Informed Consent
   Expert opinion emphasizes the need for tailored informed consent processes depending on the stem cell source (ESCs, iPSCs, or ASCs). Donors must be clearly informed about potential uses (e.g., disease modeling, drug screening, or commercialization) and whether their tissues could contribute to controversial organoids (e.g., brain organoids or synthetic embryoids). A dynamic consent model is increasingly favored to balance donor autonomy with research flexibility.
2. Moral Status of Organoids and Sensitive Research
   The development of brain organoids and embryo-like structures challenges traditional definitions of human embryos and consciousness. Experts argue for clear ethical boundaries to determine whether certain organoids warrant moral consideration, particularly as they acquire advanced functional properties (e.g., neural activity). Regulatory frameworks must address whether restrictions akin to those for human embryo research should apply.
3. Governance Gaps in Biobanking and Commercialization
   There is a lack of international standards for organoid biobanking, ownership, and data privacy. Experts highlight risks of exploitation and inequitable access, as patenting and proprietary control could limit affordability. Recommendations include global harmonization of biobanking protocols and benefit-sharing agreements to ensure ethical commercialization and equitable distribution of therapies.
4. Anonymization vs. Traceability in Organoid Research
   While anonymization was traditionally used to protect donor privacy, advances in genomics make complete de-identification nearly impossible. Experts advocate for transparent consent frameworks that allow traceability for longitudinal

studies while ensuring donors retain some control, including the right to withdraw samples from sensitive research (e.g., neuro-organoids).

5. Clinical Translation and Equity Concerns
As organoids move toward personalized medicine, experts stress the need for equitable access to prevent exacerbating healthcare disparities. Ethical frameworks must ensure that organoid-based therapies are not limited to affluent populations and that vulnerable groups (e.g., marginalized communities) are included in research benefits. Regulatory oversight should prioritize fair pricing and inclusive trial participation.

## References

1. Bredenoord AL, Clevers H, Knoblich JA. Human tissues in a dish: the research and ethical implications of organoid technology. Science. 2017 Jan 19;355(6322):eaaf9414.
2. Rothstein MA. Is deidentification sufficient to protect health privacy in research? Am J Bioeth. 2010 Sep;10(9):3–11.
3. von Thenen N, Ayday E, Cicek AE. Re-identification of individuals in genomic data-sharing beacons via allele inference. Bioinformatics. 2019 Feb 1;35(3):365–71.
4. Lensink MA, Boers SN, Jongsma KR, Carter SE, van der Ent CK, Bredenoord AL. Organoids for personalized treatment of cystic fibrosis: professional perspectives on the ethics and governance of organoid biobanking. J Cyst Fibros. 2020;20:443–51.
5. Boers SN, van Delden JJMM, Bredenoord AL. Organoids as hybrids: ethical implications for the exchange of human tissues. J Med Ethics. 2019;45:131–9.
6. Boers SN, Bredenoord AL. Consent for governance in the ethical use of organoids. Nat Cell Biol. 2018;20:642–5.
7. Mollaki V. Ethical challenges in organoid use. BioTech. 2021 Jun 28;10(3):12.
8. Boers SN, van Delden JJ, Clevers H, Bredenoord AL. Organoid biobanking: identifying the ethics: organoids revive old and raise new ethical challenges for basic research and therapeutic use. EMBO Rep. 2016;17(7):938–41.
9. O'Brien SJ. Stewardship of human biospecimens, DNA, genotype, and clinical data in the GWAS era. Annu Rev Genomics Hum Genet. 2009;10:193–209.
10. Saito Y, Muramatsu T, Kanai Y, Ojima H, Sukeda A, Hiraoka N, *et al.* Establishment of patient-derived organoids and drug screening for biliary tract carcinoma. Cell Rep. 2019 Apr 23;27(4):1265–76.e4.
11. de Poel E, Spelier SC, Hagemeijer MC, van Mourik P, Suen SWF, Vonk AM, *et al.* FDA-approved drug screening in patient-derived organoids demonstrates potential of drug repurposing for rare cystic fibrosis genotypes. J Cyst Fibros. 2023;22(3):548–59.

12. Dekkers JF, van der Ent CK, Beekman JM. Novel opportunities for CFTR-targeting drug development using organoids. Rare Dis. 2013;1(1):e26713.
13. de Jongh D, Massey EK, Berishvili E, Fonseca LM, Lebreton F, Bellofatto K, *et al.* Organoids: a systematic review of ethical issues. Stem Cell Res Ther. 2022;13(1):302.
14. Schneemann SA, Boers SN, van Delden JJM, Nieuwenhuis EES, Fuchs SA, Bredenoord AL. Ethical challenges for pediatric liver organoid transplantation. Sci Transl Med. 2020;12:eaat8471.
15. Tsuchida T, Murata S, Hasegawa S, Mikami S, Enosawa S, Hsu HC, *et al.* Investigation of clinical safety of human iPS cell-derived liver organoid transplantation to infantile patients in porcine model. Cell Transplant. 2020;29:1–13.
16. The Tokyo Medical and Dental University (TMDU) team succeeded with the world's first mini organ transplantation to a patient with ulcerative colitis. Tokyo Med Dent Univ. 2022.
17. Zhang CJ, Jin ZB. Turning point of organoid transplantation: first-in-human trial of iPSC-derived retinal organoid grafting in patients with retinitis pigmentosa. Sci China Life Sci. 2024 Feb;67(5):1082–4.
18. Lavazza A, Massimini M. Cerebral organoids: ethical issues and consciousness assessment. J Med Ethics. 2018;44:606–10.
19. Quadrato G, Nguyen T, Macosko EZ, Sherwood JL, Yang SM, Berger DR, *et al.* Cell diversity and network dynamics in photosensitive human brain organoids. Nature. 2017;545:48–53.
20. Trujillo CA, Gao R, Negraes PD, Gu J, Buchanan J, Preissl S, *et al.* Complex oscillatory waves emerging from cortical organoids model early human brain network development. Cell Stem Cell. 2019;25(4):558–69.e7.
21. Chen HI, Song H, Ming GL. Applications of human brain organoids to clinical problems. Dev Dyn. 2019;248:53–64.
22. Li S, Wang M, Zhou J. Brain organoids: a promising living biobank resource for neuroscience research. Biopreserv Biobank. 2020;18:136–43.
23. Cohen J. Neanderthal brain organoids come to life. Science. 2018;360:1284.
24. Giandomenico SL, Mierau SB, Gibbons GM, Wenger LMD, Masullo L, Sit T, *et al.* Cerebral organoids at the air–liquid interface generate diverse nerve tracts with functional output. Nat Neurosci. 2019;22:669–79.
25. Haselager DR, Boers SN, Jongsma KR, Vinkers CH, Broekman ML, Bredenoord AL. Breeding brains? Patients' and laymen's perspectives on cerebral organoids. Regen Med. 2020;15(12):2351–60.
26. Sawai T, Hayashi Y, Niikawa T, Shepherd J, Thomas E, Lee TL, Sakaguchi H. Mapping the ethical issues of brain organoid research and application. AJOB Neurosci. 2021;13(2):81–94.

27. Koplin JJ, Savulescu J. Moral limits of brain organoid research. J Law Med Ethics. 2019; 47:760–7.
28. Munsie M, Hyun I, Sugarman J. Ethical issues in human organoid and gastruloid research. Stem Cell Reports. 2017;9(5):842–5.
29. Kaye J, Whitley EA, Lund D, Morrison M, Teare H, Melham K. Dynamic consent: a patient interface for twenty-first century research networks. Eur J Hum Genet. 2015;23(2):141–6.
30. Hyun I. Reconstructing the ethics of stem cell research in cerebral organoids. Nat Rev Neurosci. 2020;21(2):89–91.
31. Blasimme A, Vayena E. Becoming partners, retaining autonomy: ethical considerations on the development of precision medicine. BMC Med Ethics. 2016;17(1):67.
32. Knoppers BM, Chadwick R. Human genetic research: emerging trends in ethics. Nat Rev Genet. 2005;6(1):75–9.
33. Casarotto S, Comanducci A, Rosanova M, Sarasso S, Fecchio M, Napolitani M, *et al.* Stratification of unresponsive patients by an independently validated index of brain complexity. Ann Neurol. 2016;80(5):718–29.
34. Chen HI, Wolf JA, Song H, Ming GL. Human organoids and the ethics of modeling human brain function. Cell Stem Cell. 2019;24(6):791–4.
35. Hoppe M, Muller P, Fuchs S, Aigner J, Bredenoord AL. A code of conduct for brain organoid research. Front Neurosci. 2023;17:1147505.
36. Hyun I, Scharf-Deering JC, Lunshof JE. Ethical issues related to brain organoid research. Nat Methods. 2020;17(7):595–8.
37. Ienca M, Andorno R. Towards new human rights in the age of neuroscience and neurotechnology. Life Sci Soc Policy. 2017;13(1):5.
38. Xiang Y, Tanaka Y, Patterson B, Kang YJ, Govindaiah G, Roselaar N, *et al.* Fusion of regionally specified hPSC-derived organoids models human brain development and interneuron migration. Cell Stem Cell. 2017;21(3):383–98.
39. Baylis F. Altered inheritance: CRISPR and the ethics of human genome editing. Harvard Univ Press. 2019.
40. International Society for Stem Cell Research. ISSCR guidelines for stem cell research and clinical translation. 2021.
41. Komeya M, Sato T, Ogawa T. Long-term ex vivo maintenance of testis tissues producing fertile sperm in a microfluidic device. Sci Rep. 2016;6:21472.
42. Rivron NC, Frias-Aldeguer J, Vrij EJ, Boisset JC, Korving J, Vivie J, *et al.* Blastocyst-like structures generated solely from stem cells. Nature. 2018;557(7703):106–11.

43. Turco MY, Gardner L, Hughes J, Cindrova-Davies T, Gomez MJ, Farrell L, *et al.* Long-term, hormone-responsive organoid cultures of human endometrium in a chemically defined medium. Nat Cell Biol. 2017;19(5):568–77.
44. Gymrek M, McGuire AL, Golan D, Halperin E, Erlich Y. Identifying personal genomes by surname inference. Science. 2013;339(6117):321–4.
45. Clevers H. Modeling development and disease with organoids. Cell. 2016;165(7):1586–97.
46. Kim J, Koo BK, Knoblich JA. Human organoids: model systems for human biology and medicine. Nat Rev Mol Cell Biol. 2020;21(10):571–84.
47. Kirk RGW. The 3Rs and the shaping of scientific culture: animal welfare in laboratory practice in the UK, 1947–1986. Soc Hist Med. 2018;31(3):501–19.
48. Lancaster MA, Renner M, Martin CA, Wenzel D, Bicknell LS, Hurles ME, *et al.* Cerebral organoids model human brain development and microcephaly. Nature. 2013;501(7467):373–9.
49. National Academies of Sciences, Engineering, and Medicine. Emerging ethical considerations for brain organoid research. Washington, DC: National Academies Press; 2021.
50. Pham MT, Pollock KM, Rose MD, Cary WA, Stewart HR, Mattis VB, *et al.* Generation of human vascularized brain organoids. Neuroreport. 2018;29(7):588–93.
51. Takebe T, Zhang B, Radisic M. Synergistic engineering: organoids meet organs-on-a-chip. Cell Stem Cell. 2017;21(3):297–300.

https://doi.org/10.1142/9789819817597_bmatter

# Index

adult stem cells (ASCs), 2–5, 16, 35, 64, 124, 311, 313, 314, 329, 331
artificial intelligence (AI), v, 35, 52, 53, 61, 71, 73, 75, 78, 79, 103, 109–112, 126, 127, 135, 142, 146, 228, 229, 269, 272, 281–306
automation, v, 19, 39, 48, 60, 61, 63, 71, 73, 75, 86, 111, 123, 132, 133, 135, 153, 154, 156, 164, 173, 175, 261, 271, 281, 282, 286, 290, 302, 303

biobank, 19, 66–69, 172, 197, 198, 206, 225, 297, 316
bio-ink, 41–43, 45–48, 50, 78, 86, 88, 89, 94–96, 98, 111
bioprinting, 18, 26, 40–43, 45–51, 53, 66, 78, 79, 85–91, 94, 96, 97, 111, 112, 130, 133, 145
brain organoid, 101, 109, 268, 301–303, 327

chemotherapy, 68–70, 110, 111, 138, 181–189, 192–198, 200, 202, 204, 236, 293

deep profiling, 78, 106
drug screening, v, 1, 6, 18, 19, 26, 27, 33, 34, 39, 40, 48, 49, 61, 64, 66, 67, 75, 82, 85, 91, 93, 101, 110, 112, 119, 122–125, 128, 130–135, 139, 142, 145, 151, 156, 183–186, 189, 194, 197, 198, 206, 208, 222, 227, 235–237, 240, 244, 285, 286, 292, 298, 311, 320, 321, 324, 326, 331
drug sensitivity testing, 138, 185, 186, 188, 189, 198, 206, 207, 220–222, 227, 297

embryonic stem cells (ESCs), 2, 16, 64, 124, 251, 313, 314, 329, 331
ethics, 306, 311, 316, 323, 324

high-throughput screening (HTS), 63, 90, 93, 102, 110, 120, 123, 124, 126, 127, 129, 130, 132–135, 143, 145, 150–157, 159, 161–167, 169, 173–175, 228, 281, 282, 286, 287, 292, 330
human, v, 2, 3, 6, 8, 16, 26, 27, 30, 32–37, 39, 40, 46–48, 52, 60, 61, 64, 71, 72, 74, 75, 80, 82, 93–98, 101, 103, 109, 111, 120–123, 131, 135, 139–146, 151–155, 157–160, 163, 167–172, 174, 182, 187, 193, 197, 199, 209, 220, 230, 232, 236, 237, 246–248, 258, 268, 271, 281–288, 305, 306, 311, 312, 315, 319, 320, 323–328, 330, 331

image analysis, 110, 126–128, 134, 228, 282, 286, 289, 292, 293
immunotherapy, 5, 7, 8, 75, 124, 138, 140, 141, 181–184, 190, 191, 199–202, 204, 220, 300
induced pluripotent stem cells (iPSCs), 16, 48, 64, 66, 82, 124, 172, 313–315, 323, 331

machine learning, 110, 126, 134, 137, 142, 221, 222, 229, 268, 269, 281–283, 288, 289
microfluidic, 18, 26, 29–32, 34–38, 49, 78, 85, 90, 91, 93, 94, 99, 100, 105, 111, 120, 125, 127, 130–133, 144, 145, 173, 249, 259, 260, 264, 320
microfluidic-on-chip, 29
multi-omics, 110, 111, 137, 138, 139, 142, 172, 208, 229, 239, 243–245, 261, 263, 265–272, 281, 282, 287, 288, 290, 292, 295–299, 306

neoadjuvant therapy, 182, 183, 186, 195

organoid engineering, 78, 80, 86, 92, 100, 101, 111, 130
organoid-on-chip, 26, 27, 29, 35, 37–39, 48
organ-on-chip (OoC), 26–28, 30, 32–35, 37–39, 131, 144–146, 174

patient-derived organoid (PDO), 68, 69, 74, 75, 182–193, 195–197, 199, 201, 203, 206–208, 236, 238, 239, 281, 282, 294–299
personalized therapy/treatment, 19, 64, 69, 75, 134, 135, 143, 182, 184, 191, 195, 199, 207, 220, 235, 237, 247, 271, 285, 286, 297, 235, 306
predictive modeling, 229, 282–284, 289
protocol, 1, 2, 3, 8, 17, 157, 172, 208, 230, 232, 239, 262, 301, 316, 321

radiotherapy, 69, 70, 181–184, 191–193, 202–205

self-organization, 3, 26, 35, 60–62, 64, 79, 81, 85, 86, 89, 120, 123–126, 171, 284
single-cell sequencing, 142, 146, 243, 244, 246, 250, 252–256, 263, 267, 268

targeted therapy, vii, 7, 67, 69, 70, 132, 141, 152, 158, 181–184, 187–189, 192, 196–198, 202, 221, 236, 247, 299
target identification, 119, 135, 138, 139, 145, 150, 151, 153, 169, 172, 287
target validation, 119
tumor organoid, 8, 9, 13, 110, 208, 223, 296

ultra-high-throughput screening (uHTS), 150, 151, 154, 156, 157, 159, 161, 164–169

www.ingramcontent.com/pod-product-compliance
Lightning Source LLC
Chambersburg PA
CBHW061603120126
37764CB00024B/187